EARLY CLINICAL INTERVENTION
AND PREVENTION IN SCHIZOPHRENIA

Early Clinical Intervention and Prevention in Schizophrenia

Edited by

William S. Stone, PhD

*Harvard Institute of Psychiatric Epidemiology and Genetics,
and Harvard Medical School Department of Psychiatry at Massachusetts Mental
Health Center, Boston, MA*

Stephen V. Faraone, PhD

*Harvard Institute of Psychiatric Epidemiology and Genetics,
and Harvard Medical School Department of Psychiatry at Massachusetts General
Hospital, Boston, MA*

Ming T. Tsuang, MD, PhD, DSc

*Harvard Institute of Psychiatric Epidemiology and Genetics, Harvard Medical
School Departments of Psychiatry at Massachusetts Mental Health Center and
Massachusetts General Hospital, and Department of Epidemiology, Harvard
School of Public Health, Boston, MA*

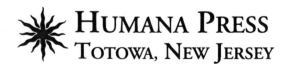

Humana Press
Totowa, New Jersey

© 2004 Humana Press Inc.
999 Riverview Drive, Suite 208
Totowa, New Jersey 07512

humanapress.com

For additional copies, pricing for bulk purchases, and/or information about other Humana titles, contact
Humana at the above address or at any of the following numbers: Tel: 973-256-1699; Fax: 973-256-8341;
E-mail: humana@humanapr.com; website at humanapress.com

This publication is printed on acid-free paper. ∞
ANSI Z39.48-1984 (American National Standards Institute)
Permanence of Paper for Printed Library Materials.

Production Editor: Robin B. Weisberg.

Cover design by Patricia F. Cleary.

Printed in the United States of America.   10 9 8 7 6 5 4 3 2 1

1-59259-729-7 (e-book)

Library of Congress Cataloging-in-Publication Data

Early clinical intervention and prevention in schizophrenia / edited by William S. Stone, Stephen V.
Faraone, Ming T. Tsuang.
     p. ; cm.
Includes index.

Additional material to this book can be downloaded from http://extras.springer.com.
ISBN 1-58829-001-8 (alk. paper)
  1. Schizophrenia--Prevention. 2. Schizophrenia--Etiology. 3. Schizophrenia--Risk factors.
  [DNLM: 1. Schizophrenia--genetics. 2. Schizophrenia--prevention & control. WM 203 E125 2004] I.
Stone, William S., PhD. II. Faraone, Stephen V. III. Tsuang, Ming T., 1931-
  RC514.E24 2004
  616.89'8205--dc21   2003014324

PREFACE

The primary goals of schizophrenia research are to understand the causes of the disorder and to attenuate its symptoms. Advances in diagnosis and treatment have produced significant progress toward these aims, but there are still many hurdles to clear before the biological, genetic, and environmental etiologies of the illness are understood fully. Similarly, much work is needed to alleviate the residual and positive symptoms associated with schizophrenia. One important consequence of our progress to date combines our understanding of the etiology of the disorder with our understanding of treatment options. There is a clear consensus that better outcomes are associated with earlier initiation of treatment.

In fact, if a list of "holy grails" could be identified in schizophrenia research, none would rank higher than the development of strategies aimed at preventing the onset of the disorder. Prevention itself, however, is a multidimensional concept, and our current distance from the grail depends on which dimension is the focus of attention. Although primary prevention remains further off on the horizon, early intervention for psychosis and the development of psychosis (i.e., the prodrome) are active areas of investigation. One of the most significant impediments to both early intervention and prevention research is that we do not yet know what the liability to schizophrenia looks like. We do not know who will develop the disorder and who will not. As a result, we do not know who should receive treatment before their clinical symptoms become overt. This becomes more evident as the distance from psychosis increases. Prodromal symptoms, which are a target of many current models of early intervention, are often nonspecific for schizophrenia. Problems that may precede prodromal symptoms, such as negative symptoms, are even less clearly points on a trajectory to psychosis, as are the absence of clinical symptoms or other abnormalities (e.g., neuropsychological, psychophysiological, or neurobiological deficits) in individuals with one or more risk factors for schizophrenic illness, such as those with a family history of the disorder, pregnancy, or obstetric complications.

Fortunately, the situation is improving. High-risk longitudinal studies and family studies now identify a range of likely clinical, biological, cognitive, and social problems in relatives of patients with schizophrenia that may represent liability/vulnerability factors. A recent reformulation of Paul Meehl•s concept of schizotaxia supports the view that one or more liability syndromes might be identified and validated. There is also growing attention to the nature and delineation of the prodrome. Because interest in the prevention of schizophrenia is high, and characterization of liability syndromes has the potential to move pre-

vention research forward, the time seems right for a volume on prevention in schizophrenia. *Early Clinical Intervention and Prevention of Schizophrenia* focuses on the status of prevention research within the broader context of our current knowledge of the causes and early treatments of schizophrenia, with the goal of determining how early we can intervene in schizophrenic illness. To accomplish this aim, we invited experts working in the field to contribute chapters in the framework of four major sections. We also emphasized our reformulation of schizotaxia to substantiate the notion that the liability to schizophrenia often manifests itself with meaningful clinical, neuropsychological, social, and neurobiological concomitants.

The first section reviews the origins of schizophrenia. In order to develop rational interventions, it is crucial to understand what causes the illness and how it develops. Thus, this section focuses on the genetic (Steve Faraone and colleagues), early environmental (Sarnoff Mednick and colleagues), and neurodevelopmental (Stefano Marenco and Daniel Weinberger) determinants of schizophrenia.

With this framework in mind, the second section characterizes current views of the vulnerability to schizophrenia. In particular, it explores the nature of the liability from several dimensions, including the prodrome (Jaak Rakfeldt and Thomas McGlashan) and our proposed pre-prodromal syndrome of schizotaxia (Steve Faraone and colleagues). More specific manifestations of schizotaxia used here in a generic sense to describe the liability to schizophrenia include cognitive deficits in high-risk populations (Allan Mirsky and Connie Duncan) and in adult, nonpsychotic, biological relatives of patients with schizophrenia (William Kremen and Anne Hoff), socioemotional deficits (Elaine Walker and Karen Hochman), neuroanatomical abnormalities (Larry Seidman and colleagues), and neurophysiological deficits (Marina Myles-Worsley). Finally, Robin Murray and colleagues review several of the dimensions considered in previous chapters to determine whether schizophrenia is actually predictable.

The most important value of characterizing the liability to develop schizophrenia involves, arguably, the identification of treatment/intervention targets. In this light, the third section addresses issues of early intervention and prevention more directly. Following a discussion of conceptual and methodological considerations necessary for the design and implementation of prevention protocols (Hendricks Brown and Steve Faraone), the focus turns to protocols for the treatment of schizotaxia (Ming Tsuang and colleagues), prodromal symptoms (Barbara Cornblatt and colleagues), and issues related to genetic counseling (Debby Tsuang and colleagues).

Finally, the last section looks ahead to the near future of prevention research from two vantage points. One involves representative neurochemical areas that are relevant for schizotaxia research, but are in need of additional investigation

(William Stone and colleagues), and the other explores the prospects of molecular biology for advancing the goals of prevention and early intervention (Will Carpenter and James Koenig).

Early Clinical Intervention and Prevention of Schizophrenia explores the multidimensional nature of the liability to schizophrenia, often in the absence of psychosis or even a schizophrenia-related clinical diagnosis. Although prodromal or psychotic symptoms are already targets of active investigations, it is clear that pre-prodromal intervention based on clinical symptoms or cognitive deficits remains premature. Yet, as many of the authors in this volume demonstrate, the field is at the point of mapping strategies and validating intervention targets. Together with current efforts to attenuate prodromal and incipient psychotic symptoms, these developments bring us closer to the threshold of prevention studies. It is hoped that the multidimensional and interdisciplinary description of these efforts will benefit everyone interested in the prevention of schizophrenia, and more broadly, anyone interested in the prevention of major mental disorders.

William S. Stone, PhD
Stephen V. Faraone, PhD
Ming T. Tsuang, MD, PhD, DSc

CONTENTS

Preface v

Contributors xi

Value-Added eBook/PDA xiv

PART I. THE ETIOLOGY AND GENETICS OF SCHIZOPHRENIA

1 The Genetic Basis of Schizophrenia 3
   Stephen V. Faraone, Stephen J. Glatt, and Levi Taylor

2 Early Environmental Determinants of Schizophrenia 23
   *Jason Schiffman, John Carter, Ricardo A. Machón,
   and Sarnoff Mednick*

3 Obstetric Risk Factors for Schizophrenia and Their
   Relationship to Genetic Predisposition: *Following Ariadne's
   Double-Stranded Thread Through Early Development* 43
   Stefano Marenco and Daniel R. Weinberger

PART II. THE VULNERABILITY TO SCHIZOPHRENIA

4 The Nature of the Prodrome in Schizophrenia 75
   Jaak Rakfeldt and Thomas H. McGlashan

5 The Nature of Schizotaxia 93
   Stephen V. Faraone, Ming T. Tsuang, and Sarah I. Tarbox

6 A Neuropsychological Perspective on Vulnerability
   to Schizophrenia: *Lessons From High-Risk Studies* 115
   Allan F. Mirsky and Connie C. Duncan

7 Neurocognitive Deficits in the Biological Relatives
   of Individuals With Schizophrenia 133
   William S. Kremen and Anne L. Hoff

8 The Nature and Origin of Socioemotional Deficits
   in Schizophrenia 159
   Elaine Walker and Karen M. Hochman

9 Neuroimaging Studies of Nonpsychotic First-Degree Relatives
   of People With Schizophrenia: *Toward a Neurobiology
   of Vulnerability to Schizophrenia* 179
   *Larry J. Seidman, Heidi E. Wencel, Colm McDonald,
   Robin M. Murray, and Ming T. Tsuang*

10 Neurophysiological Endophenotypes in Early Detection
    of Schizophrenia 211
    Marina Myles-Worsley

11 Is the Development of Schizophrenia Predictable? 225
    *Paola Dazzan, Eugenia Kravariti, Paul Fearon,
    and Robin M. Murray*

PART III. EARLY INTERVENTION AND PREVENTION OF SCHIZOPHRENIA

12 Prevention of Schizophrenia and Psychotic Behavior:
    Definitions and Methodological Issues.....................................255
    C. Hendricks Brown and Stephen V. Faraone

13 The Treatment of Schizotaxia 285
    *Ming T. Tsuang, Sarah I. Tarbox, Levi Taylor,
    and William S. Stone*

14 Treatment of the Schizophrenia Prodrome 303
    *Barbara Cornblatt, Todd Lencz, Christopher Smith,
    and Andrea Auther*

15 The Role of Genetic Counseling..325
    Debby W. Tsuang, Stephen V. Faraone, and Ming T. Tsuang

PART IV. CHALLENGES FOR THE NEAR FUTURE

16 The Biology of Schizotaxia 339
    William S. Stone, Stephen J. Glatt, and Stephen V. Faraone

17 Molecular Medicine and the Prospects for Prevention
    and Early Intervention in Schizophrenia....................................355
    William T. Carpenter, Jr. and James I. Koenig

Index 367

CONTRIBUTORS

ANDREA AUTHER, PhD • *Department of Psychiatry Research, The Zucker Hillside Hospital of the North Shore-Long Island Jewish Health System, Glen Oaks, NY*

C. HENDRICKS BROWN, PhD • *Department of Epidemiology and Biostatistics, College of Public Health, University of South Florida, Tampa, FL and Departments of Biostatistics and Mental Hygiene, The Johns Hopkins Bloomberg School of Public Health, Baltimore, MD*

WILLIAM T. CARPENTER, JR., MD • *Department of Psychiatry, University of Maryland School of Medicine and Maryland Psychiatric Research Center, Baltimore, MD*

JOHN CARTER, MA *Social Science Research Institute, University of Southern California, Los Angeles, CA*

BARBARA CORNBLATT, PhD • *Department of Psychiatry Research, The Zucker Hillside Hospital of the North Shore-Long Island Jewish Health System, Glen Oaks, NY*

PAOLA DAZZAN, MD, MSc, MRCPsych • *Division of Psychological Medicine, Institute of Psychiatry, London, United Kingdom*

CONNIE C. DUNCAN, PhD • *Clinical Psychophysiology and Pharmacology Laboratory, Department of Psychiatry, Uniformed Services University of the Health Sciences and Section on Clinical and Experimental Neuropsychology, National Institute of Mental Health, Bethesda, MD*

STEPHEN V. FARAONE, PhD • *Harvard Institute of Psychiatric Epidemiology and Genetics, and Harvard Medical School Department of Psychiatry at Massachusetts General Hospital, Boston, MA*

PAUL FEARON, MB, MSc, MRCPI, MRCPsych • *Division of Psychological Medicine, Institute of Psychiatry and Guy's, King's and St. Thomas's School of Medicine, London, United Kingdom*

STEPHEN J. GLATT, PhD • *Department of Psychiatry, Harvard Medical School, Department of Psychiatry at Massachusetts Mental Health Center; Harvard Institute of Psychiatric Epidemiology and Genetics, Boston, MA*

KAREN M. HOCHMAN, MD • *Department of Psychiatry and Behavioral Science, Emory University School of Medicine, Atlanta, GA*

ANNE L. HOFF, PhD • *Department of Psychiatry and Behavioral Sciences, University of California, Davis School of Medicine, Sacramento and Napa State Hospital, Napa, CA*

JAMES I. KOENIG, PhD • *Department of Psychiatry, University of Maryland School of Medicine and Maryland Psychiatric Research Center, Baltimore, MD*

EUGENIA KRAVARITI, MA, MSc, PhD • *Division of Psychological Medicine, Institute of Psychiatry, London, United Kingdom*

WILLIAM S. KREMEN, PhD • *Department of Psychiatry and Behavioral Sciences, University of California, Davis School of Medicine, Sacramento and Napa State Hospital, Napa, CA*

TODD LENCZ, PhD • *Department of Psychiatry Research, The Zucker Hillside Hospital of the North Shore-Long Island Jewish Health System, Glen Oaks, NY*

RICARDO A. MACHÓN, PhD • *Department of Psychology, Loyola Marymount University, Los Angeles, CA*

STEFANO MARENCO, MD • *Clinical Brain Disorders Branch, National Institute of Mental Health, Bethesda, MD*

COLM McDONALD, MB, MRCPsych • *Division of Psychological Medicine, Institute of Psychiatry, London, United Kingdom*

THOMAS H. McGLASHAN, MD • *Department of Psychiatry, Yale Psychiatric Research Center, Yale University, New Haven, CT*

SARNOFF MEDNICK, PhD, MD • *Social Science Research Institute, University of South California, Los Angeles, CA*

ALLAN F. MIRSKY, PhD • *Section on Clinical and Experimental Neuropsychology, National Institute of Mental Health, Bethesda, MD*

ROBIN M. MURRAY, MD, FRCPsych, DSc • *Division of Psychological Medicine, Institute of Psychiatry, London, United Kingdom*

MARINA MYLES-WORSLEY, PhD   *Department of Psychiatry, University of Utah School of Medicine, Salt Lake City, UT*

JAAK RAKFELDT, PhD • *Social Work Department, Southern Connecticut State University and Department of Psychiatry, Yale University, New Haven, CT*

JASON SCHIFFMAN, PhD   *Department of Psychiatry, University of Hawaii at Manoa, Honolulu, HI*

LARRY J. SEIDMAN, PhD • *Department of Psychiatry, Harvard Medical School; Department of Psychiatry at Massachusetts Mental Health Center, Brockton/West Roxbury VA Medical Center and Massachusetts General Hospital, Harvard Institute of Psychiatric Epidemiology and Genetics, Boston, MA*

CHRISTOPHER SMITH, MA   *Department of Psychiatry Research, The Zucker Hillside Hospital of the North Shore-Long Island Jewish Health System, Glen Oaks, NY*

WILLIAM S. STONE, PhD • *Harvard Institute of Psychiatric Epidemiology and Genetics, and Harvard Medical School Department of Psychiatry at Massachusetts Mental Health Center, Boston, MA*

SARAH I. TARBOX, BA *Department of Psychology, University of Pittsburgh, Pittsburgh, PA*

LEVI TAYLOR, PhD • *Department of Psychiatry, Harvard Medical School, Department of Psychiatry at Massachusetts Mental Health Center; Harvard Institute of Psychiatric Epidemiology and Genetics, Boston, MA*

DEBBY W. TSUANG, MD, MSc • *Department of Psychiatry and Behavioral Sciences, University of Washington, Mental Illness Research Education and Clinical Center, VA Puget Sound Health Care System, Seattle, WA*

MING T. TSUANG, MD, PhD, DSc • *Harvard Institute of Psychiatric Epidemiology and Genetics, Harvard Medical School Departments of Psychiatry at Massachusetts Mental Health Center and Massachusetts General Hospital, and Department of Epidemiology, Harvard School of Public Health, Boston, MA*

ELAINE WALKER, PhD • *Department of Psychology and Department of Psychiatry and Behavioral Science, Emory University, Atlanta, GA*

DANIEL R. WEINBERGER, MD • *Clinical Brain Disorders Branch, National Institute of Mental Health, Bethesda, MD*

HEIDI E. WENCEL, PhD • *Department of Psychiatry, Harvard Medical School; Department of Psychiatry at Massachusetts Mental Health Center, Boston, MA*

Value-Added eBook/PDA

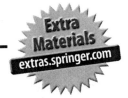

This book is accompanied by a value-added CD-ROM that contains an Adobe eBook version of the volume you have just purchased. This eBook can be viewed on your computer, and you can synchronize it to your PDA for viewing on your handheld device. The eBook enables you to view this volume on only one computer and PDA. Once the eBook is installed on your computer, you cannot download, install, or e-mail it to another computer; it resides solely with the computer to which it is installed. The license provided is for only one computer. The eBook can only be read using Adobe® Reader® 6.0 software, which is available free from Adobe Systems Incorporated at www.Adobe.com. You may also view the eBook on your PDA using the Adobe® PDA Reader® software that is also available free from Adobe.com.

You must follow a simple procedure when you install the eBook/PDA that will require you to connect to the Humana Press website in order to receive your license. Please read and follow the instructions below:

1. Download and install Adobe® Reader® 6.0 software

   You can obtain a free copy of Adobe® Reader® 6.0 software at www.adobe.com

   *Note: If you already have Adobe® Reader® 6.0 software, you do not need to reinstall it.
2. Launch Adobe® Reader® 6.0 software
3. Install eBook: Insert your eBook CD into your CD-ROM drive

   a. **PC:** Click on the "Start" button, then click on "Run"

   At the prompt, type "d:\ebookinstall.pdf" and click "OK"

   *Note: If your CD-ROM drive letter is something other than d: change the above command accordingly.

   b. **MAC:** Double click on the "eBook CD" that you will see mounted on your desktop. Double click "ebookinstall.pdf"
4. Adobe® Reader® 6.0 software will open and you will receive the message "This document is protected by Adobe DRM" Click "OK"

   *Note: If you have not already activated Adobe® Reader® 6.0 software, you will be prompted to do so. Simply follow the directions to activate and continue installation.

   Your web browser will open and you will be taken to the Humana Press eBook registration page. Follow the instructions on that page to complete installation. You will need the serial number located on the sticker sealing the envelope containing the CD-ROM.

If you require assistance during the installation, or you would like more information regarding your eBook and PDA installation, please refer to the eBookManual.pdf located on your cd. If you need further assistance, contact Humana Press eBook Support by e-mail at ebooksupport@humanapr.com or by phone at 973-256-1699.

*Adobe and Reader are either registered trademarks or trademarks of Adobe Systems Incorporated in the United States and/or other countries.

I

The Etiology and Genetics of Schizophrenia

1 The Genetic Basis of Schizophrenia

Stephen V. Faraone, PhD,
Stephen J. Glatt, PhD,
and Levi Taylor, PhD

Since early 2001, a draft of the map of the entire base-pair sequence of human DNA has been generally available to the scientific community, permitting a range of projects that would previously have been unimaginable. Among those projects will be programmatic explorations of the genetic etiology of human disease. That research will facilitate the development of tests that can identify those at risk for a variety of disorders. Innovative therapies based on genetic information can then be designed, which will provide more effective treatments, and perhaps even methods of prevention or cure. In psychiatry, the syndrome that is perhaps most likely to benefit from such research is schizophrenia.

Schizophrenia is a biphasic illness characterized on one hand by the so-called "positive symptoms," which include delusions, hallucinations, looseness of associations, blunted or inappropriate affect, disturbances in the patient's sense of self, and bizarre or inappropriate behavior. On the other hand, schizophrenia also features "negative symptoms," such as apathy, thought blocking, autism-like behavior, abulia, and blunted affect. The prevalence of schizophrenia in the United States has been estimated to range from 6 per 1000 to 11 per 1000 (1).

It has been thought for some time that schizophrenia might have at least a partial genetic underpinning. Like most foci of psychiatric genetics, research on schizophrenia began with epidemiological studies that sought to document familial transmission of the disease. A consideration of the genetic data derived from those epidemiological studies is therefore an essential first step in the effort to understand the genetic transmission of schizophrenia.

From: *Early Clinical Intervention and Prevention in Schizophrenia*
Edited by: W. S. Stone, S. V. Faraone, and M. T. Tsuang © Humana Press Inc., Totowa, NJ

GENETIC EPIDEMIOLOGICAL STUDIES OF SCHIZOPHRENIA

Family Studies

The first family studies of schizophrenia were mostly undertaken in Europe, and began as early as the second decade of the 20th century *(2)*. That body of work showed that relatives of schizophrenic patients were at considerably greater risk of contracting the disease themselves. Specifically, the approximate life-time risks to first-degree relatives were 6% for parents, 9% for siblings, 13% for offspring with one schizophrenic parent, and 46% for offspring with two schizophrenic parents. (Parents probably had the lowest rate because schizophrenic patients are less likely to reproduce than are nonaffected individuals.) The approximate risk to other relatives were 6% for half-siblings, 2% for uncles and aunts, and 2% for first cousins *(2,3)*.

As noted by Gottesman *(3)*, many of the early studies of the familial transmission of schizophrenia lacked a control group that would permit a comparison of rates within a single study. Instead, they tended to compare rates of schizophrenia among their probands with those found in the general population *(4)*. Additionally, the researchers were frequently not blind to their subjects' diagnosis, and could therefore have been biased in their diagnostic decisions. This potentially problematic feature was exacerbated by different, and sometimes rather subjective, diagnostic criteria across the family studies and research among the general population.

More modern family studies of the transmission of schizophrenia have employed more rigorous techniques and narrower criteria for a diagnosis of the disease that incorporates neurological information in addition to clinical observations. An illustration of the importance of diagnostic criteria in conducting research of the sort found here was provided by Tsuang et al. *(5)*, who reported that the risk to first-degree relatives of schizophrenics was 3.2% when using the stringent Washington University criteria, 3.7% with *DSM–III* criteria, and 7.8% when the schizophrenia category was broadened to include atypical cases (e.g., schizoaffective disorder, psychosis not otherwise specified). As that work demonstrated, when the definition of schizophrenia is broader, higher rates of risk are generated *(6)*. Similarly, within the past decades, four studies *(7–10)* confirmed the notion that first-degree relatives of schizophrenic patients are at greater risk of developing schizophrenia themselves, although the reported degree of risk varied (1..16% for relatives vs 0. 2% for controls) depending on the operational criteria used by the researchers.

Twin Studies

Another persuasive line of research demonstrating a genetic component to schizophrenia has been generated from twin studies in which concordance rates

among monozygotic (MZ) are compared with those among dizygotic (DZ) twins *(11)*. In that connection, Kendler reviewed a series of twin studies and found the rate of concordance to be approx 53% for MZ pairs as contrasted with 15% for DZ pairs *(12)*. Interestingly, Gottesman *(2)* found a remarkably similar concordance rate of 46% for MZ pairs and 14% for DZ pairs. Taken together, the studies show that MZ twins are somewhat more than three times as likely to be concordant for schizophrenia than are DZ twins, despite the fact that the two types of twin pairs are presumably similar in the extent to which they share a common environment. Perhaps even more striking is a study of 12 pairs of MZ twins who were reared separately *(13)*: despite the fact that they were raised in entirely different environments, the twins evinced a 58% rate of concordance for schizophrenia. Obviously, however, the fact that MZ twins were not found in any work to be 100% concordant demonstrates the fact that genes cannot be the only cause of the disorder. In fact, when the relative contribution of genetic and environmental factors are compared, it has been shown that 60..70% of the variance is due to heritability.

Gottesman and Bertelson *(14)* conducted a third type of twin study in which the risk of developing schizophrenia was studied in the offspring of MZ and DZ twins who were *discordant* for schizophrenia. According to their rationale, if there is a genetically transmitted susceptibility to schizophrenia that was not expressed, the children of a nonafflicted MZ twin should then manifest schizophrenia at the same rate as the offspring of the afflicted MZ co-twin. That hypothesis received support: the offspring of nonafflicted co-twins displayed a prevalence of schizophrenia of 17.4%, as contrasted with a rate of 16.8% for the offspring of the schizophrenic twins. Moreover, the risk to offspring of a schizophrenic DZ twin was 17.4%, a level similar to that of the children of the MZ twins, but the risk to an offspring of a nonafflicted DZ co-twin was much lower, at 2.1%.

As with family studies, twin research shows substantial variability in risk rates across studies. Hence, the MZ concordance reports range from 45 to 75%; with DZ concordance ranging from 4 to 15% *(15–18)*. In that connection, McGuffin et al. *(15)* asserted that a schizophrenia diagnosis based on *DSM–III* criteria yield the highest estimates of heritability with twin research.

Adoption Studies

A third method of examining whether genes influence schizophrenia is to compare its prevalence in adoptive children with the prevalence in their biologic and adoptive relatives *(11)*. In a relatively early study, the prevalence of schizophrenia in 47 children of schizophrenic mothers who were adopted at infancy by nonbiologically related individuals was compared to the rate of illness in a control group of 50 adoptees with nonschizophrenic biological mothers *(19)*. It was

found that five biological children of schizophrenic mothers (10.6%) developed schizophrenia, whereas none of the biological children of nonafflicted mothers developed the disease. Similarly, in a study with a much larger sample, it was found that 32% of 5483 children who were given up for adoption by a schizophrenic biological parent developed schizophrenia themselves, in contrast to 18% of control adoptees (20). Kety and colleagues also determined prevalence rates for schizophrenia and related disorders in the biological relatives of schizophrenic adoptees. They found that 21% of the biological relatives of 33 schizophrenic adoptees were diagnosed with schizophrenia or a related disorder, in contrast to 11% of the biological relatives of 33 nonschizophrenic adoptees. Moreover, no differences in rates of schizophrenia were observed between the adoptive relatives of the schizophrenic and nonschizophrenic adoptees. Furthermore, children born to nonschizophrenic parents but raised by a schizophrenic parent did not show rates of schizophrenia above those predicted for the general population. That pattern of findings was more recently replicated by Kety et al. (21,22) and by Kendler and Gruenberg (23).

A potential problem with designs that focus either on the adoptees themselves or on the adoptees' relatives (24,25) is that, during gestation, a schizophrenic mother could possess or transmit some nongenetically based biological/physiological defect (e.g., eclampsia) that could later result in schizophrenia. Kety et al. addressed that issue by comparing rates of schizophrenia in paternal half-siblings of schizophrenic adoptees and in paternal half-siblings of nonschizophrenic adoptees. They found that 13% of the half-siblings of schizophrenic patients had the disorder, whereas 2% of the half-siblings of nonschizophrenic patients suffered from the disorder. Inasmuch as paternal half-siblings have different mothers, the higher rate of prevalence among the schizophrenic siblings could not have been due to some effect of the uterine environment.

Summary

Epidemiological studies of the genetics of schizophrenia support the following conclusions: (a) individuals with a schizophrenic relative are more likely than others to develop the disorder themselves; (b) an MZ twin with a co-twin who develops schizophrenia is substantially more likely to develop schizophrenia than is a DZ twin with a co-twin who develops schizophrenia; and (c) adoptees with a schizophrenic biological parent are more likely than adoptees who do not have a schizophrenic biologic parent to develop schizophrenia themselves, regardless of the status of their adoptive families. As a whole, therefore, this body of research has provided consistent backing for the idea that schizophrenia is partially, but not entirely, caused by genetic factors.

SCHIZOPHRENIA SPECTRUM DISORDERS

Epidemiologic studies have shown that there is a spectrum of disorders that are similar to schizophrenia, and that appear to be caused by the same cluster of genes. In fact, a disorder is considered to be in the schizophrenia spectrum if it occurs more frequently among the biological relatives of schizophrenic patients than it does among the relatives of people without schizophrenia. Family, twin, and adoption studies have also produced evidence for a genetic component in studies of schizophrenia-spectrum conditions.

Psychotic Spectrum Disorders

Approximately 9% of the first-degree relatives of schizophrenic patients have a psychotic disorder that does not qualify as either schizophrenia or a mood disorder *(26)*, most notably "schizoaffective disorder" and "psychosis, not otherwise specified" (NOS). The term "schizoaffective disorder" refers to a condition with features of both schizophrenia and affective disorders, although it is possible for either disorder to predominate *(13)*. It should be noted, however, that "psychosis NOS" is a diagnosis that is frequently applied to patients with psychotic symptoms who do not have symptoms that permit a more precisely defined category. The diagnosis is therefore often temporary, and is changed when the symptoms of the disorder permit a more refined diagnosis.

Both schizoaffective disorder and psychosis NOS are more common among the relatives of schizophrenic patients than they are among the relatives of non-schizophrenic individuals. For example, a review of family, twin, and adoption research showed that 13 out of 15 studies provided evidence for a genetic component for schizoaffective disorder *(13)*.

Personality Disorders

It has long been observed that some relatives of patients with schizophrenia have maladaptive personality traits, such as impaired interpersonal relationships, social anxiety, and constricted emotional responses. Less frequently, mild forms of thought disorder, suspiciousness, magical thinking, illusions, and perceptual aberrations have been observed. Those characteristics have been noted most often in schizotypal, schizoid, and paranoid personality disorders; thus, most studies of familial prevalence have been performed with those disorders.

Schizotypal personality disorder (SPD) has been observed to be more common among the biological relatives of chronic schizophrenic probands than among normal controls *(27)*. That finding has been consistently reported across family studies *(28–30)*, adoption studies *(27,31)*, and twin studies *(32,33)*. Although not all studies detected a higher rate of SPD among relatives of schizophrenic probands

(34,35), investigations with larger samples reveal that, as compared to relatives of controls, relatives of schizophrenics have higher rates of SPD *(36)*. In fact, estimates of the rate of SPD in schizophrenic families range between 4.2 and 14.6% *(28,29,37)*. Moreover, when a diagnosis of "probable" SPD is used, the estimate increases to 26.8% *(29)*.

Investigations of schizoid and paranoid personality disorders (PDs) have not provided evidence for an association *(29,38)*. The results of family studies indicate that schizophrenia and delusional disorder are not genetically related *(39–41)*. Moreover, rates of paranoid traits or *DSM–III* paranoid PD have not been found to be higher among first-degree relatives of schizophrenics *(41,42)*.

Results for schizoid PD show a somewhat stronger relationship, although it is not as strong as the apparent similarities of its symptoms (e.g., affective constriction and social isolation) to those in schizophrenia and other spectrum disorders might lead one to expect. For example, Baron et al. *(29)* found a higher (but not statistically significant) rate of schizoid PD in the relatives of schizophrenics compared to the relatives of controls (1.6% vs 0%). Kendler et al. *(37)* reported significant elevations of both paranoid and schizoid PD in relatives of persons with schizophrenia as compared to relatives of control subjects; however, those conditions were uncommon in their sample, and the increases in rate were modest.

Milder Spectrum Conditions: Schizotaxia

As discussed throughout this volume, the term "schizotaxia" refers to psychiatric, neuropsychological, neurological, and psychosocial deficits among nonpsychotic, first-degree relatives of people with schizophrenia *(43)*. In contrast to schizotypal PD, which occurs in less than 10% of the adult relatives of schizophrenic individuals *(36,44)*, the core features of schizotaxia range from 20 to 50% among first-degree relatives of schizophrenic patients *(45,46)*. Because it has not yet received formal acceptance as a diagnostic category, less epidemiologic research has been conducted for schizotaxia than for other schizophrenia spectrum disorders; more studies would be useful.

MODELS OF GENETIC TRANSMISSION

Intuitively, the most straightforward explanation for the mode of inheritance of schizophrenia would involve a simple Mendelian model, wherein a single mutation causes the disorder. Faraone et al. *(47)* showed, however, that a classic Mendelian explanation is not adequate. That is because, according to a Mendelian hypothesis, if a fully penetrant dominant gene caused schizophrenia, 50% of the offspring of one parent with schizophrenia would develop the disease. As discussed above, however, epidemiological research indicates that the rate of inheritance is much lower. Furthermore, if a fully penetrant recessive gene produces schizophrenia,

all of the offspring of two schizophrenic parents would also develop schizophrenia, whereas in fact, only 36..50% of the children of two schizophrenic parents actually develop the disorder. Perhaps most crucially, the majority of individuals with schizophrenia do not have *any* first-degree relatives with the disorder. A more complex mechanism of transmission must therefore underlie the disease.

A somewhat more sophisticated explanation for the heritability of schizophrenia is the single major locus (SML) model, i.e., the pair of genes at a single locus causes the transmission of a disease. An SML model can yield predictions of the prevalence of schizophrenia in the general population, the prevalence among children of people with schizophrenia, and the concurrence of the disorder among siblings *(48)*. Nevertheless, segregation analyses do not generally provide support for models based on single gene transmission. Even studies that did not exclude an SML acknowledge that it underestimates the risk to both MZ twins and also to the offspring of two schizophrenic parents.

Another approach to the problem involves a polygenic model, whereby "schizophrenia genes" are located at two or more loci. In that connection, there are two types of polygenic models: an oligogenic model that features a specific, limited number of loci, and a multifactorial polygenic (MFP) model that involves a large, unspecified number of loci. In connection with the latter, the term "polygenic" has come to be associated with the notion of a very large number of genes, with a limited effect size for each. The term "quantitative trait loci (QTL)" refers to multiple genes with variable individual effect sizes that, as a group, can determine the quantitative level of a trait *(49–52)*.

According to an MFP model, there are numerous interchangeable risk loci, and genes at those loci have variable, additive effects on the predisposition to schizophrenia. Those models assume that everyone has some degree of genetic "vulnerability" to schizophrenia. If the combined effects of many genetic (as well as environmental) influences summate beyond a certain, as yet undefined, threshold level, the result would be phenotypic schizophrenia or a schizophreniform disorder *(50,53)*. Whereas the MFP model appears to be a promising candidate, mixed models containing SML and MFP features are probably more effective in explaining the transmission of schizophrenia *(47,54,55)*.

Conclusions

It is inconceivable that the phenotype of schizophrenia is the outcome of the effects of a single gene. It is also very unlikely that the disease is caused by several genes with rather large, even effects. Rather, there appear to be many "susceptibility genes" of small, unequal effect size, which interact with each other (and the environment) to influence susceptibility to the disorder. Moreover, as shown by Risch *(55)*, the pattern of risk can be predicted more accurately when the prediction is based on the following: (a) the assumption of a higher risk ratio for relatives

than that of the general population; (b) a multilocus model, and (c) epistasis, or gene..gene interactions. The result is a sharper decline in risk as the extent of shared genes decreases than that which would be predicted by a noninteractive, multilocus model.

A final note in connection with the nature of the transmission of schizophrenia is that, in multilocus models such as that proposed by Risch (56), it is assumed that the same loci transmit vulnerability in most human populations. An alternative is conceivable, however, as discussed by Terwilliger et al. (57). Accordingly, it is also possible that multiple loci that transmit vulnerability vary, so that a stable constellation of genes conveying risk cannot be mapped across heterogenous populations.

LINKAGE ANALYSIS

Statistical genetics has yielded some powerful tools in the search for the genetic basis of schizophrenia. One of the most valuable techniques is linkage analysis. The rationale for linkage analysis derives from the finding that, when chromosomal DNA recombines during meiosis, genetic loci that are close to each other are more likely to be coinherited (or "cosegregate") than are loci that are more distant. That fact is important to the identification of genes that cause disease because, if some unidentified "disease gene" cosegregates with a polymorphic DNA marker with a known chromosomal locus, that marker can be used to find the disease gene. The marker must be polymorphic, so that one or more forms of it can be related to a disease gene. Linkage analysis became a powerful tool when molecular geneticists developed methods to identify many DNA markers throughout the genome.

Methods of linkage analysis involve computing the probability that the cosegregation of genetic markers and disease within pedigrees exceeds what would be expected by chance. Many linkage studies have been performed under SML conditions, in which the odds for linkage are analyzed for a specified degree of linkage. If the odds against a random finding (expressed as the logarithm of the odds ratio [LOD] score) exceed 1000 to 1 (with a corresponding LOD score of 3), evidence of linkage between a gene and a trait is provided. On the other hand, an LOD score of –2 is considered to be a cutoff point used to exclude the possibility of linkage. Those statistical decision rules have proven to be reliable for single gene diseases; however, for complex disorders like schizophrenia, other factors such as the presumed mode of transmission, the definition of the phenotype, the degree of penetrance of the disease gene, the sample size, and the number of affected family members, must also be considered in evaluating evidence for linkage (58). Unfortunately, some of those factors, such as the mode of transmission and the degree of penetrance, are not yet known for schizophrenia. To com-

pensate, linkage analyses can be performed repeatedly, with different values set for each parameter (e.g., degree of penetrance). A disadvantage of that approach, however, is that positive results must be viewed conservatively, because the risk of false-positive findings increases with the number of tests performed.

Linkage analysis is most effective in uncovering variance in genes with a Mendelian pattern of inheritance; nevertheless, independent linkage studies have produced evidence that schizophrenia-risk genes reside on several chromosomal sites. Furthermore, a number of these regions have recently gained added support from the results of two meta-analyses of all genome-wide scans for linkage with schizophrenia *(59,60)*. These findings, along with some other potentially interesting linkage results, are described next.

Chromosome 1

Several lines of research have indicated a linkage between schizophrenia and a locus on chromosome 1q. For example, early studies provided evidence of linkage between schizophrenia and a balanced translocation [t(1;11)(q42.1;q14.3)] involving chromosomes 1 and 11 *(61)*, work that was subsequently replicated *(62)*. An ensuing study also provided some evidence of linkage to chromosome 1: Hovatta et al. *(63)* reported linkage between a 90% penetrant dominant locus with 2 loci on 1q, a region that is centromeric to the chromosome 1q42.1 region reported by Millar et al. Hovatta's group *(64)* also found linkage to 1q32-41 among 69 families from Finland. Furthermore, Brzustowicz et al. *(65)* showed that 75% of families with schizophrenia were linked to that region, and they also showed linkage to 1q21-22 *(66)*. Despite the fact that Levinson et al. *(60)* found no evidence for linkage on 1q in their particular large, multicenter study, this locus shows suggestive evidence for linkage when examined across many samples by meta-analysis *(59)*.

Chromosome 2

Although chromosome 2 has not been identified in any single study as the locus showing the best evidence for linkage with schizophrenia, several studies have reported milder evidence for linkage on 2q. Thus, when the results of all genome-wide scans are examined collectively by meta-analysis, the proximal region of chromosome 2q emerges as a top candidate for harboring schizophrenia-susceptibility loci *(60,67)*.

Chromosome 5

Early linkage analysis regarding schizophrenia implicated partial trisomy of the long arm of chromosome 5, where an abnormality was found among two people with schizophrenia in a single family *(68)* and among seven other individuals across three families *(69)*. McGuffin found linkage to 5q11-q13 when data from

several previous investigations were combined *(70)*. Subsequently, the MCV/ Ireland group reported a maximum heterogeneity LOD score of 3.35 on chromosome 5q11. At the same time, the U Bonn group reported maximum LOD scores of 1.8 at marker IL9 in 14 pedigrees and 1.27 at D5S399 in an additional 40 pedigrees *(71)*. Straub et al. *(72)* found linkage throughout the region of 5q22-31, and Gurling et al. *(73)* provided new evidence for linkage to the chromosome 5q33.2. The possibility of a schizophrenia-risk locus on 5q has received additional support from meta-analysis as well *(60)*.

Chromosome 6

Research concerning chromosome 6p has received a substantial amount of attention, and has yielded mixed results. An initial study *(74)* reported evidence of linkage to chromosome 6p22 in a group of 265 Irish families; however a follow-up *(75)* reevaluated and expanded the sample, finding that the likelihood of linkage was lower than originally claimed; in fact, only one LOD score (at marker D6S296) was significant among the many analyses that were performed. In addition, linkage has been reported for 6q21-22 *(76)* and at an area of about 40 cM at 6p22-24 *(77,78)*. However, Maziade et al. *(79)* did not find evidence for linkage at 6q22 in 18 large, multigenerational pedigrees from Eastern Quebec, using a range of definitions for schizophrenia. Nevertheless, there was a trend toward linkage in one large pedigree, although that locus was linked both to schizophrenia and to bipolar disorder. That report highlighted the necessity of precision and uniformity in ascribing appropriate phenotypes for linkage analyses. Similarly, Gurling et al. *(73)* also failed to uncover linkage to chromosome 6q. Of note, the telomeric regions of both 6p and 6q have received support as schizophrenia-risk loci in different meta-analyses *(60,67)*.

Chromosome 8

Linkage studies at chromosome 8p21-22 have produced some results similar to those obtained at chromosome 6. Specifically, initial reports were at odds: significant linkage findings were reported by Blouin et al. *(80)*, Kendler et al. *(81)*, and Pulver et al. *(82,83)*. However, another large, multinational study failed to find significant results, although some evidence for linkage was still indicated (Schizophrenia Linkage Collaborative Group for Chromosomes 3, 6 and 8, 1996, no. 11404) *(84)*. Subsequently, it was concluded that there is strong support, from multiple studies, for schizophrenia-susceptibility loci on 8p21-22, despite reports that it was initially falsely implicated *(73)*. This conclusion seems to be strongly supported, as both recent meta-analyses have implicated chromosome 8p as a leading candidate locus for schizophrenia (Badner, 2002, no. 9111) *(60)*.

Chromosome 10

The first linkage study of chromosome 10 failed to provide evidence of linkage to any of four markers on 10p *(85)*. All of the markers excluded linkage (LOD <–2.0) under an autosomal dominant model and three excluded linkage under a recessive model. Moises et al. *(86)* also did not find linkage with 10p, and Barr et al. *(87)* found no evidence of linkage to markers on chromosome 10q, but did not evaluate linkage to 10p. By contrast, Faraone et al. (1998 no. 5742) provided suggestive evidence for linkage to 10p11-15 among European Americans, but not among African Americans *(88)*. Those findings with Caucasians at 10p11-15 were also uncovered in two other studies reported the same year *(89,90)*. Finally, the latest research on the subject has also indicated linkage for that locus, as well as evidence for intersample heterogeneity *(91)*.

Chromosome 11

Maziade *(92)* studied the 11q21-22 region among 242 individuals from four multigenerational pedigrees with high rates of schizophrenia, but did not find linkage with schizophrenia. Several subsequent studies also failed to uncover linkage; however, Craddock and Lendon *(93)* asserted regions 11q22-q23 might bear some relationship to psychotic symptoms *per se*. More recently, Gurling et al. *(73)* uncovered at least preliminary evidence of a relationship between schizophrenia and 11q21. Meta-analysis supports this region as a promising site for further linkage analysis *(60)*.

Chromosome 13

Studies of chromosome 13q have generally provided evidence of linkage to markers at 13q14.1-q32 *(94–96)*. Interestingly, Lin et al. *(97)* did not find evidence of linkage when they combined Caucasian and Asian pedigrees under a dominant genetic model. When the pedigrees were separated, however, only the Caucasian sample provided evidence of linkage. A subsequent study of 54 Caucasian pedigrees produced promising results with a site very near those reported by Lin et al. *(80)*, as did another group of 21 Canadian pedigrees *(98)*. Finally, Levinson and colleagues' *(91)* examination of the topic failed to provide evidence in either direction. Yet, chromosome 13q remains a region of intense interest because of the relatively consistent evidence for linkage at this locus discerned by pooled data analysis *(67)*.

Chromosome 15

Freedman et al. *(99)* linked schizophrenia to a mutant allele on chromosome 15q14, in the region of the alpha 7 subunit of the nicotinic acetylcholine receptor. Similar results were reported by Coon et al. *(85)*, Adler et al. *(100)*, Leonard et

al. *(101)*, and most recently, Stober et al. *(102)*. In fact, in a review of linkage data presented at the Sixth World Congress of Psychiatric Genetics, Craddock and Lendon *(103)* asserted that sites 15q13-q15 are strongly linked specifically to the phenotype for schizophrenia. Nevertheless, Curtis et al. *(104)* failed to uncover linkage at 15q13 and 15q14. Results from meta-analysis provide only weak evidence for a schizophrenia-sucseptibility locus on this chromosome *(67)*.

Chromosome 22

Three early linkage studies of 22q11-13 provided preliminary evidence of linkage, although small sample sizes, or a wide range of modeling assumptions concerning the mode of transmission, were usually involved *(105–107)*. A subsequent project involving a larger sample *(108)* excluded linkage to those loci; although, in a follow-up of the original sample, linkage could not be excluded *(109)*, and others demonstrated positive results *(110,111)*. A combined analysis of data from 11 independent research groups *(112)*, using an affected sib pair method, again provided evidence of linkage at 22q11-13 that might account for a small proportion (approx 3.5%) of the susceptibility to schizophrenia. Finally, Stober et al. also provided moderate support for linkage at that site *(102)*. As one of the most reliably implicated loci for schizophrenia from both meta-analyses, chromosome 22q remains as one of the most likely harbors for schizophrenia-risk genes *(60,67)*.

X Chromosome

The Finnish study described earlier by Hovatta et al. *(64)* reported a moderately significant linkage finding at Xp11, the site at which the monoamine oxidase B gene is found. Two other groups also reported significant findings at DXS7, a region that is close to Xp11 *(113,114)*, although two more recent studies have failed to do so *(115,116)*.

Summary

Despite the large amount of research that has already been done on the topic, linkage in schizophrenia has yet to be definitively established *(117)*. Nevertheless, linkage analysis has provided persuasive evidence for linkage at multiple sites, including, 1q21-22, 1q32-41, 2q, 5p13-14, 5q22-31, 6p22-24, 6q21-22, 8p21-22, 10p11-15, 13q14-32, 15q15, 22q11-13, and Xp11.

Conclusions

Few (if any) scientists would argue that genes do not play an important role in the etiology of schizophrenia, nor that genetic research has not contributed substantially to the understanding of the disease. Schizophrenia is almost certainly

caused by the interaction of many genes with a small, unequal effect size; however, research has not yet uncovered the specific genes that underlie the disease, and the relative contributions of those genes therefore remain unknown *(118)*.

Molecular geneticists are still in the early stages of identifying the complicated modes of inheritance that underlie schizophrenia. In order for schizophrenia research in psychiatric genetics to continue to advance, the following should be made high priorities: (a) an improvement of psychiatric genetic nosologies to specify useful phenotypes for linkage studies; (b) a focus on neurobiological dysfunctions that reflect more proximal effects of aberrant genes, which can serve as phenotypes in linkage studies; (c) an improvement in statistical models that account for the multifactorial etiology and heterogeneous nature of schizophrenia, including possible epistasis and intergenerational changes; and (d) continued large-scale studies with well-defined pedigrees to detect involved loci. As the relationship between genes and schizophrenia becomes better understood, improvements in traditional psychotherapeutic treatment techniques as well as pharmacotherapy will almost certainly ensue, as will important ethical debates regarding the study of so crucial a disease gene and, ultimately, the dissemination of these findings.

ACKNOWLEDGMENTS

Preparation of this chapter was supported in part by grants RO1MH43518, R01MH59624, and R01MH60485 from the National Institute of Mental Health to Dr. Ming T. Tsuang. This work was completed when Drs. Glatt and Taylor were trainees in the National Institute of Mental Health funded Psychiatric Genetics Training Program at the Harvard Institute of Psychiatric Epidemiology and Genetics (R25MH60485, M. Tsuang, PI).

REFERENCES

1. Tsuang MT, Faraone SV, Green AI. Schizophrenia and other psychotic disorders. In: Armand M, Nicholi J, eds. The Harvard Guide to Psychiatry. Cambridge, MA: Harvard University Press, 1999.
2. Gottesman II. Schizophrenia Genesis: The Origin of Madness. New York: Freeman, 1991.
3. Gottesman II. Origins of schizophrenia: past as prologue. In: Plomin R, McClearn GE, eds. Nature, Nurture, and Psychology. Washington, DC: American Psychological Association, 1993:231..244.
4. Kendler KS, Gruenberg AM, Tsuang MT. A family study of the subtypes of schizophrenia. Am J Psychiatry 1988; 145:57..62.
5. Tsuang MT, Vandermey R. Genes and the Mind: Inheritance of Mental Illness. London: Oxford University Press, 1980.
6. Faraone SV, Tsuang MT. Familial links between schizophrenia and other disorders: application of the multifactorial polygenic model. Psychiatry: Interpersonal and Biological Processes 1988; 51:37..47.

7. Parnas J, Cannon TD, Jacobsen B, Schulsinger H, Schulsinger F, Mednick SA. Lifetime DSM.III.R diagnostic outcomes in the offspring of schizophrenic mothers. Results from the Copenhagen high-risk study. Arch Gen Psychiatry 1993; 50:707..714.

8. Kendler KS, McGuire M, Gruenberg AM, O'Hare A, Spellman M, Walsh D. The Roscommon Family Study. I. Methods, diagnosis of probands, and risk of schizophrenia in relatives. Arch Gen Psychiatry 1993; 50:527.540.

9. Maier W, Lichtermann D, Minges J, et al. Continuity and discontinuity of affective disorders and schizophrenia. Results of a controlled family study. Arch Gen Psychiatry 1993; 50: 871..883.

10. Cornblatt BA, Keilp JG. Impaired attention, genetics, and the pathophysiology of schizophrenia. Schizophr Bull 1994; 20:31..46.

11. Faraone SV, Tsuang D, Tsuang MT. Psychiatric Genetics: A Guide for Mental Health Professionals. New York: Guilford, 1999.

12. Kendler KS. Overview: a current perspective on twin studies of schizophrenia. Am J Psychiatry 1983; 140:1413..1425.

13. Prescott CA, Gottesman II. Genetically mediated vulnerability to schizophrenia. Psychiatr Clin North Am 1993; 16:245.267.

14. Gottesman II, Bertelsen A. Confirming unexpressed genotypes for schizophrenia. Risks in the offspring of Fischer's Danish identical and fraternal discordant twins. Arch Gen Psychiatry 1989; 46:867..872.

15. McGuffin P, Farmer AE, Gottesman II, Murray RM, Reveley AM. Twin concordance for operationally defined schizophrenia. Confirmation of familiality and heritability. Arch Gen Psychiatry 1984; 41:541..545.

16. Farmer AE, McGuffin P, Gottesman II. Twin concordance for DSM.III schizophrenia: scrutinizing the validity of the definition. Arch Gen Psychiatry 1987; 44:634..641.

17. Onstad S, Skre I, Torgersen S, Kringlen E. Twin concordance for DSM.III.R schizophrenia. Acta Psychiatr Scand 1991; 83:395..401.

18. Cannon T, Kaprio J, Lonnqvist J, Huttunen M, Koskenvuo M. The genetic epidemiology of schizophrenia in a Finnish twin cohort. Arch Gen Psychiatry 1998; 55:67..74.

19. Heston LL. Psychiatric disorders in foster home-reared children of schizophrenic mothers. Br J Psychiatry 1966; 112:819..825.

20. Kety SS, Rosenthal D, Wender PH, Schulsinger F. The types and prevalence of mental illness in the biological and adoptive families of adopted schizophrenics. J Psychiatr Res 1968; 1:345..362.

21. Kety SS. Schizophrenic illness in the families of schizophrenic adoptees: findings from the Danish national sample. Schizophr Bull 1988; 14:217..222.

22. Kety SS, Wender PH, Jacobsen B, et al. Mental illness in the biological and adoptive relatives of schizophrenic adoptees. Replication of the Copenhagen study in the rest of Denmark. Arch Gen Psychiatry 1994; 51:442..455.

23. Kendler KS, Gruenberg AM, Kinney DK. Independent diagnoses of adoptees and relatives as defined by DSM.III in the provincial and national samples of the Danish adoption study of schizophrenia. Arch Gen Psychiatry 1994; 51:456..468.

24. Tienari P, Wynne L. Adoption studies of schizophrenia. Ann Med 1994; 26:233..237.

25. McGue M, Gottesman II. The genetic epidemiology of schizophrenia and the design of linkage studies. Eur Arch Psychiatry Clin Neurosci 1991; 240:174..181.

26. Gottesman II, Shields J. Schizophrenia: The Epigenetic Puzzle. Cambridge, England: Cambridge University Press, 1982.

27. Siever LJ, Kalus OF, Keefe RSE. The boundaries of schizophrenia. Psychiatr Clin North Am 1993; 16:217..244.
28. Baron M, Gruen R, Asnis L, Kane J. Familial relatedness of schizophrenia and schizotypal states. Am J Psychiatry 1983; 140:1437..1442.
29. Baron M, Gruen R, Asnis L, Lord S. Familial transmission of schizotypal and borderline personality disorders. Am J Psychiatry 1985; 142:927..934.
30. Kendler KS, Masterson CC, Ungaro R, Davis KL. A family history study of schizophrenia-related personality disorders. Am J Psychiatry 1984; 141:424..427.
31. Gunderson JG, Siever LJ, Spaulding E. The search for a schizotype: crossing the border again. Arch Gen Psychiatry 1983; 40:15..22.
32. Siever LJ, Gunderson JG. Genetic determinants of borderline conditions. Schizophr Bull 1979; 5:59..86.
33. Torgersen S. Relationship of schizotypal personality disorder to schizophrenia: genetics. Schizophr Bull 1985; 11:554..563.
34. Coryell WH, Zimmerman M. Personality disorder in the families of depressed, schizophrenic, and never-ill probands. Am J Psychiatry 1989; 146:496..502.
35. Squires-Wheeler E, Skodol AE, Bassett A, Erlenmeyer-Kimling L. DSM.III.R schizotypal personality traits in offspring of schizophrenic disorder, affective disorder, and normal control parents. J Psychiatr Res 1989; 23:229..239.
36. Battaglia M, Torgersen S. Schizotypal disorder: at the crossroads of genetics and nosology. Acta Psychiatr Scand 1996; 94:303..310.
37. Kendler KS, McGuire M, Gruenberg AM, O'Hare A, Spellman M, Walsh D. The Roscommon Family Study. III. Schizophrenia-related personality disorders in relatives. Arch Gen Psychiatry 1993; 50:781..788.
38. Rogers KL, Winokur G. The genetics of schizoaffective disorder and the schizophrenia spectrum. In: Tsuang MT, Simpson JC, eds. Handbook of Schizophrenia: Vol. 3. Nosology, Epidemiology, & Genetics. New York: Elsevier, 1988.
39. Kendler KS, Tsuang MT. Nosology of paranoid, schizophrenic, and other paranoid psychoses. Schizophr Bull 1981; 7:594..610.
40. Kendler KS, Hayes P. Paranoid psychosis (delusional disorder) and schizophrenia. Arch Gen Psychiatry 1981; 38:547..551.
41. Winokur G. Familial psychopathology in delusional disorder. Compr Psychiatry 1985; 26:241..248.
42. Kendler K. Diagnostic approaches to schizotypal personality disorder: a historical perspective. Schizophr Bull 1985; 11:538..553.
43. Faraone SV, Green AI, Seidman LJ, Tsuang MT. "Schizotaxia": clinical implications and new directions for research. Schizophr Bull 2001; 27:1..18.
44. Battaglia M, Bernardeschi L, Franchini L, Bellodi L, Smeraldi E. A family study of schizotypal disorder. Schizophr Bull 1995; 21:33..45.
45. Faraone SV, Kremen WS, Lyons MJ, Pepple JR, Seidman LJ, Tsuang MT. Diagnostic accuracy and linkage analysis: how useful are schizophrenia spectrum phenotypes? Am J Psychiatry 1995; 152:1286..1290.
46. Faraone SV, Seidman LJ, Kremen WS, Pepple JR, Lyons MJ, Tsuang MT. Neuropsychological functioning among the nonpsychotic relatives of schizophrenic patients: a diagnostic efficiency analysis. J Abnorm Psychol 1995; 104:286..304.
47. Faraone SV, Tsuang MT. Quantitative models of the genetic transmission of schizophrenia. Psychol Bull 1985; 98:41..66.

48. Tsuang MT, Gilbertson MW, Faraone SV. The genetics of schizophrenia: Current knowledge and future directions. Schizophr Res 1991; 4:157..171.
49. Crabbe JC, Belknap JK, Buck KJ. Genetic animal models of alcohol and drug abuse. Science 1994; 264:1715..1723.
50. Gottesman II. Twins: en route to QTLs for cognition. Science 1997; 276:1522..1523.
51. Plomin R, Pedersen NL, Lichtenstein P, McClearn GE. Variability and stability in cognitive abilities are largely genetic later in life. Behav Genet 1994; 24:207..215.
52. Takahashi JS, Pinto LH, Vitaterna MH. Forward and reverse approaches to behavior in the mouse. Science 1994; 264:1724..1732.
53. McGue M, Bouchard TJ Jr, Iacono WG, Lykken DT. Behavioral genetics of cognitive ability: a life-span perspective. In: Plomin R, McClearn GE, eds. Nature, Nurture, and Psychology. Washington, DC: American Psychological Association, 1993:59..76.
54. Risch N, Baron M. Segregation analysis of schizophrenia and related disorders. Am J Hum Genet 1984; 36:1039..1059.
55. Vogler GP, Gottesman II, McGue MK, Rao DC. Mixed model segregation analysis of schizophrenia in the Lindelius Swedish pedigrees. Behav Genet 1990; 20:461..472.
56. Risch N. Genetic linkage and complex diseases, with special reference to psychiatric disorders. Genet Epidemiol 1990; 7:3..7.
57. Terwilliger JD, Zollner S, Laan M, Paabo S. Mapping genes through the use of linkage disequilibrium generated by genetic drift: "drift mapping" in small populations with no demographic expansion. Hum Hered 1998; 48:138..154.
58. Lander E, Kruglyak L. Genetic dissection of complex traits: Guidelines for interpreting and reporting linkage results. Nat Genet 1995; 11:241..247.
59. Badner J, Gershon E. Meta-analysis of whole-genome linkage scans of bipolar disorder and schizophrenia. Mol Psychiatry 2002; 7:405..411.
60. Levinson DF, Lewis CM, Wise LH. 16 contributing groups. Meta-analysis of genome scans for schizophrenia. Am J Med Genet (Neuropsychiatric Genetics) 2002; 114:700..701.
61. St. Clair D, Blackwood D, Muir W, et al. Association within a family of a balanced autosomal translocation with major mental illness. Lancet 1990; 336:13..16.
62. Millar JK, Christie S, Semple CA, Porteus DJ. Chromosomal location and genomic structure of the human translin-associated factor X gene (TRAX; TSNAX) revealed by intergenic splicing to DISC1, a gene disrupted by a translocation segregating with schizophrenia. Genomics 2000; 67:69..77.
63. Hovatta L, Terwilliger J, Lichtermann D, et al. Schizophrenia in the genetic isolate of Finland. Am J Med Genet (Neuropsychiatric Genetics) 1997; 74:353..360.
64. Hovatta I, Varilo T, Suvisaari J, et al. A genomewide screen for schizophrenia genes in an isolated Finnish subpopulation, suggesting multiple susceptibility loci. Am J Hum Genet 1999; 65:1114..1124.
65. Brzustowicz LM, Hodgkinson KA, Chow EWC, Honer WG, Basett AS. Location of a major susceptibility locus for familial schizophrenia on chromosome 1q21-q22. Science 2000; 288: 678..682.
66. Shaw SH, Kelly M, Smith AB, et al. A genome-wide search for schizophrenia susceptibility genes. Am J Med Genet (Neuropsychiatric Genetics) 1998; 81:364..376.
67. Badner JA, Gershon ES, Berrettini WH, et al. Evidence of linkage disequilibrium between bipolar disorder and D18S53. Psychiatr Genet 1995; 5:S16.
68. Bassett AS, McGillivray BC, Jones BD, Pantzar JT. Partial trisomy of chromosome 5 cosegregating with schizophrenia. Lancet 1988; 1:799..801.

69. Sherrington R, Brynjolfsson J, Petursson H, et al. Localization of a susceptibility locus for schizophrenia on chromosome 5. Nature 1988; 336:164..167.
70. McGuffin P, Sargeant M, Hetti G, Tidmarsh S, Whatley S, Marchbanks RM. Exclusion of a schizophrenia susceptibility gene from the chromosome 5q11-q13 region: new data and a reanalysis of previous reports. Am J Hum Genet 1990; 47:524..535.
71. Schwab SG, Eckstein GN, Hallmayer J, et al. Evidence suggestive of a locus on chromosome 5q31 contributing to susceptibility for schizophrenia in German and Israeli families by multipoint affected sib-pair linkage analysis. Mol Psychiatry 1997; 2:156..160.
72. Straub RE, MacLean CJ, O'Neill FA, Walsh D, Kendler KS. Support for a possible schizophrenia vulnerability locus in region 5q21-q31 in Irish families. Mol Psychiatry 1997; 2:148..155.
73. Gurling HM, Kalsi G, Brynjolfson J, et al. Genomewide genetic linkage analysis confirms the presence of susceptibility loci for schizophrenia, on chromosomes 1q32.2, 5q33.2, and 8p21-22 and provides support for linkage to schizophrenia, on chromosomes 11q23.3-24 and 20q12.1-11.23. Am J Hum Genet 2001; 68:661..673.
74. Wang S, Sun CE, Walczak CA, et al. Evidence for a susceptibility locus for schizophrenia on chromosome 6pter-p22. Nat Genet 1995; 10:41..46.
75. Straub RE, MacLean CJ, O'Neill FA, et al. A potential vulnerability locus for schizophrenia on chromosome 6p24-22: evidence for genetic heterogeneity. Nat Genet 1995; 11:287..293.
76. Cao Q, Martinez M, Zhang J, et al. Suggestive evidence for a schizophrenia susceptibility locus on chromosome 6q and a confirmation in an independent series of pedigrees. Genomics 1997; 43:1..8.
77. Antonarakis SE, Blouin J-L, Pulver AE, et al. Schizophrenia susceptibility and chromosome 6p24-22. Nat Genet 1995; 11:235..236.
78. Schwab SG, Albus M, Hallmayer J, et al. Evaluation of a susceptibility gene for schizophrenia on chromosome 6p by multipoint affected sib-pair linkage analysis. Nat Genet 1995; 11: 325..327.
79. Maziade M, Bissonnette L, Rouillard E, et al. 6p24-22 region and major psychoses in the eastern Quebec population. Am J Med Genet (Neuropsychiatric Genetics) 1997; 74:311..318.
80. Blouin J, Dombroski BA, Nath SK, et al. Schizophrenia susceptibility loci on chromosomes 13q32 and 8p21. Nat Genet 1998; 28:70..73.
81. Kendler KS, MacLean CJ, O'Neill FA, et al. Evidence for a schizophrenia vulnerability locus on chromosome 8p in the Irish Study of High-Density Schizophrenia Families. Am J Psychiatry 1996; 153:1534..1540.
82. Pulver AE. Search for schizophrenia susceptibility genes. Biol Psychiatry 2000; 47:221..230.
83. Pulver AE, Mulle J, Nestadt G, et al. Genetic heterogeneity in schizophrenia: stratification of genome scan data using co-segregating related phenotypes. Mol Psychiatry 2000; 5:650..653.
84. Kunugi H, Curtis D, Vallada HP, et al. A linkage study of schizophrenia with DNA markers from chromosome 8p21-p22 in 25 multiplex families. Schizophr Res 1996; 22:61..68.
85. Coon H, Jensen S, Holik J, et al. Genomic scan for genes predisposing to schizophrenia. Am J Med Genet (Neuropsychiatric Genetics) 1994; 54:59..71.
86. Moises HW, Yang L, Kristbjarnarson H, et al. An international two-stage genome-wide search for schizophrenia susceptibility genes. Nat Genet 1995; 11:321..324.
87. Barr CL, Kennedy JL, Pakstis AJ, et al. Progress in a genome scan for linkage in schizophrenia in a large Swedish kindred. Am J Med Genet (Neuropsychiatric Genetics) 1994; 54:51..58.
88. Kaufmann CA, Suarez B, Malaspina D, et al. NIMH genetics initiative Millennium schizophrenia consortium: linkage analysis of African-American pedigrees. Am J Med Genet (Neuropsychiatric Genetics) 1998; 81:282..289.

89. Straub RE, MacLean CJ, Martin RB, et al. A schizophrenia locus may be located in region 10p15-p11. Am J Med Genet (Neuropsychiatric Genetics) 1998; 81:296..301.
90. Schwab SG, Hallmayer J, Albus M, et al. Further evidence for a susceptibility locus on chromosome 10p14-p11 in 72 families with schizophrenia by non-parametric linkage analysis. Am J Med Genet (Neuropsychiatric Genetics) 1998; 81:302..307.
91. Levinson DF, Holmans P, Straub RE, et al. Multicenter linkage study of schizophrenia candidate regions on chromosomes 5q, 6q, 10p, and 13q: schizophrenia linkage collaborative group III. Am J Hum Genet 2000; 67:652..663.
92. Maziade M, Raymond V, Cliche D, et al. Linkage results on 11Q21-22 in Eastern Quebec pedigrees densely affected by schizophrenia. Am J Med Genet (Neuropsychiatric Genetics) 1995; 60:522..528.
93. Craddock N, Lendon C. New susceptibility gene for Alzheimer's disease on chromosome 12? Lancet 1998; 352:1720..1721.
94. Lin MW, Curtis D, Williams N, et al. Suggestive evidence for linkage of schizophrenia to markers on chromosome 13q14.1-q32. Psychiatr Genet 1995; 5:117..126.
95. Antonarakis SE, Blouin JL, Curran M, Luebbert H, Kazazian HH, Dombroski B, et al. Linkage and sibpair analysis reveal a potential schizophrenia susceptibility gene on 13q32. Am J Hum Genet 1996; 59:A210.
96. Kalsi G, Chen C-H, Smyth C, Brynjolfsson J, Sigmundsson T, Curtis D, et al. Genetic linkage analysis in an Icelandic/British family fails to exclude the putative chromosome 13q14.1-q32 schizophrenia susceptibility locus. Am J Hum Genet 1996; 59:A388.
97. Lin MW, Sham P, Hwu HG, Collier D, Murray R, Powell JF. Suggestive evidence for linkage of schizophrenia to markers on chromosome 13 in Caucasian but not Oriental population. Hum Genet 1997; 99:417..420.
98. Brzustowicz LM, Honer WG, Chow EW, et al. Linkage of familial schizophrenia to chromosome 13q32. Am J Hum Genet 1999; 65:1096..1103.
99. Freedman R, Coon H, Myles-Worsley M, et al. Linkage of a neurophysiological deficit in schizophrenia to a chromosome 15 locus. Proc Natl Acad Sci USA 1997; 94:587..592.
100. Adler LE, Freedman R, Ross RG, Olincy A, Waldo MC. Elementary phenotypes in the neurobiological and genetic study of schizophrenia. Biol Psychiatry 1999; 46:8..18.
101. Leonard S, Gault J, Moore T, et al. Further investigation of a chromosome 15 locus in schizophrenia: analysis of affected sibpairs from the NIMH Genetics Initiative. Am J Med Genet (Neuropsychiatric Genetics) 1998; 81:308.312.
102. Stober G, Saar K, Ruschendorf F, et al. Splitting schizophrenia: periodic catatonia-susceptibility locus on chromosome 15q15. Am J Hum Genet 2000; 67:1201..1207.
103. Craddock N, Lendon C. Chromosome Workshop: chromosomes 11, 14, and 15. Am J Med Genet (Neuropsychiatric Genetics) 1999; 88:244.254.
104. Curtis D. Chromosome 21 workshop. Am J Med Genet (Neuropsychiatric Genetics) 1999; 88:272.275.
105. Coon H, Holik J, Hoff M, et al. Analysis of chromosome 22 markers in 9 schizophrenia pedigrees. Am J Med Genet (Neuropsychiatric Genetics) 1994; 54:72..79.
106. Pulver AE, Karayiorgou M, Wolyneic P, et al. Sequential strategy to identify a susceptibility gene for schizophrenia: report of potential linkage on on chromosome 22q12-q13.1: part 1. Am J Med Genet (Neuropsychiatric Genetics) 1994; 54:36.43.
107. Polymeropoulos MH, Coon H, Byerley W, et al. Search for a schizophrenia susceptibility locus on human chromosome 22. Am J Med Genet (Neuropsychiatric Genetics) 1994; 54: 93..99.

108. Pulver AE, Karayiorgou M, Lasseter VK, et al. Follow-up of a report of a potential linkage for schizophrenia on chromosome 22q12-q13.1: part 2. Am J Med Genet (Neuropsychiatric Genetics) 1994; 54:44..50.

109. Lasseter VK, Pulver AE, Wolyniec PS, et al. Follow-up report of potential linkage for schizophrenia on chromosome 22q: part 3. Am J Med Genet (Neuropsychiatric Genetics) 1995; 60:172..173.

110. Moises HW, Yang L, Havsteen B, et al. Evidence for linkage disequilibrium between schizophrenia and locus D22S278 on the long arm of chromosome 22. Am J Med Genet (Neuropsychiatric Genetics) 1995; 60:465..467.

111. Vallada HP, Collier D, Sham P, et al. Linkage studies on chromosome 22 in familial schizophrenia. Am J Med Genet (Neuropsychiatric Genetics) 1995; 60:139..146.

112. Schizophrenia Collaborative Linkage Group (Chromosome 22). A combined analysis of D22S278 marker alleles in affected sib-pairs: support for a susceptibility locus at chromosomen 22q12. Am J Med Genet (Neuropsychiatric Genetics) 1996; 67:40..45.

113. Dann J, DeLisi LE, Devoto M, et al. A linkage study of schizophrenia to markers within Xp11 near the *MAOB* gene. Psychiatry Res 1997; 70:131..143.

114. DeLisi LE, Friedrich U, Wahlstrom J, et al. Schizophrenia and sex chromosome anomalies. Schizophr Bull 1994; 20:495..505.

115. Kalsi G, Gamble D, Curtis D, et al. No evidence for linkage of schizophrenia to DXS7 at chromosome Xp11. Psychiatr Genet 1999; 9:197..199.

116. DeLisi LE, Shaw S, Sherrington R, et al. Failure to establish linkage on the X chromosome in 301 families with schizophrenia or schizoaffective disorder. Am J Med Genet (Neuropsychiatric Genetics) 2000; 96:335..341.

117. Moldin SO, Gottesman, II. At issue: genes, experience, and chance in schizophrenia   positioning for the 21st century. Schizophr Bull 1997; 23:547..561.

118. Tsuang MT. Genetics, epidemiology and the search for the causes of schizophrenia. Am J Psychiatry 1994; 151:3..6.

2

Early Environmental Determinants of Schizophrenia

Jason Schiffman, PhD,
John Carter, MA, Ricardo A. Machón, PhD,
and Sarnoff Mednick, PhD, MD

Modern research conceptualizes schizophrenia as a disorder stemming from multiple sources of risk. Genetic vulnerability (having parents with schizophrenia) is the single strongest liability for schizophrenia. Researchers also identify early environmental determinants contributing to the later development of schizophrenia. Some of these early risk factors include maternal health during pregnancy, obstetrical complications through pregnancy, and later rearing circumstances through childhood. This chapter discusses each of these early environmental risk factors in turn.

To help explain the origins of schizophrenia, Mednick and colleagues propose a "two-hit model" *(1)*. The theory suggests that two stressors, or "hits," result in increased risk for schizophrenia. The *first hit* stems from a genetic liability for schizophrenia that may increase risk for disruptions of fetal neural development. In cases with low genetic risk, teratogens such as influenza, or maternal stress, during a critical period of gestation (e.g., second trimester), may cause disruptions of fetal neural development that contributes to later schizophrenia. According to the theory, the *second hit* is an environmental stressor; examples of second hits include high levels of family stress, unstable rearing circumstances, and possibly obstetrical complications. When the first and second hits occur, risk for schizophrenia increases.

THE FIRST HIT: SECOND-TRIMESTER DISRUPTION AND ADULT MENTAL HEALTH

In 1988, we reported an increase in the rate of schizophrenia among Helsinki residents exposed to the 1957 influenza virus. Individuals were at greater risk for

From: *Early Clinical Intervention and Prevention in Schizophrenia*
Edited by: W. S. Stone, S. V. Faraone, and M. T. Tsuang © Humana Press Inc., Totowa, NJ

schizophrenia if they were exposed to the virus during the second trimester (or more precisely, the sixth month) of fetal development *(2)*. Since 1988, most research continues to support the hypothesis that a teratogen experienced during the second trimester increases risk for schizophrenia *(3–6)*. There have been some failures to replicate *(7)*. In a follow-up of our original 1988 report, we reported that 86.7% of schizophrenia patients whose second-trimester gestation overlapped the height of the epidemic had mothers who *actually contracted* influenza (not simply exposed) *(8)*.

Sixth-Month Studies

Timing of exposure may impact later psychopathological outcome. Five prenatal influenza infection studies similar to our own suggest that the schizophrenia-relevant teratogen occurred during the sixth month of gestation *(9–13)*.

In addition to schizophrenia, affective disorders, as well as violent offending, relate to maternal influenza infection *(14,15)*. Results suggest increases in affective disorders among individuals exposed to the 1957 Helsinki influenza during the second trimester. The authors compared the precise timing of exposure of patients with schizophrenia to the exposure of patients with affective disorders. The majority of individuals with affective disorders experienced influenza exposure during the fifth month of gestation, whereas the majority of individuals with schizophrenia experienced influenza exposure during the sixth month of gestation *(8)*.

Examining this same cohort also reveals a relation between violent offending and second-trimester exposure to the influenza epidemic. Mednick and Tehrani contend that late sixth-month and early seventh-month exposure to the influenza epidemic increases risk for violent criminal offending, but not property offending *(16)*. These data suggest that specific behavioral deviance may differentially relate to specific brain systems. If the development of a specific brain system is compromised, then risk for a specific behavioral disorder may be increased. Which brain region is at risk may depend on which fetal brain area is experiencing rapid development at the time of the impact of the teratogen.

EFFECTS OF A FIRST HIT:
SCHIZOTYPAL PERSONALITY DISORDER
AND SECOND-TRIMESTER DISRUPTION

Schizotypal personality disorder (SPD) resembles schizophrenia in nature, but is lesser in terms of severity of symptoms. Researchers often consider SPD as a less severe condition on a continuum toward schizophrenia. SPD is more common and less debilitating than schizophrenia, therefore, studying individuals with SPD offers a more convenient population to derive information regarding the determinants of schizophrenia.

As mentioned earlier, we have suggested that schizophrenia is a "two-hit" disorder. We posit that the first hit alone, without a second hit, may increase risk for neural disorganization leading to cognitive and perceptual distortions observed in people with SPD.

The Finnish Recruit Study

We predict that a severe influenza epidemic may constitute increased risk for a first hit and may correlate with an increase of births of individuals who later develop SPD. (Some of these individuals will suffer a second hit, which will increase risk for schizophrenia.) We determined to test the hypothesis that a second-trimester maternal influenza exposure would correlate with an elevation in the number of SPD individuals. We exploited the fact that almost all Finnish young men must serve in the military. All new recruits are given the Minnesota Multiphasic Personality Inventory (MMPI). We defined an MMPI scale score pattern that would relate to an SPD diagnosis. We hypothesized that recruits exposed to an influenza epidemic during their sixth month of gestation would more often evidence a pattern of MMPI scales scores reflecting a diagnosis of SPD than would nonexposed recruits.

All Finnish draftees are given a standardized battery of psychological tests, including the MMPI. In 1969, a pandemic of type A influenza struck Helsinki, Finland, between January 12 and January 26. We analyzed the adult MMPI results of individuals *in utero* during the pandemic ($N = 2339$). As a comparison group, we examined the adult MMPI results of a noninfluenza-exposed group born 2 years later ($N = 2151$). An individual's week of birth provided an estimate of the week of exposure to the pandemic. The influenza group had an average of 58 individuals born each week ($SD = 8.8$). (Note that the exposed and nonexposed subjects were tested with the MMPI at the same age.)

To provide a relative index of schizotypal personality disorder, we combined scales 7 (Pt, Psychasthenia) and 8 (Sc, Schizophrenia) of the MMPI to construct the SPD scale score *(17)*. (The original formulation of the SPD composite included scale 2 [D, depression] in the index of SPD. The Army psychological evaluation of subjects in this study did not include the administration of scale 2 of the MMPI.) We hypothesized that individuals exposed to the influenza virus during the sixth month of gestation (weeks 21.24) would show elevated SPD scale scores as compared to control subjects born during the same week, 2 years later, in an epidemic-free year. Results suggest that fetuses exposed during the 23rd week of gestation have a significantly higher mean schizotypal scale score ($M = 9.2$, $SD = 3.9$) than control subjects born during the same week of the year, 2 years later ($M = 7.7$, $SD = .1$). Weeks 21, 22, and 24 show no differences between exposed and nonexposed. In exploratory analysis we find no other week evidencing an increase in the SPD scale score. The isolated effect of week 23 suggests the possibility of

a narrow window for developmental disruptions impacting adult development of schizotypal traits.

BEHAVIORAL INDICANTS
OF FIRST-HIT FETAL BRAIN DAMAGE

Research has uncovered various behavioral abnormalities more common among individuals who later develop schizophrenia. Preschizophrenia patients have been shown to evidence premorbid behavioral disturbances, as well as premorbid cognitive deficits. We suggest that some premorbid neuromotor and neurocognitive deficits reported in the literature may reflect second-trimester disruptions in fetal-neural development.

Childhood Neuromotor Deficits Are Related to Adult Schizophrenia

In a study of childhood behavior and adult brain morphology in patients with schizophrenia, Walker and colleagues found that neuromotor deficits and negative affect during infancy linked with greater ventricular enlargement in adulthood *(18)*. Also, parental ratings of the severity of "externalized" childhood behavior problems (likely associated with a difficult temperament) showed an inverse relation with adult cortical volume.

Infant Neuro-Behavioral Deficits Are Related to Adult Schizophrenia

Researchers consistently find ventricular enlargement and decreased cortical volume in patients with schizophrenia *(19)*. Prenatal and perinatal stressors have been linked to ventricular enlargement in humans *(20)*, and to hippocampal structural and cellular abnormalities in rats *(21)*. These brain abnormalities relate to schizophrenia later in life. Furthermore, Walker asserts that schizotypal adolescents with high rates of dysmorphic signs (reflecting prenatal stress), as well as heightened cortisol responses to stress, demonstrate more adjustment problems than controls *(22)*.

Infants at high risk for neurological disorders, such as schizophrenia, have been found to evidence greater numbers of attentional and cognitive deficits as well. In addition, specific abnormalities in neuromotor functioning, as early as 6 months of age, seem to reflect the developmental neuropathology underlying these disorders *(23)*.

One subtype of motor abnormality, excessive involuntary movements (clinical and subclinical hyperkinesias or dyskinesias), may uniquely link with schizophrenia and spectrum disorders (e g., schizotypal personality disorder). Khot and Wyatt observed elevated rates of involuntary movements in treatment-naive and medicated schizophrenia patients *(24)*. Similar to adult schizophrenia patients, children who subsequently manifest the disorder show heightened involuntary

movements (e.g., hand posturing and irregular, writhing movements of the hands) as observed in home movies of preschizophrenia children from birth to 2 years of age *(25)*. Furthermore, the severity of premorbid dyskinesia predicts the severity of psychiatric symptoms in adulthood *(26)*. Motor abnormalities such as these may result from early disruption of neural development that leaves the individual vulnerable to not only motor disturbances, but perceptual and cognitive deficits as well.

OBSTETRICAL COMPLICATIONS IN SCHIZOPHRENIA

Researchers have identified obstetrical complications (OCs) as an early risk factor for schizophrenia. McNeil and Cantor-Graae define OCs as deviations from a normal course of development during pregnancy, delivery, and the early neonatal period *(27)*. Examples of OCs include deviations in gestational age; low birthweight; deviation in size; small head circumference; oxygen deprivation during pregnancy, labor, or delivery; preeclampsia; placental abnormality; and instrumental interventions during labor.

A great deal of research supports a relation between early OCs and the later development of schizophrenia. One convincing study by Jones and colleagues examined a Finnish cohort of 11,017 subjects born in 1966 *(28)*. The authors found schizophrenia patients six times more likely to be born prematurely and seven times more likely to have perinatal brain damage. Additionally, a recent study by Hultman and colleagues also lends support to the relation between OCs and later schizophrenia. The authors compared the rate of OCs of a large sample of schizophrenia patients to various control groups *(29)*. Schizophrenia patients evidenced an increase in OCs compared to the controls.

Literature reviews of the OCs and schizophrenia also lend cogent support to role of OCs as an early determinant of schizophrenia. In a 1995 review, McNeil reported that seven of eight prospective studies found higher rates of OCs in schizophrenia patients than in normal comparison subjects *(30)*. In a more recent meta-analysis, pooling data from 12 independent studies, Geddes and colleagues report a twofold increased risk for developing schizophrenia among subjects suffering from Ocs *(31)*.

Specific OCs and Schizophrenia

OCs vary in terms of type and severity. Recently, researchers have attempted to identify particular OCs specific to later schizophrenia. In their meta-analysis, Geddes and colleagues identify premature rupture of membranes, prematurity, and use of an incubator or resuscitation as significant risk factors for the later development of schizophrenia *(31)*. McNeil and Cantor-Graae cite other OCs typically related to schizophrenia, such as bleeding during pregnancy, prolonged labor,

umbilical cord complications, and asphyxia. These OCs often result in oxygen deprivation in the offspring, thus leading McNeil and Cantor-Graae to suggest that oxygen deprivation may underlie the relation between OCs and schizophrenia (27). In a large birth cohort study, Dalman and colleagues found preeclampsia to be the strongest risk factor for schizophrenia, but also noted the independent contributions of prematurity and hypoxia/ischemia factors (32). This suggests that a number of mechanisms, including abnormal fetal blood flow and oxygen deprivation, may act together to increase vulnerability to schizophrenia.

OCs and Brain Abnormalities

In addition to a relation between OCs and later schizophrenia, OCs also relate to brain abnormalities found in schizophrenia patients. In a study of monozygotic twins discordant for schizophrenia, McNeil, Cantor-Graae, and Weinberger report that smaller hippocampi and larger ventricles found in the affected twin relate to OCs (specifically, labor. delivery complications) (33). Stefanis and colleagues report similar findings (34). In their study of 27 schizophrenia patients, they report that OCs significantly contribute to hippocampal abnormalities common in schizophrenia. Similar to McNeil and Cantor-Graae's assertion (27), Stefanis and colleagues conclude that OCs leading to oxygen deprivation may account for reduced hippocampal volume associated with schizophrenia.

Discrepant Findings in OC/Schizophrenia Research

Despite a majority of evidence supporting a link between OCs and later schizophrenia, several studies do not find this association. Using a prospective design, Done and colleagues failed to find an association between schizophrenia and Ocs (35). Gunduz and colleagues also do not find an association between OCs and schizophrenia (36). Information regarding OCs in this study, however, was mostly obtained through retrospective maternal reports, considered less reliable than prospectively obtained hospital records.

Some researchers who accept the OC relation with schizophrenia, question the direction of effects between OCs and schizophrenia (37,38). In an alternative line of reasoning, some researchers suggest that OCs may be an epiphenomenal result of some other factors that relate more directly to schizophrenia. From this perspective, OCs may result from preexisting abnormalities in the fetus; these abnormalities also account for the later development of schizophrenia. McNeil and Cantor-Graae empirically address the hypothesis that preexisting abnormalities cause OCs in fetuses who later develop schizophrenia. They report that schizophrenia patients with signs of early abnormal fetal maldevelopment (e.g., minor physical anomalies, reduced head size) do not evidence more OCs than patients without early abnormal fetal development. They conclude that OCs do not result from preexisting fetal abnormalities (39).

OCs Among Vulnerable Children

As mentioned earlier, the interaction between a "first" and a "second hit(s)" leading to schizophrenia offers some promise toward understanding the etiology of schizophrenia. The role that OCs play in the "two-hit" model of schizophrenia remains unclear. Various research investigating OCs and schizophrenia among subjects at genetic risk for schizophrenia (generally considered "high risk" due to at least one parent with schizophrenia) suggests discrepant findings. In a study from our lab, we found that OC more closely correlated with increased ventricular volume as genetic risk increased. Those subjects with the highest genetic risk *and* with high OCs most often developed schizophrenia, thus suggesting that OCs serve as a "second hit" leading toward schizophrenia *(20)*. To the contrary, DeLisi and associates found no differences in the hippocampi of high- and low-risk schizophrenia patients with and without OCs *(40)*. Their sample, however, consisted of only seven subjects. The majority of studies described here do not specify the genetic liability of subjects; therefore, whether OCs are more likely "first" or "second" hits remains undetermined.

EARLY-REARING FACTORS IN SCHIZOPHRENIA

Researchers report mixed findings regarding the relationship between risk of developing schizophrenia and early-rearing factors such as family dysfunctioning and parental loss or separation. These relationships, however, seem clearer when research designs consider the vulnerability resulting from a first hit. It appears that when combined with the occurrence of a first hit, disruptive early-rearing circumstances contribute significantly to the later development of schizophrenia.

Family Disharmony and Schizophrenia: Low-Risk Studies

Early theories attempted to explain an apparent relation between family dysfunction and schizophrenia in offspring *(41–43)*. Many of these theories have been psychoanalytic in nature and tended to focus attention on the •schizophrenogenic mother *(44,45)*. With a later acceptance of the strong role of genetics in the etiology of schizophrenia *(46–48)*, the role of the family tended to be discredited *(49)*. Early empirical reports were criticized for inadequate control groups, small sample sizes, inconsistent operationalization of "family dysfunctioning," failure to include possible confounding factors, and retrospective bias.

Some recent work has lent renewed credence to family theories of schizophrenia. In a prospective design of troubled adolescents and their families, Goldstein found that parental disturbance in general, and communication deviance (CD) and negative affective style in particular, predict schizophrenia-spectrum outcome in at least one of the children *(50)*. Rund found a similar pattern of CD and hostility in Norse families whose children later develop schizophrenia *(51)*. Despite

these findings, the relation between family functioning and schizophrenia remains controversial. Other researchers point to negative findings *(49,52)*, and the lack of close correspondence between the pattern of findings and a coherent theoretical model *(53)*. In this light, many contemporary scholars are quick to echo Roff and Knight's suggestion that the etiological significance of family functioning to schizophrenia is unknown *(54)*.

Parental Loss and Schizophrenia

Numerous studies examine parental loss and the development of general psychopathology, as well as schizophrenia specifically. Two reviews note mixed finding from investigations of parental absence and schizophrenia *(55,56)*. Many of the included studies suffer from methodological limitations that may have influenced findings.

Whether parental loss serves as a general risk factor for later psychiatric problems or whether such an experience has a specific impact on outcomes of schizophrenia is another issue researchers attempt to address. Overall, the research does not provide clear results regarding the specific effects of separation and an outcome of schizophrenia *(57–59)*.

Researchers also consider type of loss in relation to schizophrenia. The majority of parental loss studies only consider loss through death. Parental separation, through divorce, however, may have a unique effect on child development. The limited studies that do address this issue are inconclusive regarding the relation between type of loss and later schizophrenia *(60–62)*.

Age of separation is another important factor that may moderate the relationship between schizophrenia and early parental absence. Children at different developmental stages may have different levels of vulnerability to stress associated with parental loss. Most studies generally consider early parental loss as including loss before the ages of 16 to 19. Consistent with other studies of parental loss and schizophrenia, studies of age of separation reveal mixed results *(58,63)*.

The Impact of Rearing Environment on Genetically Vulnerable Children

The reviews presented here do not reveal a consistent pattern of findings regarding the relation between early negative rearing factors and schizophrenia in the general population. These findings remain unclear even when moderators such as type of loss and age of separation are taken into consideration. By contrast, investigations into the relationship between early-rearing stress and later schizophrenia *among genetically vulnerable individuals* find consistent significant effects. In most cases, studies define genetically vulnerable children as children with a parent with schizophrenia ("high risk" [HR]).

Family Discord and Schizophrenia: High-Risk Studies

A wide range of reports, utilizing diverse designs, point to family stress as a prominent risk factor within HR samples *(64–68)*. In the Finnish adoption study, Tienari contrasts a group of HR children raised by their biological (i.e., schizophrenic) parents with a similar group of HR children raised by adoptive (and non-schizophrenic) parents *(69,70)*. Across both groups, parental emotional disturbance is a powerful predictor of eventual decompensation in the children. In Marcus and colleagues' analysis of the 13-year diagnostic outcomes of the National Institute of Mental Health (NIMH) Israeli Kibbutz-City study, poor parenting appears to be a strong predictor of schizophrenia-spectrum outcome among HR children *(65)*. Of the 19 HR children subject to poor parenting (defined as having at least one parent whose parenting combined at least two of three negative styles: overinvolvement, inconsistency, and/or hostility), 9 (47%) developed a schizophrenia-spectrum disorder; none of the 31 HR children with relatively healthy parents did so. It is unknown if this finding is replicated with the most recent 23-year follow-up diagnoses, although a reduction in the number of lifetime schizophrenia-spectrum cases from nine to four (because of criteria changes) make this less likely *(71,72)*.

The UCLA Family Study notes a high likelihood of schizophrenia-spectrum outcome in at least one child (71%) given a combination of both family history of severe mental illness and parental communication deviance *(50)*. In his review of the family relations literature, Asarnow concludes that the evidence "points to the highest rates of schizophrenia spectrum disorders in individuals exposed to both disturbed rearing environments and genetic risk *(73)*.

Our own findings support these general trends in the HR literature. The Copenhagen High-Risk Project, begun in 1962, assessed the rearing environments of 207 children of mothers with schizophrenia, as well as 104 children of parents without a psychiatric history. Rearing variables were drawn from both the retrospective accounts of the child (average age = 15) and their mother (or primary caregiver) and data from the mother's hospital records. These variables have shown consistent success in predicting both 10-year and 25-year outcomes. In an early study of the mother's hospital data, maternal social instability (a composite of items rating the mother's sexual promiscuity, substance abuse, unreliable employment, and premorbid antisocial tendencies) increased the risk for schizophrenia among the HR children *(67)*.

A recent report from this same project suggests that those HR children who later manifested schizophrenia reported less satisfactory relationships with their parents than those who did not later manifest schizophrenia *(68)*. The parent… child relationship scales contained items that relate to the children's attitudes toward their mothers and fathers, the nature of the relationship as perceived by

the parents, and current frequency of contact. Results tentatively suggest that getting along well with both parents may protect HR individuals from developing schizophrenia, whereas not getting along with both parents may increase the likelihood of schizophrenia. This report uses lifetime diagnosis (defined as the more severe of 10-year and 25-year diagnoses), and essentially replicates a finding by Burman and colleagues for 10-year outcome *(64)*.

We began a second longitudinal study in 1971, assessing 72 children with a schizophrenic parent, 72 children with a mentally ill (but nonschizophrenic) parent, and 121 children of parents without a psychiatric condition at an average age of 11 *(74)*. These children were selected from a birth cohort of 9125, consisting of all children born between September 1, 1959, and December 31, 1961, at Rigshospitalet in Copenhagen *(75)*. Rearing variables were assessed through a social worker interview with the child and their parents. In a recent analysis of these data together with 20-year psychiatric outcome, a stressful rearing environment was found characteristic of the families of HR subjects who later decompensated to schizophrenia. In this study, rearing stress was indexed by father's negative attitude toward child, mother's negative attitude toward child, low social class, poor living conditions, and child's negative opinion of family health *(76)*.

High-Risk Studies of Parental Loss and Schizophrenia

Accounting for genetic liability for schizophrenia may also help clarify the previously reported equivocal relationships between schizophrenia and parental absence *(77,78)*. An early report from the Copenhagen High-Risk Project finds that genetically vulnerable children experiencing maternal and paternal separation in the form of child institutionalization (but not supportive foster homes) during the first 3 years of life more often developed schizophrenia at 10-year follow-up than those who were not institutionalized *(78)*. This finding was recently confirmed using 25-year diagnostic outcomes *(79)*. Using a different model, Cannon, Mednick, and Parnas found that a family instability variable (combining separation from one or both parents, institutionalization, and changes in the family constellation in the first 5 years) specifically predicted positive-symptom schizophrenia among children at genetic risk *(80)*.

In the Danish birth cohort of 9125 children described earlier, parental separations were recorded through the first year of life. Separation from parents (resulting from death, hospitalization, and/or children's institutionalization) during the first year was found to predict schizophrenia, but only for children with a family history of schizophrenia *(81)*. Because data were not available on parental separation after the first year, it is uncertain whether this effect is specific to losses in infancy, or whether early separations predict a pattern of losses throughout childhood (death, illness, divorce) that exert a cumulative effect.

Comparison of Rearing Factors Within a High-Risk Design

In our work with the Copenhagen High-Risk Project and the Danish Perinatal Project, we have found that both family discord and parental absence variables increase the risk for genetically predisposed individuals. Building on this, we can consider the relationship among different rearing variables in the prediction of schizophrenia. Which is more predictive: parental absence or family discord? What type of parental absence most affects the vulnerable child: is it inconsistency in who their parents are, or is it periods of isolation from parents in an impersonal rearing environment? Is it the misbehavior and hostility of the mother or the father that affects the child more? Conversely, are the measures we have of the rearing environment perhaps not so much independent variables, as indicators of a global stress factor?

In an attempt to resolve these issues, we recently used the Copenhagen High-Risk Project data to create five variables measuring different aspects of the rearing environment *(82)*. Number of upheavals in the parental dyad was composed of instances of parental death and divorce, as well as changes in single parents' domestic partners. Length of time spent in a children's institution was measured in months. Negative personality and parenting qualities of the mother were brought together in a maternal conflict scale; a similar paternal conflict scale pertained to the father (or father figure). We also included a measure of the peer environment, tapping the number and closeness of the child's peer contacts, owing to literature that suggests that a positive peer network is a possible buffer to negative family dynamics *(83)*.

Within the HR sample, institutionalization was the single variable most predictive of lifetime schizophrenia diagnosis (contrasted with no mental illness), followed by paternal conflict, and upheavals in the parental dyad. Maternal conflict showed a trend toward predicting schizophrenia, and the peer environment appeared to have no impact. These findings suggest that changes in the family unit, whether because of death, divorce, or dating, appear to increase the risk of schizophrenia in a vulnerable child. Also, father's negative behavior appears to have a greater impact than mother's negative parenting (alternately, the behavior of the mothers with schizophrenia was already poor, whereas the variation in the father's behavior was greater). Furthermore, it seems that children's institutions are a far less favorable place to grow up than even the unstable family environment. These three aspects appear to predict relatively independently because when each is entered in a hierarchical regression equation, the others remain significant (with the exception that paternal conflict is no longer significant when institutionalization is considered first).

The greatest predictive efficacy, however, is achieved if the relationship between genetic risk and global rearing stress is modeled as a true multiplicative

interaction. Within the HR group, multiplying the number of schizophrenia-spectrum parents (e.g., one or two) by the equally weighted sum of the five rearing variables results in an interaction term that strongly predicts schizophrenia vs no mental illness outcome. If this model is applied to the entire sample (with low-risk individuals assigned an interaction score of 0), the interaction term accounts for 26% of the variance, almost twice as much as genetic risk alone (16%) and two-and-a-half times as much as any single rearing variable (upheavals in parental dyad   11%).

This may indicate that a global, diffuse "rearing stress" variable, although criticized at times for being too vague *(84)*, may be the specific variable of interest. This is consistent with the general robustness of the rearing findings despite the use of different methods of assessment. For example, within the Copenhagen High-Risk sample alone, the following variables have *all* been noted to predict schizophrenia: institutionalization before age 3 *(78)*, institutionalization before age 10 *(79,85)*; an index combining parental absence, constellation changes, and institutionalization *(80)*; number of upheavals in parental dyad; mother's social instability *(67)*; perceived relationship with parents *(68)*, and maternal and paternal conflict *(85)*.

It may be that our search for the most specifically deleterious rearing event for HR youth is a case of missing the forest for the trees. Although it is true that individuals differ in their ability to process stress *(84,86)*, this does not prohibit us from drawing general conclusions regarding the ill effects of rearing stress on a predisposition for schizophrenia, as individual differences will tend to cancel each other out with increased numbers and diversity of samples.

Rival Interpretations

The research reviewed here supports an interactive relationship between rearing stressors and HR status impacting later schizophrenia. Another interpretation of these results suggests that mothers and fathers with greater genetic liability for schizophrenia tend to have poorer relationships with their children; thus the observed relationship between poor parenting and schizophrenic outcome in the offspring may be only an artifact of the underlying genetic transmission. Although our design does not control for severity of parental illness, it remains unlikely that parents' genetic loading would have such a direct impact on the parental absence and institutionalization variables, which also predict later schizophrenia. In addition, the Finnish Adoption Study separates rearing from genetic parenting, and finds that emotional disturbance in the rearing parents, whether biological or adoptive, increases the risk of schizophrenia-spectrum breakdown *(69)*.

Another interpretation identifies family discord and parental absence as markers of a more general predisposing factor: low socioeconomic status (SES). This reading is grounded in evidence of increased schizophrenia associated with

poorer neighborhoods, urban residence, and more crowded living quarters (87, 88). The schizophrenogenic effects of low SES may operate through either the general stress of chronic poverty or an increased frequency of adverse events such as obstetrical complications and viral infections. However, at least within the Copenhagen High-Risk sample, the data dispute this interpretation, as rearing variables remain predictive even after we accounted for the effects of SES.

A third hypothesis holds that the direction of implied causality between rearing stress and later schizophrenia should be reversed: that a disturbed child, already on a trajectory toward schizophrenia, negatively impacts the family (49). Thus, we are asked to believe that all (or most) rearing disruptions that occur in pre-schizophrenia childhoods are external effects of an insidious disease process, and that the rearing environment itself exerts little influence. That this seems unlikely is bolstered by evidence that premorbid behavior disturbances are typically noted in only a subset of schizophrenia cases, and tend to be subtle before adolescence (89). Also, parents are not noted to be especially accurate in predicting which of their children will eventually develop schizophrenia. Finally, this "disturbed child" hypothesis is not supported by the Copenhagen data: even when personality in adolescence is factored in as a precursor of schizophrenia, rearing environment exerts a significant effect.

In summary, the literature and data from HR designs is most consistent with a multiplicative interaction between the level of genetic vulnerability and the cumulative effect of stress and disruptions in the rearing milieu. In other words, the impact of traumas and other painful events experienced during childhood will be magnified in the vulnerable individual and contribute to eventual development of schizophrenia.

THE TWO-HIT THEORY

The findings presented here suggest that the likelihood of developing schizophrenia is increased by an interaction between prenatal disruptions of fetal neural development and early environmental stress. We have proposed a "two-hit model" to help explain this interaction (1). As mentioned earlier, the two-hit model suggests that two events, or "hits," are associated with increased risk for schizophrenia. The first hit can stem from a genetic liability for schizophrenia. It is hypothesized that this genetic liability may be transmitted from a parent with schizophrenia, and may result in a preprogrammed disruption of fetal neural development. The disruption of fetal neural development may interfere with neural migration, connections, or cell death, and correlate with later cognitive and perceptual disturbances. These disturbances may later increase risk for schizophrenia. Events during gestation may also cause neural developmental disruption. These prenatal events (potential first hits) might include maternal influenza or maternal stress during a critical period of gestation (e.g., second trimester).

Examinations of this model, however, generally focus on having a parent with schizophrenia as the indication of a first hit.

The second hit is modeled as an environmental stressor. Possible second hits include separation from parents, institutional rearing, and high levels of family stress. Although still undetermined, our investigation of OCs and schizophrenia among HR individuals suggests that OCs may also serve as a second hit *(19)*. According to the theory, a second hit in the absence of a first hit does not increase the risk for schizophrenia. In conjunction with a first hit, however, a second hit increases the likelihood of later schizophrenia *(90)*.

As a whole, the two-hit model accounts for several consistent findings, but is far from verified. In its support, it seems evident that rearing trauma acts as a second hit when genetic risk is present. Although unreplicated, results from our lab suggest that OCs may also interact with genetic predisposition in a manner consistent with the model. Additionally, the weight of evidence points to a consistent elevation of risk among the general population when exposed to prenatal teratogens (e.g., maternal influenza) or perinatal stressors (e.g., hypoxia).

The question remains as to whether the etiological mechanisms of genetic transmission and prenatal insult are interchangable (as "first hits"), or even similar. In our most recent results, we find that we can account for one-quarter of the total variance in eventual outcome of schizophrenia using the two-hit model in a HR setting; however, the proportion of variance explained by the pre- and perinatal events proposed as first and/or second hits in the general population is typically much smaller (probably only 0.5%). To our knowledge, no studies have yet explicitly addressed the extent to which second hits may increase the risk of those exposed to an *environmental* first hit. It is unknown whether certain disruptions in the fetal environment mimic the neurological changes wrought by schizophrenic genes; or whether pre- and perinatal irregularities may either reflect or enhance an underlying genetic process. We noted that the timing of in utero insults plays a role in determining what disorder develops, but the specificity and predictive efficacy of particular gestational "windows" awaits further research. In any case, the vast majority of the population exposed to early environmental stressors does *not* develop a schizophrenia-spectrum disorder. For the many cases of schizophrenia that appear to be without genetic precedent, then, we are left with a puzzle as to what chain of events or combination of factors abrupt normal development in favor of schizophrenogenesis.

REFERENCES

1. Mednick SA, Watson JB, Huttunen M, et al. A two-hit working model of the etiology of schizophrenia. In: Lenzenweger M, Dworkin RH, eds. Origins and Development of Schizophrenia: Advances in Experimental Psychopathology. Washington DC: American Psychological Association, 1998.

2. Mednick SA, Machon RA, Huttunen MO, Bonnet D. Adult schizophrenia following prenatal exposure to an influenza epidemic. Arch Gen Psychiatry 1988; 45:189..192.
3. Adams W, Kendell RE, Hare HH, Munk-Jorgensen P. Epidemiological evidence that maternal influenza contributes to the aetiology of schizophrenia: an analysis of Scottish, English, and Danish data. Brit J Psychiatry 1993; 163:522.534.
4. Fahy TA, Jones PB, Sham PC, Takei N, Murray RM. Schizophrenia in Afro-Caribbeans in the UK following prenatal exposure to the 1957 A2 influenza pandemic. Schizophr Res 1993; 9:132.
5. Machón RA, Mednick SA. Adult schizophrenia and early neurodevelopmental disturbances. In: Confrontations psychiatrigues: Epidemiologie et psychiatrie. No. 35. Specia Rhone-Poulenc Rore, 1994.
6. Waddington JL. The declining incidence of schizophrenia controversy: a new approach in rural Irish Population. Paper presented at the annual meeting of the Royal College of Psychiatrists, July 24..27, 1992, Dublin, Ireland.
7. Brown AS. Prenatal infection and adult schizophrenia: a review and synthesis. Int J Ment Health 2001; 29:22..37.
8. Machón RA, Mednick SA, Huttunen MO. Fetal viral infection and adult schizophrenia: empirical findings and interpretation. In: Mednick SA, Hollister JM, eds. Neural Development and Schizophrenia. New York: Plenum Press, 1995.
9. Barr C, Mednick SA, Munk-Jorgensen P. Exposure to influenza epidemics during gestation and adult schizophrenia. Arch Gen Psychiatry 1990; 47:869..874.
10. Kendell RE, Kemp IW. Maternal influenza in the etiology of schizophrenia. Arch Gen Psychiatry 1989; 46:878..882.
11. Kunugi H, Nankos S, Takei N. Influenza and schizophrenia in Japan. Brit J Psychiatry 1992; 160:274..275.
12. O'Callaghan E, Sham P, Takei N, Glover G, Murray RM. Schizophrenia after prenatal exposure to 1957 A2 influenza epidemic. Lancet 1991; 337:1248..1250.
13. Sham PC, O'Callaghan E, Takei N, Murray GK, Hare H, Murray RM. Schizophrenia following pre-natal exposure to influenza epidemics between 1939 and 1960. Brit J Psychiatry 1992; 160:461..466.
14. Machón RA, Mednick SA, Huttunen MO. Adult major affective disorder following prenatal exposure to an influenza epidemic. Arch Gen Psychiatry 1997; 54:322..328.
15. Tehrani JA, Brennan PA, Hodgins S, Mednick SA. Mental illness and criminal violence. Soc Psychiatry Psychiatr Epidemiol 1998; 33:S81..S85.
16. Mednick SA, Tehrani JA. Prenatal disturbances and criminal violence. In: Gottesman R, ed. Encyclopedia of Violence in the United States. New York: Charles Scribner's Sons, 1999.
17. Meyer RG. The Clinician's Handbook: Integrated Diagnostics, Assessment, and Intervention in Adult and Adolescent Psychopathology, 3rd ed. Needham Heights, MA: Allyn and Bacon, 1993.
18. Walker EF, Lewine FJ, Neumann C. Childhood behavioral characteristics and adult brain morphology in schizophrenia. Schizophr Res 1996; 22:93..101.
19. Harrison PJ. The neuropathology of schizophrenia. A critical review of the data and their interpretation. Brain 1999; 122:593..624.
20. Cannon TD, Mednick SA, Parnas J, Schulsinger F, Praestholm J, Vestergaard A. Developmental brain abnormalities in the offspring of schizophrenic mothers. I. Contributions of genetic and perinatal factors. Arch Gen Psychiatry 1993; 50:551..564.
21. Hayashi A, Nagaoka M, Yamada K, Ichitani Y, Miake Y, Okado, N. Maternal stress induces synaptic loss and developmental disabilities of offspring. Int J Dev Neurosci Special 1998; 16:209..216.

22. Brennan PA, Walker EF. Vulnerability to schizophrenia: risk factors in childhood and adolescence. In: Ingram RE, Price JM, ed. Vulnerability to Psychopathology: Risk Across the Lifespan. New York: Guilford, 2001.
23. Hollister MJ, Mednick SA, Brennan PA. Impaired autonomic nervous system habituation in those at genetic risk for schizophrenia. Arch Gen Psychiatry 1994; 51:552.558.
24. Khot V, Wyatt R J. Not all that moves is tardive dyskinesia. Am J Psychiatry 1991; 148: 661..666.
25. Walker EF, Savoie T, Davis D. Neuromotor precursors of schizophrenia. Schizophr Bull 1994; 20:441.451.
26. Neumann CS, Walker EF. Childhood neuromotor soft signs, behavior problems, and adult psychopathology. In: Ollendick T, Prinz R, eds. Advances in Clinical Child Psychology, Vol. 18. New York: Plenum, 1996.
27. McNeil TF, Cantor-Graae E. Obstetric complications as risk factors for schizophrenia. Int J Ment Health 2000; 29:73..83.
28. Jones P, Rantakallio P, Hartikaninen AL, Isohanni M, Sipila P. Schizophrenia as a long term outcome of pregnancy and delivery complications: a 28 year follow-up of the 1966 North Finland general population birth cohort. Am J Psychiatry 1998; 155:355..364.
29. Hultman CM, Sparen P, Takei N, Murray R, Cnattingius S. Prenatal and perinatal risk factors for schizophrenia, affective psychosis, and reactive psychosis. BMJ 1999; 310:421..425.
30. McNeil TF. Perinatal risk factors and schizopohrenia: selective review and methodological concerns. Epidemiol Rev 1995; 17:107..112.
31. Geddes JR, Verdoux H, Takei N, et al. Schizophrenia and complications of pregnancy and labor: an individual patient data meta-analysis. Schizophr Bull 1999; 25:413..423.
32. Dalman C, Allebeck P, Cullberg J, Grunewald C, Koster M. Obstetrical complications and the risk of schizophrenia: a longitudinal study of a national birth cohort. Arch Gen Psychiatry 1999; 56:234..240.
33. McNeil TF, Cantor-Graae E, Weinberger DR. Relationship of obstetric complications and differences in size of brain structures in monozygotic twin pairs discordant for schizophrenia. Am J Psychiatry 2000; 157:203..212.
34. Stefanis N, Frangou S, Yakeley J, et al. Hippocampal volume reduction in schizophrenia: effects of genetic risk and pregnancy and birth complications. Biol Psychiatry1999; 46:697..702.
35. Done DJ, Johnstone EC, Frith CD, Golding J, Shepherd PM, Crow TJ. Complications of pregnancy and delivery in relation to psychosis in adult life: data from the British perinatal mortality survey sample. BMJ 1991; 302:1576..1580.
36. Gunduz H, Woerner MG, Alvir JM, Degreef G, Lieberman JA. Obstetrical complications in schizophrenia, schizoaffective disorder and normal comparison subjects. Schizophr Res 1999; 40:237.243.
37. Goodman R. Obstetric complications and schizophrenia. Brit J Psychiatry 1988; 153:850.
38. Owen M, McGuffin P. Obstetric complications and schizophrenia. Lancet 1990; 336:122.
39. McNeil TF, Cantor-Graae E. Does preexisting abnormality cause labor-delivery complications in fetuses who will later develop schizophrenia? Schizophr Bull 1999; 25:425..435.
40. DeLisi LE, Dauphinais ID, Gershon ES. Perinatal complications and reduced size of brain limbic structures in familial schizophrenia. Schizophr Bull 1988; 14:185..191.
41. Lidz T, Cornelison A, Terry D, Fleck S. The intrafamilial environment of schizophrenic patients: II. Marital schism and marital skew. Am J Psychiatry 1957; 114:241.248.
42. Wynne LC, Ryckoff I, Day J, Hirsch S. Pseudomutuality in the family relations of schizophrenics. Psychiatry Res 1958; 21:205..220.

43. Wynne LC. Family transactions and schizophrenia: II. Conceptual considerations for a research strategy. In: Romano J, ed. The Origin of Schizophrenia. Amsterdam: Excerpta Medica, 1967.

44. Lukoff D, Snyder K, Ventura J, Neuchterlein KH. Life events, familial stress, and coping in the developmental course of schizophrenia. Schizophr Bull 1984; 10:258..292.

45. Mahler M. On child psychosis and schizophrenia. Psychoanal Study Child 1952; 7:286..305.

46. Shields J, Slater E. Heredity and psychological abnormality. In: Eysenck HJ, ed. Handbook of abnormal psychology. New York: Basic Books, 1961.

47. Gottesman II, Shields J. Schizophrenia and genetics: a twin study vantage point. New York: Academic, 1972.

48. Gottesman II, Shields J. Schizophrenia: the Epigenetic Puzzle. New York: Cambridge University Press, 1982.

49. Wender PH, Rosenthal D, Rainer JD, Greenhill L, Sarlin B. Schizophrenics' adopting parents: psychiatric status. Arch Gen Psychiatry 1977; 34:777..784.

50. Goldstein MJ. The UCLA High-Risk Project. Schizophr Bull 1987; 13:505..514.

51. Rund BR. The relationship between psychosocial and cognitive functioning in schizophrenic patients and expressed emotion and communication deviance in their parents. Acta Psychiatr Scand 1994; 90:133..140.

52. Moldin SO, Gottesman II. At issue: genes, experience, and chance in schizophrenia positioning for the 21st century. Schizophr Bull 1997; 23:547..561.

53. Byrne CP, Velamoor VR, Cernovsky ZZ, Cortese L, Losztyn S. A comparison of borderline and schizophrenic patients for childhood life events and parent-child relationships. Can J Psychiatry 1990; 35:590..595.

54. Roff JD, Knight R. Family characteristics, childhood symptoms, and adult outcome in schizophrenia. J Abnorm Psychol 1981; 90:510..520.

55. Granville-Grossman K. Early bereavement and schizophrenia. Brit J Psychiatry 1966; 112:1027.

56. Ragan PV, McGlashan TH. Childhood parental death and adult psychopathology. Am J Psychiatry 1986; 143:153..157.

57. Gay M, Tonge W. The late effects of loss of parents in childhood. Brit J Psychiatry 1967; 113:753..759.

58. Hilgard J, Newman M. Parental loss by death in childhood as an aetiological factor among schizophrenic and alcoholic patients compared with a non-patient community sample. J Nerv Ment Dis 1963; 137:14..28.

59. Munro A, Griffiths A. Some psychiatric non-sequelae of childhood bereavement. Brit J Psychiatry 1969; 115:305..311.

60. Brill N, Liston, E. Parental loss in adults with emotional disorders. Arch Gen Psychiatry 1966; 14:307..314.

61. Furukawa T, Mizukawa R, Hirai T, Fujihara S, Kitamura T, Takahashi K. Childhood parental loss and schizophrenia: evidence against pathogenic but for some pathoplastic effects. Psychiatry Res 1998; 81:353..362.

62. Maekikyroe T, Sauvola A, Moring J, et al. Hospital-treated psychiatric disorders in adults with a single-parent and two-parent family background: a 28-year follow-up of the 1966 Northern Finland Birth Cohort. Fam Process 1998; 37:335..344.

63. Watt NF, Nicholi A. Early death of a parent as an etiological factor in schizophrenia. Am J Orthopsychiatry 1979; 49:465..473.

64. Burman B, Mednick SA, Machon RA, Parnas J, Schulsinger F. Children at high risk for schizophrenia: parent and offspring perceptions of family relationships. J Abnorm Psychol 1987; 96:364..366.

65. Marcus J, Hans S, Nagler S, Auerbach J, Mirsky A, Aubrey A. Review of the NIMH Israeli Kibbutz-City Study and Jerusalem Infant Development study. Schiz Bull 1987; 13:425.438.
66. Singer MT, Wynne LC, Toohey ML. Communication disorders and the families of schizophrenics. In: Wynne LC, Cromwell RL, Matthysse S, eds. The Nature of Schizophrenia: New Approaches to Research and Treatment. New York: Wiley, 1978.
67. Talovic A. High-risk for schizophrenia: Father's contribution to child outcome. Unpublished doctoral dissertation, University of Southern California, 1984.
68. Schiffman J, LaBrie J, Carter J, et al. Perception of parent-child relationships in high-risk families, and adult schizophrenia outcome of offspring. J Psychiatry Res 2002; 36:41.47.
69. Tienari P. Interaction between genetic vulnerability and family environment: the Finnish adoptive family study of schizophrenia. Acta Psychiatr Scand 1991; 84:460.465.
70. Tienari P, Lahti I, Sorri A, Naarala M, Moring J, Wahlberg KE. The Finnish adoptive family study of schizophrenia: possible joint effects of genetic vulnerability and family environment. Brit J Psychiatry 1989; 155:29.32.
71. Mirsky AF, Kugelmass S, Ingraham LJ, Frenkel E, Nathan M. Overview and summary: twenty-five-year followup of high risk children. Schizophr Bull 1995; 21:227.239.
72. Nathan M, Frenkel E, Kugelmass S. From adolescence to adulthood: development of psychopathology in kibbutz and town subjects. J Youth and Adolescence 1993; 22:605.621.
73. Asarnow JR. Children at risk for schizophrenia: converging lines of evidence. Schizophr Bull 1988; 14:613.631.
74. Mednick S, Mura E, Schulsinger F, Mednick B. Perinatal conditions and infant development in children with schizophrenic parents. Soc Biol 1971; 18:5103.5113.
75. Zachau-Chistiansen B, Ross EM. Babies: Human Development During the First Year. New York: Wiley, 1975.
76. Schiffman J, LaBrie J, Mednick S, Cannon T, Parnas J, Schulsinger F. The two-hit model: a prospective investigation. Unpublished manuscript, University of Southern California, 1999.
77. Parnas J, Teasdale T, Schulsinger H. Institutional rearing and diagnostic outcome in children of schizophrenic mothers. Arch Gen Psychiatry 1995; 42:762.769.
78. Walker EF, Cudek R, Mednick SA, Schulsinger F. The effects of parental absence and institutionalization on the development of clinical symptoms in high-risk children. Acta Psychiatr Scand 1981; 63:95.109.
79. Gutkind D, Mednick B, Cannon T, Parnas J, Schulsinger F, Mednick SA. Parental absence and schizophrenia a 27-year follow-up of the Copenhagen High-Risk Cohort. University of Southern California, 1996, submitted.
80. Cannon TD, Mednick SA, Parnas J. Antecedents of predominantly negative- and predominantly positive-symptom schizophrenia in a high-risk population. Arch Gen Psychiatry 1990; 47:622.632.
81. Schiffman J, Barr CE, Mednick SA, et al. Very early parental separation: a risk factor for schizophrenia and other psychiatric disorders. Unpublished manuscript, 1999.
82. Carter JW, Schulsinger F, Parnas J, Cannon T, Mednick SA. A multivariate prediction model of schizophrenia. Schiz Bull 2002; 28:649.682.
83. Price JM. Friendships of maltreated children and adolescents: contexts for expressing and modifying relationship history. In: Bukowski WM, Newcomb AF, Hartup WW, eds. The Company They Keep: Friendship in Childhood and Adolescence. New York: Cambridge University Press, 1996.
84. Strauss JS, Hafez H, Lieberman P, Harding CM. The course of psychiatric disorders: III. Longitudinal principles. Am J Psychiatry 1985; 142:289.296.

85. Carter JW, Mednick SA. Premorbid intervention: identification of those at risk. In: Miller T, Mednick SA, McGlashan T, eds. Early Intervention in Psychiatric Disorders. Dordrecht, Netherlands: Kluwer Academic, 2001.
86. Weintraub S. Risk factors in schizophrenia: the Stony Brook High-Risk Project. Schizophr Bull 1987; 13:439.450.
87. Torrey EF, Yolken RH. Is household crowding a risk factor for schizophrenia? Paper presented at the Ninth Biennial Winter Workshop on Schizophrenia, Davos, Switzerland, 1998.
88. Harrison G, Glazebrook C, Page K, Brewin J. Social deprivation at birth and increased risk of psychosis: evidence from a first episode study. Paper presented at the Ninth Biennial Winter Workshop on Schizophrenia, Davos, Switzerland, 1998.
89. Watt NF. Longitudinal changes in the social behavior of children hospitalized for schizophrenia as adults. J Nerv Ment Dis 1972; 155:42.54.
90. Walker E F, Diforio D. Schizophrenia: a neural diathesis-stress model. Psychol Rev 1997; 104:667..685.

3

Obstetric Risk Factors for Schizophrenia and Their Relationship to Genetic Predisposition

Following Ariadne's Double-Stranded Thread Through Early Development

Stefano Marenco, MD
and Daniel R. Weinberger, MD

INTRODUCTION

The literature on early life environmental risk factors for schizophrenia is a labyrinth of enormous extent, and it is growing. A literature search on obstetric and pregnancy complications and schizophrenia yields more than 1000 papers. In the arduous attempt to provide a compass, we have been struck by the tension between genes and early environment that is present throughout this literature. We do not promise to find the exit to the labyrinth, we only hope to show that following both threads will be necessary to start to understand the pathophysiology of the illness.

We review here some of the evidence for a role of early environmental factors in causing schizophrenia, but we refer often to the confounder of genetic causation. The general framework to understand early environmental causation comes in part from the neurodevelopmental hypothesis of schizophrenia *(1)*, which posits a disease process affecting the brain during early development, and reaching full-blown consequences during adolescence or early adulthood. There is ample evidence for this hypothesis spanning from epidemiological studies to clinical characteristics of the illness, to evidence from post mortem studies (reviewed in ref. *2*).

From: *Early Clinical Intervention and Prevention in Schizophrenia*
Edited by: W. S. Stone, S. V. Faraone, and M. T. Tsuang © Humana Press Inc., Totowa, NJ

This chapter focuses on obstetric developmental risk factors as the prototype for an early environmental causation of schizophrenia. In addition, we dedicate a section of this chapter to animal models that have tried to reproduce the role of clearly environmental factors in producing later-onset aberrant behaviors. The analogy to schizophrenia is strengthened by the fact that abnormal behaviors occur only after puberty (although the "risk factor" occurs during pregnancy or shortly after birth) and by the responsivity of these behaviors to neuroleptic treatment.

We do not address risk factors during childhood and adolescence in this review, partly because of space constraints, and partly because the information that allows separation of genetic and environmental factors is more limited. Suffice it to say that schizophrenia has antecedents in childhood and adolescence ranging from neurological and coordination deficits, to abnormalities in social interactions, to reduced IQ and cognitive abilities such as attention, to positive symptoms well before disease onset. These, however, may also reflect earlier developmental risk factors. In addition, events that are more likely to be environmental in origin such as traumatic brain injury, malnutrition and infections in infancy, and substance abuse in adolescence may also constitute independent risk factors, although their role is not well established.

The goals of this review are to show the following: (a) environment has a role in causing schizophrenia, (b) environmental causes act on a fertile genetic background, (c) familial transmission of schizophrenia may depend on a different genetic background from sporadic cases, and (d) a genetic predisposition to affective disorders and altered stress responsivity may constitute the key background for environmental insults to result in schizophrenia in "sporadic" cases.

Obstetric Complications

Many studies have shown that obstetric complications (OCs) are significant, although small risk factors for schizophrenia. Multiple obstetric risk factors have been linked with schizophrenia, including preeclampsia *(3,4)*, small head circumference *(5,6)*, low birthweight *(7–9)*, Rh incompatibility *(10)*, fetal distress *(11)*, weight heavy for length *(12)*, multiparity, maternal bleeding during pregnancy *(13)*, and abnormal presentations *(14–16)*. Most of these reports are from case-control studies and many have relied exclusively on maternal recall of events occurring 20.30 years earlier. However, there is further recent evidence based on large cohort studies and contemporaneous obstetric records that strongly support the role of OCs.

A particularly noteworthy recent study *(17)* determined the impact of OCs from an unselected sample of more than 500,000 births in Sweden. The authors identified 238 cases with a diagnosis of schizophrenia and, importantly, controlled in their analysis for the excess risk conferred by the mother having a psychotic illness. The relative risk for schizophrenia was increased up to 2.5 times by pre-

eclampsia, gestational age below 33 weeks, inertia of labor, vacuum extraction, respiratory illness, and low birthweight. Diagnostic outcomes were assessed at age 22, so we might expect even more patients to be diagnosed in the next 10 years. After logistical regression, preeclampsia, an indicator of fetal malnutrition, remained the strongest risk factor, increasing the risk for schizophrenia between 2 and 2.5 times. Extreme prematurity also increased risk for schizophrenia by more than two times whereas several mechanisms responsible for fetal hypoxia increased risk less consistently (with the exception of cesarean section because of fetal distress, which also increased risk by 2.5-fold). OCs seemed to be associated with schizophrenia more frequently in males than in females, but this finding might be a consequence of the earlier median age of onset for males and their consequent overrepresentation in this sample (about 60% of the sample). It should also be noted that despite the statistical significance of the results, the absolute increase in risk is small. Indeed, only 11 cases involved preeclampsia, 5 extreme prematurity, and 2 very low birthweight.

Another study that offers strong support to the role of OCs was conducted in Finland (9). This study included 76 cases with schizophrenia out of a cohort of 11,000 whose pregnancy records were collected in the 1960s. Low birthweight as well as short gestation conferred an increased risk for schizophrenia, whereas being small for gestational age did not. No other OC was significantly associated with schizophrenia. Prior studies linking low birthweight and schizophrenia (7, 18,19) had not controlled for gestational age. An interesting association found in this study (9) was that mothers of patients with schizophrenia reported being depressed during pregnancy more frequently than mothers of probands without the disorder.

A case-control study based on about 100 cases (12) reported that subjects with multiple complications had about five times the likelihood of developing schizophrenia than subjects with less severe forms of OCs. This provides some evidence in favor of a "dose. response" relationship. Also supporting this relationship between OC severity and illness course is the study by Robinson et al. (20), indicating that first-episode patients who are refractory to treatment and who continue to have disabling positive symptoms even after aggressive attempts at treatment are more likely to have OCs in their history. Similarly, OCs have been found to correlate with a chronic course (21), with predominant negative symptomatology (22), and with younger age at onset (11,23), which are in turn related to poorer outcome.

The literature is not uniform in supporting the role of OCs in schizophrenia. In particular, two recent large case-control studies based on contemporaneous birth records invite caution: Byrne et al. (24) found that OCs were more frequent and more severe only in males presenting for psychiatric treatment before the age of 30. They analyzed 431 cases. In contrast, Kendell et al. (25) found almost no

association between OCs and schizophrenia in an even larger (almost 500 cases) case-control study. These results were in conflict with those obtained 4 years earlier on the same group of subjects *(3)* when fewer schizophrenia cases had traversed the period at risk. The authors identified an erroneous case-control matching algorithm in the first positive study as the culprit for findings that kept the controls' rate of OCs artificially low. Some older cohort studies based on obstetric records also did not show a significant association *(26,27)*, although Buka et al. *(26)* found that preterm subjects had significantly higher rates of cognitive impairment just as adults and subjects who had experienced chronic fetal hypoxia had higher rates of psychosis and cognitive impairment (not significant because of the small number of cases with psychosis). However, a successive re-analysis of the Done et al. *(27)* study *(28)*, found that schizophrenia was associated with a higher likelihood of risk behavior during pregnancy by the mothers, including smoking, drinking, poorer prenatal care, and the like. Perhaps, these should be considered as full-fledged OCs, although they are not included in the scales that have been most frequently used in case-control studies. In addition to this, replication studies by the Harvard group *(29)*, based on the National Collaborative Perinatal Project (NCPP), did show significant associations between schizophrenia and OCs.

Two meta-analyses of this literature have recently been conducted. Geddes and Lawrie *(30)* found that the overall risk of schizophrenia may be doubled by an OC. However, they also found evidence for a publication bias against smaller negative studies. In an effort to correct this, they selected studies that all used the Lewis scale for OCs (which does not offer a quantitative range for multiple or severe complications and may therefore be less sensitive) and collected individual data from several authors *(31)*. This re-analysis led to a sample of 700 schizophrenia cases and 835 controls, showing a significantly elevated risk of schizophrenia for subjects with at least one definite complication. The odds ratio, however, was only 1.38, a 40% increase in risk. The single complications that appeared to be most important were premature rupture of membranes, prematurity, birthweight below 2500 g, and use of an incubator or resuscitation, all indexes of fetal malnourishment. An important detail is that out of 491 patients for whom psychiatric information on the parents was available, 38% had a parent who had experienced psychosis. Most of this information derived from patient reports and might have been misleading. No correction for this was applied in the analysis, therefore it remains unclear whether OCs were related to family history.

Several notes of caution in interpreting the literature on OCs are in order. The scales most commonly used *(16,32)* lump together OCs occurring at different times during gestation, delivery, and the neonatal period. Recently, more detailed and differentiated scales have been developed *(33)* that promise to be more sensitive, but often information from birth records or maternal recall is insufficient

to truly capture the spectrum of possible insults to the fetus during pregnancy. There has been no agreement on what scales to use and whether multiple OCs should be considered as a measure of increasing severity (*see* refs. *34,35* for critique). Maternal recall recently has been shown to underestimate the occurrence of OCs, especially when mothers of patients with schizophrenia are the source of information *(36–38)*. These recent results are in contrast to an initial study on this subject, which was quite optimistic *(39)*. This study was quite small and the frequency of occurrence of complications such as preeclampsia might have been too low for a fair assessment. OCs do not appear to be specific for schizophrenia. For example, an increased frequency of OCs has been reported in association with bipolar disorder *(27,40–43)*, although Verdoux and Bourgeois *(44)* found that OCs were more frequent in patients with schizophrenia than in patients with bipolar disorder and Bain et al. *(45)* found that it was unlikely that OCs play a role in the etiology of affective psychosis in a fairly large case-control study with documentation of OCs obtained at birth. Also, data from Browne et al. *(46)* indicate that mania cases are not associated with increased rates of OCs, however, birth records were available only for one-third of the initially identified cases. Birth complications also have been related to disruptive behavior in adolescents *(47)*, antisocial behaviors *(48)*, autism *(49)*, and "minimal brain dysfunction" *(50)*. Most of these studies, however, have been in small samples. Nelson showed a very strong association of OCs with neurological complications such as cerebral palsy, and this is a well-established finding *(51–56)*. It may well be that many psychiatric disorders have this antecedent and that OCs are just a generic risk factor for many behavioral complications.

Another caveat is that most of the studies addressing this theme do not differentiate according to the timing of OCs during pregnancy. One of the problems in interpreting the implications of OCs therefore, is, understanding how causes acting in the second or third trimester or in the perinatal period end up with a similar outcome. A disruption in brain development at different times might be expected to result in different outcomes. Indeed, one of the perplexing aspects of the OC literature is the variability from one study to another of which OC confers increased risk.

Another technical issue that is quite surprising is that almost none of the studies cited here consider tobacco, drugs, and alcohol use in pregnancy as possible risk factors. Tobacco use is considered as a confounder only in the study by Jones et al. *(9)*. It is clear that tobacco and alcohol use are very likely to increase the frequency of OCs and to affect the developing brain of the fetus. For example, recent studies *(57,58)* show that tobacco use during pregnancy is associated with a higher risk for violent criminal behavior in the offspring. A very thorough review by Bennedsen *(59)* provides further reading on the importance of several environmental risk factors to pregnancy outcomes.

Based on this literature, there is little doubt that OCs play a role in the causation of schizophrenia. The following examines the genetic background with which they interact.

Linking Genetic Load and Obstetric Complications

OCs affect a much larger proportion of the population than does schizophrenia or any other psychiatric disturbance. It is probably fair to say that most OCs do not result in any permanent damage to the individual. Therefore, it seems likely that on the one hand, genetic endowment operates to protect against the negative effects of OCs in some subjects and that on the other, it is likely to play a role in exaggerating the developmental consequences of OCs in others. But are there genes and possibly other environmental factors involved? One possibility is that the same genes that are responsible for the familial transmission of schizophrenia also predispose to OCs. In this case, OCs should be more frequent in relatives of patients with schizophrenia as well as in the patients themselves as compared to the general population or to matched normal controls. If this is not the case, then there might be other recognizable genetic contributions that predispose to OCs. For example, the data by Sacker et al. (28) indicate that the genetics of risk behavior during pregnancy may be associated with OCs and then schizophrenia. Although these genes may partially overlap with those of familial schizophrenia proper, they might also be quite distinct. To render matters even more complex, some OCs and particularly those causing anoxia in the fetus might be related to genetic characteristics of the fetus or to interactions between the mother's and the fetus's histocompatibility genes (29). In this review, we use OCs as the prototype for environmental causation and family history of psychosis as the hallmark of "genetic" etiology; however, this is an oversimplification, useful only to start making hypotheses about what genes are involved and what interactions with the environment are necessary to get to the schizophrenia outcome.

Some studies have found an increase in OCs only for cases without a family history of psychosis (60–64), or the absence of a relationship between family history and OCs (11,65,66). A recent study by Cannon et al. (67), based on the Philadelphia site of the NCPP (a mainly African American population) found that although there was a clear dose. effect relationship between OCs and risk of schizophrenia, the siblings of schizophrenia patients were no more likely than controls to have suffered from OCs. Another investigation by Rosso et al. (68) in the 1955 Helsinki birth cohort (80 patients with schizophrenia sampled randomly out of more than 250, the result of a cohort consisting of more than 11,000 people) also found that although perinatal hypoxia-related OCs more than doubled the risk of early-onset schizophrenia (but not of late-onset schizophrenia), there was no excess of these OCs in a group of 61 nonpsychotic siblings.

A recent study by Zornberg et al. *(29)* requires a more detailed description. The authors interviewed 693 persons (about 75% of the sample who originally participated in NCPP). Of these, 12 had developed schizophrenia or another non-affective psychosis by the time the interview was conducted (mean age of 23) and 7 had developed a psychotic mood disorder. Zornberg et al. focused on hypoxia-causing OCs and constructed specific categories of OCs based on hunches from the literature. Compared to prior literature, their groupings combine different OCs and are therefore more stringent categories (or more severe OCs). They attempted to control for family history, gender, race, age, prenatal care, and socioeconomic status at birth, however they were unable to control for more than one of these factors at a time. They found a fivefold elevated risk of developing schizophrenia in subjects who had experienced hypoxic-ischemic OCs. When the most severe complications were considered, the odds ratio increased to 19. Adjustment for family history of schizophrenia did not change the stunning increase in risk, however there was a nonsignificant trend for family history to be associated with a 12 times higher risk of schizophrenia in people exposed to hypoxic injuries vs a doubling of risk for those without a family history. This points to an association between family history and risk of hypoxia, which is consistent with the studies by Bennedsen et al. *(69,70)*. Although this study is consistent with other literature, and in a way makes sense of the prior nonsignificant findings by Buka et al. *(26)* conducted on a subsample deriving from the same cohort, a note of caution is needed because the age at interview was young and the numbers of subjects were quite small. This is especially true for the category of affective psychosis, where no firm conclusions are possible in our view. Also, the extreme variability in the confidence intervals for the odds ratios and the inability to control for multiple confounders contemporarily, should caution one not to draw definitive conclusions from this otherwise important study. The lesson to be derived is that genetic and environmental variables are clearly in a complex relationship.

Marcelis et al. *(43)* asked the inverse question: they identified patients with schizophrenia and controls who had been exposed to OCs to determine if there was any difference in the risk for psychiatric illness in their first-degree relatives. If the same genes that predispose to familial transmission of schizophrenia also influence the rate of OCs, then the risk of schizophrenia should be more elevated in the relatives of patients with schizophrenia who have undergone OCs. The study identified 151 patients and 100 controls whose mothers could be contacted for an interview. OCs as well as psychiatric family history were determined by maternal recall. In addition to this, about 50% of more than 1000 relatives were directly interviewed to establish a psychiatric diagnosis. Familial risk for affective disorders, but not for psychosis or schizophrenia was increased in those with a history of OCs. A family history of *affective disorders* was associated with pre-

eclampsia and breech presentation, and this association was even more marked when affective illness occurred in the mother of the probands. There is evidence supporting the fact that affective disorders also are linked to poor pregnancy outcomes *(71,72)*. Poor compliance with antenatal visits due to affective disorder can predispose to preeclampsia and breech presentation *(73)*.

Previously it was shown that OCs survive as a risk factor even when family history of psychosis is covaried out *(17)*, Jones et al. *(9)* found that depression in the mother (not psychosis) was a risk factor for schizophrenia, and that psychological problems and risk behaviors in the mother increased the risk of schizophrenia in the British birth cohort *(28)*. The latter finding indicates that psychological variables during pregnancy are important but does not differentiate between psychosis and other psychiatric or behavioral disturbances.

Finally, there is some even more indirect evidence that OCs and the genetics of schizophrenia are independently determined. Orr et al. *(74)* studied the frequency of mixed-handedness and OCs in patients with schizophrenia and their relatives. They found an excess of mixed-handedness in patients with schizophrenia and their relatives compared to controls and patients with affective illness, but no association with OCs. Although their data support a genetic determination of mixed-handedness, they are also consistent with OCs being determined independent of genetic background for handedness or schizophrenia.

There are studies, however, that show poorer pregnancy outcomes in mothers with schizophrenia. Sacker et al. *(75)* did a meta-analysis of 15 studies mostly conducted in the 1970s where data were available about parental diagnosis of schizophrenia and frequency of OCs. Mothers who suffered from schizophrenia had a higher frequency of OCs than did control cases, but when the father suffered from schizophrenia the children were not more likely to have OCs, indicating that the increased risk was somewhat independent of family history. The authors hypothesize that the increased risk may be mediated by increased stressful life circumstances in the mothers with schizophrenia. The limitations of this meta-analysis lie mostly in the extremely heterogeneous and sometimes poorly defined criteria for schizophrenia found in the studies. Moreover, publication bias was not assessed adequately. A more definitive answer to this issue comes from the studies of Bennedsen et al. *(69,70)*. All births occurring in Denmark between 1973 and 1993 were sampled, and mothers who had been admitted to any hospital in Denmark with a diagnosis of schizophrenia between 1969 and 1993 were identified as cases. These studies deserve particular attention because they are free of bias, include large numbers of subjects (more than 2000 births to about 1500 mothers with schizophrenia and more than 120,000 births to 72,000 women in the control group), have prospectively collected data on smoking, pregnancy complications, health-related beaviors during pregnancy, and many other confounding variables. The findings reveal that children of women with schizophrenia are at increased risk

for preterm delivery, low birthweight, and being small for gestational age. There was also an increased incidence of Cesarean sections (C-sections) and of other interventions during delivery. Children born to mothers with schizophrenia tended to have lower APGAR scores, however this was statistically significant only for scores below 10 at 1 minute, a measure that is not predictive of poor long-term outcome from an obstetrical standpoint. Interestingly, pregnancy complications themselves were not more frequent in women with schizophrenia, and in fact they had a lower risk of preeclampsia. Smoking, poorer prenatal care attendance, and low socioeconomic status explained at least part of the differences between births to schizophrenic mothers and controls. In conclusion, it appears that genetic factors alone cannot explain any of the OC findings and that the behavior of the mother during pregnancy (with particular emphasis on smoking) remains an important contributor to OCs.

Another question of relevance to this debate is whether mothers whose children will develop schizophrenia are more likely to experience OCs in other pregnancies. The evidence in favor of this should be considered weak, as it is currently supported by a single small case-control study (76). Another case-control study (11) and the previously cited cohort study by Jones et al. (9) have found no evidence of this.

In summary, there is converging evidence, although still incomplete and methodologically weak, that OCs and the genetics of familial schizophrenia are independent risk factors, whereas genetic risk for affective disorders seems to be more important in causing OCs and possibly later schizophrenia in a subgroup of patients. Because only a minority of children with OCs will have psychiatric outcomes, for an OC to result in later psychopathology, there has to be an interaction with a yet unknown genetic and developmental substrate (i.e., the timing of the OC relative to the stage of development of the individual brain must have some relevance, although this is one of the most obscure areas of investigation). Some proof of this principle is seen in the animal studies.

The preponderance of the evidence supporting a role for environmental factors points to a disturbance occurring during gestation, particularly reduced nutrients to the fetus during the third trimester of pregnancy or an insult occurring during birth or shortly thereafter. However, good longitudinal studies in large populations, with follow-ups in childhood and adolescence prior to illness onset are lacking, and the contribution of later factors cannot be excluded. This caveat is especially timely in light of emerging research indicating the importance of early childhood experiences in determining risk for mental illness.

Exposure to Infections During Pregnancy

One possible etiological factor that has been a subject of considerable discussion and investigation as a cause of *in utero* damage is exposure to viruses. An

association has been found between some influenza epidemics, especially the one in Europe in 1957, and an excess of births that would later develop schizophrenia *(77,78)*. This observation has been replicated in several countries, both in the northern *(79–81)* and the southern *(82)* hemispheres. According to these studies, the fetus, judging from its date of birth, should have been in the second trimester of pregnancy when exposed to the virus. There are only a few studies where an attempt was made to verify whether mothers had actually suffered from a viral infection during their second trimester *(83–85)* and results of these studies are controversial. In particular, whereas Mednick et al. *(83)*, found an association between influenza exposure and schizophrenia in their original 1988 cohort, Crow and Done *(84)*, using the British birth cohort of 1957, found no evidence of such an effect (for other studies that failed to support the hypothesis, *see* refs. *86–91*).

In studies that reviewed the effect of epidemics other than the one in 1957, there is less consistency in identifying influenza as the only potential etiological agent: diphteria and pneumonia were implicated by Watson et al. *(92)*, measles, polio, varicella, and zoonoses by Torrey et al. *(86,93)*. Also, some influenza epidemics had an association with excess schizophrenia births and others did not *(82)*. Most importantly, even considering only the positive studies, influenza can account only for a minority of the cases of schizophrenia. For example Barr *(94)* calculated that only 4% of schizophrenia cases could be accounted for by influenza exposure. A thoughtful review by McGrath and Castle *(95)* concludes that the strength and specificity of the association between *in utero* exposure to influenza and schizophrenia remain weak.

A recent study on a very large cohort of subjects in Denmark *(96)* found no association between influenza rates and schizophrenia risk. They found instead that belonging to a large family and having siblings up to 2 years older or younger tended to increase the risk of schizophrenia by 15.20% (a small increase, which could account for about 10% of the total number of schizophrenia patients). The authors were able to account for multiple confounders: age and psychiatric status of the parents (therefore making the finding more likely related to environmental variables), degree of urbanization, and season of birth. However, they did not correct for the socioeconomic level of the families, which could be an important factor in large families with short intervals between children.

The pathogenetic mechanism by which influenza *in utero* might produce schizophrenia is unclear, as there is little evidence for direct cytotoxicity of the influenza virus in the fetus *(97)* and influenza viral markers have not been found in cerebrospinal fluid (CSF) or in postmortem brains of patients with schizophrenia *(98,99)*. In addition, influenza exposure *in utero* has also been linked to affective disorders in a recent study by Machon et al. *(100)*. This study was performed on the

same population of cases exposed to the 1957 epidemic in Finland that generated the initial data for schizophrenia.

Recent data have shown that rubella is another pathogen that could result in adulthood schizophrenia outcomes when the fetus is exposed *(101,102)*. These results derive from a cohort established in the 1960s to study the short- and long-term effects of rubella exposure during pregnancy. Of 254 cases originally present in the cohort, only 53 could be located, but 20% of these had schizophrenia-spectrum disorders, a rate almost 20 times higher than the prevalence of nonaffective psychoses in the general population. Interestingly, there also was a reduction in IQ, increased prevalence of neuromotor dysfunction, mannerisms, and deviant behaviors during assessments in childhood and adolescence in the subjects who later developed schizophrenia-spectrum disorders as compared to those who had been exposed to rubella *in utero* but did not have psychiatric dysfunction. Moreover, eight of the nine subjects who went on to exhibit schizophrenia-spectrum disorders were exposed during the first 3 months of gestation, a substantially different timing than influenza. It may be important to note also that affective disorders, especially unipolar major depressive disorder, were quite elevated in frequency (24%), however, the childhood and adolescence concomitants of affective disorders were not explored in more detail.

Infections from poliovirus during the second trimester of pregnancy also have been associated with schizophrenia *(103)*. The cited study is based on a large population sample and constitutes strong evidence in favor of this effect, although prior lower-quality studies were controversial.

No information is available on the possible interaction of *in utero* infections with genetic contributions; i.e., it is not known whether infections during pregnancy are more likely to result in a schizophrenia adult outcome if occurring in mothers with a strong family history vs those without such a genetic predisposition.

Malnutrition During Pregnancy

Another potential specific causative agent that has been explored is malnutrition. Exposure to malnutrition during the Dutch famine of 1944 *(104–106)* has been reported to increase schizophrenia cases, especially if the exposure was in the first trimester. Also the risk for affective psychoses was increased, but for exposures in the last two trimesters *(107,108)*. Further evidence of poor nutrition during pregnancy as a risk factor for schizophrenia has emerged from the 1958 UK birth cohort *(27)*, and from two other studies *(68,109)*. They found that low maternal weight, anorexia during pregnancy, and low maternal body mass, respectively, were related to schizophrenia in the offspring.

There is not enough information in these studies to sort out genetic from environmental causes.

Being Born in Winter–Spring

The study described in more detail in the following section *(110)* constitutes strong evidence in favor of birth in late winter. early spring as a risk factor for schizophrenia. Multiple studies have shown this effect *(111–115)* and have been reviewed by Cotter et al. *(116)* and the most likely explanation still seems to be increased rates of infection during the winter, possibly at a critical period of gestation. However, there is little research linking directly infection rates and season of birth in the same population and fluctuations in epidemic infection rates are unlikely to account for the whole effect *(117)*. There may be some inter-action between the seasonal variation of schizophrenia births and urban births *(118)*, but this has not been replicated in a much larger sample *(119)*. In general, there appears to be no consensus in the literature regarding the correlates of seasonal variation in schizophrenia births (*see* ref. *116* for review). Moreover, seasonal variation in births may be present in the population as a whole *(120)* and in other psychiatric conditions such as bipolar disorder, autism, dyslexia, and others *(116)*. There are also discrepancies in the degree of variation in season-ality of birth according to the country where it is measured, with similar data in Japan *(121)* and Finland *(119)* and a quite different pattern in Scotland *(122)*.

O'Callaghan et al. *(79)* found in a rather large case-control study that only patients without a family history of schizophrenia had an excess of winter births, suggesting an environmental etiology to this variability. Two very recent papers *(119,123)* explored seasonality of birth in more than 15,000 patients with schizo-phrenia and 37,000 of their siblings born in Finland between 1950 and 1969. The very large sample size and the lack of bias render this the definitive study to dis-criminate whether seasonal effects are environmental or genetic in nature. One would expect that if seasonality of schizophrenia births was determined by gene-tic factors or by a tendency of parents of children with schizophrenia to reproduce at certain times of the year, the frequency of births during late winter. early spring for patients and their siblings should be similar and higher than for the general population. This was indeed the case overall, although siblings seemed to have a pattern of seasonality of birth intermediate between controls and patients. The authors attribute their findings to differences in conception patterns in the parents of children who later develop schizophrenia or to a higher risk of preterm deliv-eries in these children. However, in addition to this, the pattern of seasonal births was much more accentuated for patients compared to their siblings in the 1955... 1959 time period only. This points quite clearly to an irregular environmental contribution, which the authors attribute to influenza and polio epidemics, which were more severe and frequent during that time period. These papers illustrate beautifully the complexity of gene. environment interactions.

A further recent investigation *(124)* shows that in a Japanese population there is an association between a surface antigen expressed on leukocytes (human leu-

kocyte antigen [HLA]-DR1) and birth during February and March. This antigen, which has frequently been reported to be overrepresented in patients with schizophrenia, is suspected of conferring a protection from rheumatoid arthritis in this population. It is also an antigen that is very important in many immune functions. The reasons for this association are unknown, the study is preliminary and not replicated, but these are exactly the types of studies that promise to open new avenues of interpretation for the discovery of interacting factors in schizophrenia etiology.

Being Born and Raised in a City

Urban residence had been identified as a risk factor for schizophrenia by several studies (125–128), however, it was unclear from these studies at what point in time the urban environment was exerting its maximal effect: was it an effect on the pregnancy or was it an effect of being reared in the city?

A recent epidemiological survey (110) has argued for the importance of city birth as a risk factor for schizophrenia. The authors identified more than 2 million people born in Denmark between 1935 and 1978. All were at least 25 years old at the time of the survey, therefore constituting a group well within the age at risk. Of these, about 2700 patients with schizophrenia were identified. About 180 had family histories of schizophrenia (a first-degree relative with schizophrenia) and about 860 were born in a major city. Whereas the overall risk to an individual of developing schizophrenia was more strongly predicted by family history than by environmental factors (a relative risk between 5 and 9 for family history vs relative risks between 2.4 and 3.5 for being born in a large town or outside of Denmark proper), the number of cases explained by environmental factors was in excess of 45% (adding period and location of birth) vs only 5.5% explained by family history. Other environmental risk factors found in this study were an unknown father and migration of the mother outside of Denmark prior to the birth of the proband. Moreover, very little interaction was present between genetic and environmental risk factors. Therefore, this study seems to support independent genetic and environmental causation of schizophrenia. Another implication is that although it may be easier to predict who will develop schizophrenia based on family history, interventions aimed at reducing environmental causes of schizophrenia are likely to have a much more profound impact on the incidence of schizophrenia. On the other hand, the biology underlying the risk factors identified (migration of the parents, unknown father, period and place of birth) remains unclear. Could there be a tendency for parents with specific genes predisposing to schizophrenia to move in the large urban centers or to migrate? Or is there a higher risk of infections during pregnancy or of perinatal complications for people who live in the city, or, as has been proposed, are migrants more susceptible to infections they have not been exposed to in their original environment (129)? Yet

another possibility could be that mothers who have emigrated into substantially different cultures, or who experienced a more stressful social environment because of living in the city, are more likely to suffer from depression or other affective disorders that may substantially alter the biological environment of the fetus. This, in turn, could have negative consequences on brain development. All these hypotheses will need to be tested in the future.

The same group *(130)*, using a part of the same register as Mortensen et al. *(110)*, showed that urban place of birth remains a strong risk factor despite adjustment for OCs. Their data on OCs, however, is incomplete and only multiparity (three children or more) and a mother less than 20 years old had significantly increased odds ratios for schizophrenia. This is inconsistent with much of the literature reviewed earlier. Nevertheless, this study suggests that urban birth is not necessarily linked to schizophrenia through an increased rate of OCs.

The Mortensen et al. study may also put to rest the notion that patients with schizophrenia "drift" to the city due to the prodrome of the illness, therefore increasing the number of patients diagnosed in cities. An earlier study of about 50,000 Swedish conscripts to the army *(125)* showed that there was an excess of people brought up in larger cities among patients diagnosed with schizophrenia. Therefore, any "drift" toward the city would have to have occurred in the mother of the unborn child or shortly after birth. Two other points of interest are noted in the paper by Lewis et al. *(125)*. The first is that adjustment of the rates for family history (defined as a family member taking medication) did not alter the results to any significant extent, again an indication of the relative independence of genetic and environmental contributions. The second is that other psychoses and psychiatric diagnoses all revealed the same trend, although to a lesser extent: people raised in the cities were at higher risk for mental illnesses period. The authors also indicate that living in the city is associated with increased stressful life events, childhood head trauma, viral infections, and poorer mental health in general. Finally, it should be noted that the increase in risk reported in this study was quite small (an odds ratio of 1.65, which means a probability increase of about 60% for being raised in a city vs a rural area, compared with and increased risk of 900% for having a first-degree relative with schizophrenia).

Data from Marcelis et al. *(131)* collected in Holland seem to confirm that urban environment tends to act distal from illness onset: the risk for schizophrenia was highest for those born in the city, regardless of their residence in the city around the time of illness onset. The broad definition of schizophrenia had the strongest increase in risk, whereas a narrow schizophrenia definition showed a more moderate increase. Being born in the city conferred roughly a doubling of schizophrenia risk as compared to persons born and raised in "rural" areas.

These results should invite reflection upon the specificity of the phenomenon we are exploring. Is schizophrenia really a separate entity from other psychoses

or even from other psychiatric disturbances, or is it just a similar phenomenon of poor social adaptation only more severe? This question emerges again when considering many other data relating to gene. environment interactions.

In summary, being born in the city appears to be a risk factor for schizophrenia. Therefore, there is something about the city that adversely affects pregnancy. Although there is little direct evidence in this literature to differentiate genetic and environmental contributions, it is entirely conceivable that city environments may cause disproportionate stress in the mother during pregnancy.

Stress During Pregnancy and Geographical Migration

We have seen here that affective disturbance and poor health-related behaviors during pregnancy have been associated with higher rates of schizophrenia in the offspring. Is there any evidence that particularly stressful conditions during pregnancy can increase the incidence of schizophrenia? If this were the case, it would increase the likelihood that the genetics of stress responsivity may modulate the effects of environmental variables on brain development.

Van Os and Selten (132) showed an association between exposure to World War II bombings during the first trimester of pregnancy and subsequent development of schizophrenia. Again, this represents weak evidence given the possible confounders associated with the deprivations of war operating during pregnancy and early childhood. Another study by Selten et al. (133) used the example of a flood in the Netherlands to look at the effects of a severe stressor during pregnancy on the development of schizophrenia in the offspring. Again, risk for schizophrenia-related disorders was almost doubled for those children born to mothers exposed to the flood as opposed to those who were not, although this result was not statistically significant (most likely due to insufficient power).

Another stressful situation is migration to a different culture. Odegaard (134) had first noticed an increase in psychotic disorders among Norwegian immigrants to the United States. He thought that this was caused by selective migration of patients in prodromal stages. Since then, several studies have confirmed that migration constitutes a risk factor for schizophrenia and related disorders not only in the first generation but also in the offspring. This has been shown in Carribean immigrants to the UK (135), in Morocccan and Surinamese immigrants to the Netherlands (136,137), in some European immigrants to Denmark (138), and we also saw some evidence of this in Danish people who migrated out of Denmark proper (110). Although some ethnic groups do not seem to show an increased incidence of schizophrenia (e.g., Yugoslavian and Turkish people emigrating to Denmark [138] or Turkish immigrants to Germany [139] and to the Netherlands [137]), this is not sufficient to ignore migration as a possible risk factor. The results from Selten et al. (137) indicate that second-generation immigrants from Surinam and Morocco had higher risk of schizophrenia than the first generation (relative

risk of 5.5 and 8 for the second generation vs 3.2 and 4.5 for the first generation, respectively). This clearly indicates an interaction between environmental and genetic factors, with the environmental variable exerting a stronger effect in pregnancy than in childhood or adulthood. The hypothesis is that certain populations are more sensitive to the stress of acculturation (and of poverty, especially for some of these ethnic groups) because of a genetic predisposition or because of less cohesion within their ethnic community in the host country. This may cause a higher incidence of depression or affective disturbance in the mothers, and this in turn could affect brain development of the fetus during pregnancy. This hypothesis remains weak, however, given the importance of relatively more adverse environments during childhood development in ethnic minorities (e.g., *see* ref. *140*).

Although intriguing, the studies on geographic migration have to be viewed cautiously for several reasons: the rates of schizophrenia in the countries of origin are usually not well characterized, the number of immigrants from a certain ethnicity (which constitutes the denominator of relative risk for a certain population) is never exactly known, family history of psychosis is rarely accounted for, and there may be selective referral, treatment, or diagnostic bias toward minority populations. Although some studies have addressed these issues, this area of investigation still remains fraught with difficulties.

To summarize this section, we think there may be significant commonalities among the risk factors that have been identified as acting during pregnancy. We believe that the literature reviewed so far demonstrates that environmental factors during pregnancy are important in causing schizophrenia. An attractive hypothesis that could link most of the putative causation mechanisms is that genetic predispostion to respond to stress with depression and lack of good mental care may lead to OCs and to an increase in schizophrenia rates in the offspring. This genetic predisposition may overlap only in part with the genes responsible for familial transmission of the disorder, where environmental causation may have a lesser role.

Animal Studies

Several animal models have been developed in an attempt to reproduce the type of environmental insult that could derail development so as to result in abnormal behaviors in adulthood that are not observed prior to puberty. The behaviors in question are mainly hypermotility induced by dopamimetic substances such as amphetamine. These behaviors are considered to be the analog of positive symptoms in the animal model world because they can be dampened by neuroleptics, both typical and atypical (e.g., ref. *141*). The models we mention here also generally find alterations in other neurophysiological paradigms that are also thought to be associated with schizophrenia such as prepulse inhibition deficits or reduced performance on delayed alternation tasks, which are conceptually equivalent to

working memory in humans (e.g., ref. *142*). An excellent road map to this literature can be found in Lipska and Weinberger *(143)*. We reiterate here a few points that are relevant to the epidemiologic literature reviewed previously.

Among the several animal models that have been proposed to mimic behavioral, neuropathologic, or neurostransmission aspects of schizophrenia, the one that appears to reproduce with more fidelity dopaminergic dysfunction and other neurophysiological parameters that are found in schizophrenia was developed by Lipska et al. *(144)*. It consists of a bilateral lesion of the ventral hippocampus in the first days of life of a rat. The rat will develop hypermotility in response to amphetamine and to novel stimuli only in adulthood. These abnormalities in behavior appear to be related to hyperdopaminergia in the basal ganglia. A similar intervention (a bilateral neonatal hippocampal lesion) has been shown to cause increased dopamine release in the basal ganglia in primates *(145)*. This is likely due to a disconnection between the hippocampus and the prefrontal cortex, which regulates under normal circumstances dopamine release in the basal ganglia. The prefrontal cortex, which been shown to mature late in adolescence and this could explain why the aforementioned deficits arise only after puberty. The analogy to schizophrenia has been made even more marked by the recent discovery that N-acetyl-aspartate (NAA) concentrations (a supposed marker of neuronal integrity) in the prefrontal cortex of patients with schizophrenia correlate negatively with the amount of dopamine released in the basal ganglia under amphetamine stimulation *(146)*.

The weakness of this rat model is that the damage to the hippocampus is quite extensive and difficult to reconcile with the absence of a clear medial temporal lesion in postmortem studies of schizophrenia. However, multiple magnetic resonance imaging (MRI) studies show a reduction in hippocampal size (e.g., ref. *147*) and evidence from different sources indicates that hippocampal neuropil loss may be a critical component of the pathology of schizophrenia (reviewed in ref. *148*), indicating that the medial temporal lobe is certainly implicated in the pathogenesis of the disorder. The data by Suddath et al. *(147)* in monozygotic twins discordant for schizophrenia also support the role of environmental causation because the affected twins had smaller hippocampi than their genetically identical well twins. A recent PET study also showed failure of hippocampal activation during a mnemonic task in patients with schizophrenia *(149)*, further supporting hippocampal dysfunction.

The fact that the medial temporal lobe is dysfunctional in schizophrenia is important in the context of this review for at least two reasons: (a) the part of the brain that is most vulnerable to the effects of hypoxia during pregnancy (and afterward) is the hippocampus and parahippocampal area (*see* references in ref. *29*), and this makes it plausible that OCs based on fetal malnutrition/hypoxia are involved in the pathogenesis of the disorder, and (b) the hippocampus is particularly rich

in steroid receptors, and is therefore exquisitely sensitive to fluctuations in hypo-thalamo..pituitary..adrenal (HPA)-axis hormonal cascade *(150)*. This latter point may constitute a link to the indirect evidence reviewed earlier that genes involved in affective disorder and possibly in stress regulation may constitute a fertile sub-strate for OCs to exert their long-term effects.

Other animal models of schizophrenia have been developed attempting to mimic the OCs discussed earlier. Models based on malnutrition during pregnancy *(151)* have been characterized in a more limited fashion than the model by Lipska et al. *(114)* and suffer from a similar lack of neuropathological similarity to schizo-phrenia. Models based on C-sections and brief anoxia during birth *(152)* have also been developed: pups delivered via C-sections exhibited hypermotility to amphetamine as adults, as compared to rats delivered vaginally. Surprisingly, however, when a short period of hypoxia was combined with the C-section, the hypermotility was less evident than with the C-section alone *(153)*. Some models have tried to disrupt cellular migration and proliferation during particular stages of pregnancy that appear to be particularly important in the development of the temporal lobe *(154–157)*. All of these have some value and reproduce aspects of behavior in adult animals that are related to dopaminergic dysfunction.

One other important observation is that a series of studies directed at develop-ing a rat model for anxiety and depression have shown that repeated stress during the last week of a rat's pregnancy (corresponding roughly to the last trimester of gestation in humans) has far-reaching implications for the offspring, especially when the pups reach adulthood. The HPA axis of the offspring is modified per-manently, the number of hippocampal corticosteroid receptors is reduced *(158)*, the synaptic density of the hippocampus is reduced *(159)* and memory deficits appear *(160)*. In particular, the difficulties in hippocampal-dependent learning that these pups experience bear some resemblance with the cognitive deficits that patients with schizophrenia exhibit as a stable and premorbid trait *(161–167)*. Even more interestingly, recent research has suggested that these memory deficits may relate to an abnormality in learning-related neurogenesis in the dentate gyrus *(168)*. In this study, the total number of granule cells in the dentate gyrus was not altered in juvenile pups, but was reduced in adulthood for the prenatally stressed rats as compared to the controls. Finally, there was no indication of increased cell necrosis in the hippocampus, which is in keeping with the overall lack of cell number reduction or gliosis that has been found in neuropathological studies of schizophrenia. Another finding that could be construed as a similarity between the schizophrenia body of knowledge and the model of prenatal stress in rats is that prefrontal NAA of prenatally stressed rats appears to be reduced as compared to controls *(169)*.

We are not suggesting that the model of prenatal stress may be a model for schiz-ophrenia on its own, but that it would be worthwhile to explore the effect of such

a manipulation on different strains of rats with differential sensitivity to stress, while adding an additional environmental insult similar to an OC. If the hypothesis we have put forth that sensitivity to stress in the mother combines with OCs to yield a schizophrenia-like phenotype is true, then one would expect that prenatal stress and an OC in a species shown to be more sensitive to stress would produce more severe damage to the offspring, possibly involving also measures of prefrontal function in addition to hippocampal related deficits. Although we are not aware of studies combining an OC with prenatal stress or comparing tests of frontal lobe abilities in rats of different species subjected to prenatal stress, a recent study by Stohr et al. (170) is worth mentioning. They compared the long-term effects of prenatal stress in Fischer and Lewis rats. Lewis rats stressed prenatally showed a range of behavioral changes that were consistent with improved adaptation to a series of measures of responsivity to stressful stimuli in adulthood. Female Fischer rats developed hyperlocomotion in response to novelty, but this was not observed in males.

In fact, there are two studies that have already addressed the issue of inflicting an environmental lesion on different rat strains. Lipska and Weinberger (171) made neonatal ventral hippocampal lesions of different sizes in rats of three different species, on a continuum of stress reactivity. Fischer 344 rats are known to be very sensitive to stress, which includes having excess HPA axis responsivity (172), whereas Lewis rats are "hyporesponsive" to the same stressful stimuli. Sprague Dawley rats lie somewhere between the two other species and are the most commonly used strain for this kind of research. Lipska and Weinberger (171) showed that the Fisher strain had increased hypermotility to amphetamine and to a novel environment as compared to the Sprague Dawley or the Lewis strain. They also found that the size of the lesion was not as important in determining the extent of hypermotility as the rat strain itself.

A more recent study (173) applied the same construct on their model of C-section as an environmental insult. Fischer rats had hypermotility as adults when delivered by C-section and the mother was anesthetized, but not when the mother was decapitated. Sprague Dawley rats developed hypermotility as adults when delivered by C-section of either anesthetized or decapitated mothers, whereas Lewis rats developed hypomotility in both cases. These results are somewhat puzzling and the reasons for such differences between decapitated and anesthetized mothers remain obscure; nevertheless the point is made again that variations in genetic background can lead to important changes in long-term outcomes of environmental manipulations during pregnancy.

These results appear to be in complete agreement with the hypothesis formulated from the human evidence. Of course, until the genetics of schizophrenia are better known, one cannot extrapolate from animal models to humans without caution, but noting the analogies is a first step for formulating hypotheses to be

tested in epidemiological studies. For example, variables that may be important to collect in future studies may be family history of affective disorder besides family history of psychosis, or testing HPA responsivity in relatives of patients with "sporadic" forms of schizophrenia.

Conclusion

The neurodevelopmental hypothesis of schizophrenia offers a framework for investigation that prompts us to focus on early antecedents and in particular on events during pregnancy. Several perturbations of pregnancy and early life have been implicated as environmental risk factors for schizophrenia. The genetic background on which they occur is an essential requirement for further development of the illness. From our reading of the literature, it appears that a strong family history of schizophrenia (high genetic loading) is insufficient, with or without OCs, to cause schizophrenia. There is multiple circumstantial evidence from human studies and significant analogies to animal studies that suggest that something about depression or stress responsivity of the mother may be an important genetic substrate for OCs to become a key causal ingredient in "sporadic" cases. However, even in sporadic cases, OCs and stress-response gene interactions are insufficient to explain causation for the majority of patients. It is possible that environmental effects during childhood and adolescence may play a further role (e.g., early head trauma *[174,175]* early central nervous system infection *[176]*, or substance abuse *[177,178]*) and that these may be in a specific kind of relationship to other genetic backgrounds (e.g., the genetics of poor cognitive function, especially for genes regulating frontal lobe function *[179]*). Genes and environment have a complex relationship in determining schizophrenia; we have to follow both threads in order to understand the labyrinth of deviant neurodevelopment in schizophrenia.

REFERENCES

1. Weinberger DR. The pathogenesis of schizophrenia: a neurodevelopmental theory. In: Nasrallah HA, Weinberger DR, ed. The Neurology of Schizophrenia. Amsterdam: Elsevier, 1986:397..406.
2. Marenco S, Weinberger DR. The neurodevelopmental hypothesis of schizophrenia: following a trail of evidence from cradle to grave. Dev Psychopathol 2000; 12:501..527.
3. Kendell RE, Juszczak E, Cole SK. Obstetric complications and schizophrenia: a case control study based on standardised obstetric records. Br J Psychiatry 1996; 168:556..561.
4. O'Dwyer JM. Schizophrenia in people with intellectual disability: the role of pregnancy and birth complications. J Intellect Disab Res 1997; 41:238..251.
5. Kunugi H, Takei N, Murray RM, Saito K, Nanko S. Small head circumference at birth in schizophrenia. Schizophr Res 1996; 20:165..170.

6. McNeil TF, Cantorgraae E, Cardenal S. Prenatal cerebral development in individuals at genetic risk for psychosis   head size at birth in offspring of women with schizophrenia. Schizophr Res 1993; 10:1..5.

7. Lane EA, Albee GW. The birth weight of children born to schizophrenic women. J Psychology 1970; 74:157..160.

8. Torrey EF. Birth weights, perinatal insults, and HLA types: return to "original din." Schizophr Bull 1977; 3:347.351.

9. Jones PB, Rantakallio P, Hartikainen AL, Isohanni M, Sipila P. Schizophrenia as a long-term outcome of pregnancy, delivery, and perinatal complications: a 28-year follow-up of the 1966 North Finland general population birth cohort. Am J Psychiatry 1998; 155:355..364.

10. Hollister JM, Laing P, Mednick SA. Rhesus incompatibility as a risk factor for schizophrenia in male adults. Arch Gen Psychiatry 1996; 53:19..24.

11. O'Callaghan E, Gibson T, Colohan HA, et al. Risk of schizophrenia in adults born after obstetric complications and their association with early onset of illness   a controlled study. BMJ 1992; 305:1256..1259.

12. Hultman CM, Ohman A, Cnattingius S, Wieselgren IM, Lindstrom LH. Prenatal and neonatal risk factors for schizophrenia. Br J Psychiatry 1997; 170:128..133.

13. Hultman CM, Sparen P, Takei N, Murray RM, Cnattingius S. Prenatal and perinatal risk factors for schizophrenia, affective psychosis, and reactive psychosis of early onset: case-control study. BMJ 1999; 318:421.426.

14. Gunthergenta F, Bovet P, Hohlfeld P. Obstetric complications and schizophrenia   a case-control study. Br J Psychiatry 1994; 164:165..170.

15. Verdoux H, Geddes JR, Takei N, et al. Obstetric complications and age at onset in schizophrenia: an international collaborative meta-analysis of individual patient data. Am J Psychiatry 1997; 154:1220..1227.

16. Parnas J, Schulsinger F, Teasdale TW, Schulsinger H, Feldman PM, Mednick SA. Perinatal complications and clinical outcome within the schizophrenia spectrum. Br J Psychiatry 1982; 140:416.420.

17. Dalman C, Allebeck P, Cullberg J, Grunewald C, Koster M. Obstetric complications and the risk of schizophrenia   a longitudinal study of a national birth cohort. Arch Gen Psychiatry 1999; 56:234.240.

18. Foerster A, Lewis SW, Owen MJ, Murray RM. Low-birth-weight and a family history of schizophrenia predict poor premorbid functioning in psychosis. Schizophr Res 1991; 5:13..20.

19. Rifkin L, Lewis S, Jones P, Toone B, Murray R. Low-birth-weight and schizophrenia. Br J Psychiatry 1994; 165:357.362.

20. Robinson DG, Woerner MG, Alvir JMJ, et al. Predictors of treatment response from a first episode of schizophrenia or schizoaffective disorder. Am J Psychiatry 1999; 156:544.549.

21. Wilcox JA, Nasrallah HA. Perinatal distress and prognosis of psychotic illness. Neuropsychobiology 1987; 17:173..175.

22. Cannon TD, Mednick SA, Parnas J. Antecedents of predominantly negative-symptom and predominantly positive-symptom schizophrenia in a high-risk population. Arch Gen Psychiatry 1990; 47:622..632.

23. Smith GN, Kopala LC, Lapointe JS, et al. Obstetric complications, treatment response and brain morphology in adult-onset and early-onset males with schizophrenia. Psychol Med 1998; 28:645..653.

24. Byrne M, Browne R, Mulryan N, et al. Labour and delivery complications and schizophrenia. Case-control study using contemporaneous labour ward records. Br J Psychiatry 2000; 176:531..536.

25. Kendell RE, McInneny K, Juszczak E, Bain M. Obstetric complications and schizophrenia. Two case-control studies based on structured obstetric records. Br J Psychiatry 2000; 176: 516..522.
26. Buka SL, Tsuang MT, Lipsitt LP. Pregnancy/delivery complications and psychiatric diagnosis. A prospective study. Arch Gen Psychiatry 1993; 50:151..156.
27. Done DJ, Johnstone EC, Frith CD, Golding J, Shepherd PM, Crow TJ. Complications of pregnancy and delivery in relation to psychosis in adult life   data from the British Perinatal-Mortality Survey Sample. BMJ 1991; 302:1576..1580.
28. Sacker A, Done DJ, Crow TJ, Golding J. Antecedents of schizophrenia and affective-illness obstetric complications. Br J Psychiatry 1995; 166:734..741.
29. Zornberg GL, Buka SL, Tsuang MT. Hypoxic-ischemia-related fetal/neonatal complications and risk of schizophrenia and other nonaffective psychoses: a 19-year longitudinal study. Am J Psychiatry 2000; 157:196..202.
30. Geddes JR, Lawrie SM. Obstetric complications and schizophrenia: a meta-analysis. Br J Psychiatry 1995; 167:786..793.
31. Geddes JR, Verdoux H, Takei N, et al. Schizophrenia and complications of pregnancy and labor: an individual patient data meta-analysis. Schizophr Bull 1999; 25:413..423.
32. Lewis G, McKeigue P, David A, Malmberg A. Obstetric complications and schizophrenia. BMJ 1993; 306:268..268.
33. McNeil TF, Sjostrom K. McNeil-Sjostrom Scale for Obstetric Complications. Lund, Sweden: University of Lund, 1996.
34. McNeil TF. Obstetric Complications. In: Waddington JL, Buckley PF, eds. The Neurodevelopmental Basis of Schizophrenia. Georgetown, TX: R.G. Landes, 1996:61..78.
35. McNeil TF, CantorGraae E, Nordstrom LG, Rosenlund T. Does choice of scale for scoring obstetric complications influence their relationship to other etiological risk factors in schizophrenia? J Nerv Ment Dis 1997; 185:27..31.
36. Cantor-Graae E, Cardenal S, Ismail B, McNeil TF. Recall of obstetric events by mothers of schizophrenic patients. Psychol Med 1998; 28:1239..1243.
37. Tomeo CA, Rich-Edwards JW, Michels KB, et al. Reproducibility and validity of maternal recall of pregnancy-related events. Epidemiology 1999; 10:774..777.
38. Buka SL, Goldstein JM, Seidman LJ, Tsuang MT. Maternal recall of pregnancy history: accuracy and bias in schizophrenia research. Schizophr Bull 2000; 26:335 350.
39. Ocallaghan E, Larkin C, Waddington JL. Obstetric complications in schizophrenia and the validity of maternal recall. Psychol Med 1990; 20:89..94.
40. Kinney DK, Yurgelun-Todd DA, Tohen M, Tramer S. Pre- and perinatal complications and risk for bipolar disorder: a retrospective study. J Affect Disord 1998; 50:117..124.
41. Guth C, Jones P, Murray R. Familial psychiatric-illness and obstetric complications in early-onset affective-disorder   a case-control study. Br J Psychiatry 1993; 163:492..498.
42. Lewis SW, Murray RM. Obstetric complications, neurodevelopmental deviance, and risk of schizophrenia. J Psychiatr Res 1987; 21:413..421.
43. Marcelis M, van Os J, Sham P, et al. Obstetric complications and familial morbid risk of psychiatric disorders. Am J Med Genet 1998; 81:29..36.
44. Verdoux H, Bourgeois M. A comparative-study of obstetric history in schizophrenics, bipolar patients and normal subjects. Schizophr Res 1993; 9:67..69.
45. Bain M, Juszczak E, McInneny K, Kendell RE. Obstetric complications and affective psychoses. Two case-control studies based on structured obstetric records. Br J Psychiatry 2000; 176:523..526.
46. Browne R, Byrne M, Mulryan N, et al. Labour and delivery complications at birth and later mania. An Irish case register study. Br J Psychiatry 2000; 176:369..372.

47. Allen NB, Lewinsohn PM, Seeley JR. Prenatal and perinatal influences on risk for psychopathology in childhood and adolescence. Dev Psychopathol 1998; 10:513..529.
48. Szatmari P, Reitsma-Street M, Offord DR. Pregnancy and birth complications in antisocial adolescents and their siblings. Can J Psychiatry 1986; 31:513..516.
49. Bolton PF, Murphy M, Macdonald H, Whitlock B, Pickles A, Rutter M. Obstetric complications in autism: consequences or causes of the condition? J Am Acad Child Adolesc Psychiatry 1997; 36:272..281.
50. Rao JM. A population-based study of mild mental handicap in children: preliminary analysis of obstetric associations. J Mental Deficiency Res 1990; 34:59..65.
51. Nelson KB, Ellenberg JH. Obstetric complications as risk factors for cerebral palsy or seizure disorders. JAMA 1984; 251:1843..1848.
52. Rantakallio P, von Wendt L. A prospective comparative study of the aetiology of cerebral palsy and epilepsy in a one-year birth cohort from Northern Finland. Acta Paediatr Scand 1986; 75:586..592.
53. Rantakallio P, von Wendt L, Koivu M. Prognosis of perinatal brain damage: a prospective study of a one year birth cohort of 12,000 children. Early Hum Dev 1987; 15:75..84.
54. Stanley FJ, Watson L. Trends in perinatal mortality and cerebral palsy in Western Australia, 1967 to 1985. BMJ 1992; 304:1658..1663.
55. Grether JK, Nelson KB. Maternal infection and cerebral palsy in infants of normal birth weight. JAMA 1997; 278:207..211.
56. Eschenbach DA. Amniotic fluid infection and cerebral palsy focus on the fetus. JAMA 1997; 278:247..248.
57. Rasanen P, Hakko H, Isohanni M, Hodgins S, Jarvelin MR, Tiihonen J. Maternal smoking during pregnancy and risk of criminal behavior among adult male offspring in the northern Finland 1966 birth cohort. Am J Psychiatry 1999; 156:857..862.
58. Brennan PA, Grekin ER, Mednick SA. Maternal smoking during pregnancy and adult male criminal outcomes. Arch Gen Psychiatry 1999; 56:215..219.
59. Bennedsen BE. Adverse pregnancy outcome in schizophrenic women: occurrence and risk factors. Schizophr Res 1998; 33:1..26.
60. Cantorgraae E, McNeil TF, Sjostrom K, Nordstrom LG, Rosenlund T. Obstetric complications and their relationship to other etiologic risk factors in schizophrenia a case-control study. J Nerv Ment Dis 1994; 182:645..650.
61. Reveley AM, Reveley MA, Murray RM. Cerebral ventricular enlargement in non-genetic schizophrenia: a controlled twin study. Br J Psychiatry 1984; 144:89..93.
62. Ocallaghan E, Larkin C, Kinsella A, Waddington JL. Obstetric complications, the putative familial sporadic distinction, and tardive-dyskinesia in schizophrenia. Br J Psychiatry 1990; 157:578..584.
63. Lewis SW, Owen MJ, Murray RM. Obstetric complications and schizophrenia: methodology and mechanisms. In: Schultz SC, Tamminga CA, eds. Schizophrenia: Scientific Progress. New York: Oxford University Press, 1989:56..68.
64. Lewis SW, Owen MJ, Murray RM. Obstetric complications and schizophrenia: methodology and mechanisms. In: Tamminga CA, ed. Schizophrenia: Scientific Progress. New York: Oxford University Press, 1989:56..68.
65. Nimgaonkar VL, Wessely S, Tune LE, Murray RM. Response to drugs in schizophrenia the influence of family history, obstetric complications and ventricular enlargement. Psychol Med 1988; 18:583..592.
66. Reddy R, Mukherjee S, Schnur DB, Chin J, Degreef G. History of obstetric complications, family history, and CT scan findings in schizophrenic patients. Schizophr Res 1990; 3: 311..314.

67. Cannon TD, Rosso IM, Hollister JM, Bearden CE, Sanchez LE, Hadley T. A prospective cohort study of genetic and perinatal influences in the etiology of schizophrenia. Schizophr Bull 2000; 26:351..366.
68. Rosso IM, Cannon TD, Huttunen T, Huttunen MO, Lonnqvist J, Gasperoni TL. Obstetric risk factors for early-onset schizophrenia in a Finnish birth cohort. Am J Psychiatry 2000; 157: 801..807.
69. Bennedsen BE, Mortensen PB, Olesen AV, Henriksen TB, Frydenberg M. Obstetric complications in women with schizophrenia. Schizophr Res 2001; 47:167..175.
70. Bennedsen BE, Mortensen PB, Olesen AV, Henriksen TB. Preterm birth and intra-uterine growth retardation among children of women with schizophrenia. Br J Psychiatry 1999; 175: 239..245.
71. Hedegaard M, Henriksen TB, Sabroe S, Secher NJ. Psychological distress in pregnancy and preterm delivery. BMJ 1993; 307:234..239.
72. Orr ST, Miller CA. Maternal depressive symptoms and the risk of poor pregnancy outcome. Review of the literature and preliminary findings. Epidemiol Rev 1995; 17:165..171.
73. Rayl J, Gibson PJ, Hickok DE. A population-based case-control study of risk factors for breech presentation. Am J Obstet Gynecol 1996; 174:28..32.
74. Orr KG, Cannon M, Gilvarry CM, Jones PB, Murray RM. Schizophrenic patients and their first-degree relatives show an excess of mixed-handedness. Schizophr Res 1999; 39:167..176.
75. Sacker A, Done DJ, Crow TJ. Obstetric complications in children born to parents with schizophrenia: a meta-analysis of case-control studies. Psychol Med 1996; 26:279..287.
76. Preti A, Cardascia L, Zen T, Marchetti M, Favaretto G, Miotto P. Risk for obstetric complications and schizophrenia. Psychiatry Res 2000; 96:127..139.
77. Mednick SA, Machon RA, Huttunen MO, Bonett D. Adult schizophrenia following prenatal exposure to an influenza epidemic. Arch Gen Psychiatry 1988; 45:189..192.
78. Mednick SA, Machon RA, Huttunen MO, Barr CE. Influenza and schizophrenia Helsinki vs Edinburgh. Arch Gen Psychiatry 1990; 47:875..876.
79. O'Callaghan E, Sham P, Takei N, Glover G, Murray RM. Schizophrenia after prenatal exposure to 1957 A2-influenza epidemic. Lancet 1991; 337:1248..1250.
80. Kendell RE, Kemp IW. Maternal influenza in the etiology of schizophrenia. Arch Gen Psychiatry 1989; 46:878..882.
81. Kunugi H, Nanko S, Takei N, Saito K, Hayashi N, Kazamatsuri H. Schizophrenia following in-utero exposure to the 1957 influenza epidemics in Japan. Am J Psychiatry 1995; 152: 450..452.
82. McGrath JJ, Pemberton MR, Welham JL, Murray RM. Schizophrenia and the influenza epidemics of 1954, 1957 and 1959 a southern-hemisphere study. Schizophr Res 1994; 14:1..8.
83. Mednick SA, Huttunen MO, Machon RA. Prenatal influenza infections and adult schizophrenia. Schizophr Bull 1994; 20:263..267.
84. Crow TJ, Done DJ, Johnstone EC. Schizophrenia is not due to maternal influenza in the 2nd (or other) trimester of pregnancy. Schizophr Res 1992; 6:99..99.
85. Cannon M, Cotter D, Coffey VP, et al. Prenatal exposure to the 1957 influenza epidemic and adult schizophrenia: a follow-up study. Br J Psychiatry 1996; 168:368..371.
86. Torrey EF, Rawlings R, Waldman IN. Schizophrenic births and viral diseases in two states. Schizophr Res 1988; 1:73..77.
87. Selten J, Slaets JPJ. Evidence against maternal influenza as a risk factor for schizophrenia. Br J Psychiatry 1994; 164:674..676.
88. Susser E, Lin SP, Brown AS, Lumey LH, Erlenmeyerkimling L. No relation between risk of schizophrenia and prenatal exposure to influenza in holland. Am J Psychiatry 1994; 151: 922..924.

89. Cannon M, Cotter D, Sham PC, et al. Schizophrenia in an Irish sample following prenatal exposure to the 1957 influenza epidemic a case-controlled, prospective follow-up study. Schizophr Res 1994; 11:95..95.
90. Erlenmeyerkimling L, Folnegovic Z, Hrabakzerjavic V, Borcic B, Folnegovicsmalc V, Susser E. Schizophrenia and prenatal exposure to the 1957 A2 influenza epidemic in Croatia. Am J Psychiatry 1994; 151:1496..1498.
91. Morgan V, Castle D, Page A, et al. Influenza epidemics and incidence of schizophrenia, affective disorders and mental retardation in Western Australia: no evidence of a major effect. Schizophr Res 1997; 26:25..39.
92. Watson CG, Kucala T, Tilleskjor C, Jacobs L. Schizophrenic birth seasonality in relation to the incidence of infectious diseases and temperature extremes. Arch Gen Psychiatry 1984; 41:85..90.
93. Torrey FE, Rawlings R, Yolken RH. The antecedents of psychoses: a case-control study of selected risk factors. Schizophr Res 2000; 46:17..23.
94. Barr CE, Mednick SA, Munkjorgensen P. Exposure to influenza epidemics during gestation and adult schizophrenia a 40-year study. Arch Gen Psychiatry 1990; 47:869..874.
95. McGrath J, Castle D. Does influenza cause schizophrenia a 5-year review. Aust N Z J Psychiatry 1995; 29:23..31.
96. Westergaard T, Mortensen PB, Pedersen CB, Wohlfahrt J, Melbye M. Influenza rates, birth order and risk of schizophrenia: a population-based cohort study. Schizophr Res 1998; 29: 18..18.
97. Cotter D, Takei N, Farrell M, et al. Does prenatal exposure to influenza in mice induce pyramidal cell disarray in the dorsal hippocampus. Schizophr Res 1995; 16:233..241.
98. Sierrahonigmann AM, Carbone KM, Yolken RH. Polymerase chain-reaction (Pcr) search for viral nucleic-acid sequences in schizophrenia. Br J Psychiatry 1995; 166:55..60.
99. Taller AM, Asher DM, Pomeroy KL, et al. Search for viral nucleic acid sequences in brain tissues of patients with schizophrenia using nested polymerase chain reaction. Arch Gen Psychiatry 1996; 53:32..40.
100. Machon RA, Mednick SA, Huttunen MO. Adult major affective disorder after prenatal exposure to an influenza epidemic. Arch Gen Psychiatry 1997; 54:322..328.
101. Brown AS, Cohen P, Harkavy-Friedman J, et al. Prenatal rubella, premorbid abnormalities, and adult schizophrenia. Biol Psychiatry 2001; 49:473..486.
102. Brown AS, Cohen P, Greenwald S, Susser E. Nonaffective psychosis after prenatal exposure to rubella. Am J Psychiatry 2000; 157:438..443.
103. Suvisaari J, Haukka J, Tanskanen A, Hovi T, Lonnqvist J. Association between prenatal exposure to poliovirus infection and adult schizophrenia. Am J Psychiatry 1999; 156:1100..1102.
104. Susser ES, Lin SP. Schizophrenia after prenatal exposure to the Dutch hunger winter of 1944..1945. Arch Gen Psychiatry 1992; 49:983..988.
105. Hoek HW, Susser E, Buck KA, Lumey LH, Lin SP, Gorman JM. Schizoid personality disorder after prenatal exposure to famine. Am J Psychiatry 1996; 153:1637..1639.
106. Susser E, Neugebauer R, Hoek H, et al. Schizophrenia after prenatal famine: further evidence. Dev Psychobiol 1996; 29:8..8.
107. Brown AS, van Os J, Driessens C, Hoek HW, Susser ES. Prenatal famine and the spectrum of psychosis. Psychiatric Annals 1999; 29:145..150.
108. Brown AS, van Os J, Driessens C, Hoek HW, Susser ES. Further evidence of relation between prenatal famine and major affective disorder. Am J Psychiatry 2000; 157:190..195.
109. Wahlbeck K, Forsen T, Osmond C, Barker DJ, Eriksson JG. Association of schizophrenia with low maternal body mass index, small size at birth, and thinness during childhood. Arch Gen Psychiatry 2001; 58:48..52.

110. Mortensen PB, Pedersen CB, Westergaard T, et al. Effects of family history and place and season of birth on the risk of schizophrenia. N Engl J Med 1999; 340:603..608.
111. Bradbury TN, Miller GA. Season of birth in schizophrenia: a review of evidence, methodology, and etiology. Psychol Bull 1985; 98:569..594.
112. Hafner H, Haas S, Pfeifer-Kurda M, Eichhorn S, Michitsuji S. Abnormal seasonality of schizophrenic births. A specific finding? Eur Arch Psychiatry Neurol Sci 1987; 236:333..342.
113. Kendell RE, Kemp IW. Winter-born v summer-born schizophrenics. Br J Psychiatry 1987; 151:499..505.
114. Kendell RE, Adams W. Unexplained fluctuations in the risk for schizophrenia by month and year of birth. Br J Psychiatry 1991; 158:758..763.
115. Torrey EF, Bowler AE, Rawlings R, Terrazas A. Seasonality of schizophrenia and stillbirths. Schizophr Bull 1993; 19:557..562.
116. Cotter D, Larkin C. Season of birth in schizophrenia: clue or cul-de-sac? In: Buckley PF, ed. The Neurodevelopmental Basis of Schizophrenia. Georgetown, TX: R.G. Landes, 1996: 17..30.
117. Sham PC, Takei N, Murray RM, Ocallaghan E. Schizophrenia following prenatal exposure to influenza epidemics between 1939 and 1960   Reply. Br J Psychiatry 1992; 161:713..714.
118. Ocallaghan E, Cotter D, Colgan K, Larkin C, Walsh D, Waddington JL. Confinement of winter birth excess in schizophrenia to the urban-born and its gender specificity. Br J Psychiatry 1995; 166:51..54.
119. Suvisaari JM, Haukka JK, Tanskanen AJ, Lonnqvist JK. Decreasing seasonal variation of births in schizophrenia. Psychol Med 2000; 30:315..324.
120. Russell D, Douglas AS, Allan TM. Changing seasonality of birth   a possible environmental effect. J Epidemiol Community Health 1993; 47:362..367.
121. Kunugi H, Nanko S, Hayashi N, Saito K, Hirose T, Kazamatsuri H. Season of birth of schizophrenics in a recent Japanese sample. Psychiatry Clin Neurosci 1997; 51:213..216.
122. Eagles JM, Hunter D, Geddes JR. Gender-specific changes since 1900 in the season-of-birth effect in schizophrenia. Br J Psychiatry 1995; 167:469..472.
123. Suvisaari JM, Haukka JK, Lonnqvist JK. Season of birth among patients with schizophrenia and their siblings: evidence for the procreational habits hypothesis. Am J Psychiatry 2001; 158:754..757.
124. Narita K, Sasaki T, Akaho R, et al. Human leukocyte antigen and season of birth in Japanese patients with schizophrenia. Am J Psychiatry 2000; 157:1173..1175.
125. Lewis G, David A, Andreasson S, Allebeck P. Schizophrenia and city life. Lancet 1992; 340: 137..140.
126. Takei N, Sham PC, O'Callaghan E, Murray RM. Cities, winter birth, and schizophrenia. Lancet 1992; 340:558..559.
127. Torrey EF, Bowler AE, Clark K. Urban birth and residence as risk factors for psychoses: an analysis of 1880 data. Schizophr Res 1997; 25:169..176.
128. Marcelis M, Navarro-Mateu F, Murray R, Selten JP, Van Os J. Urbanization and psychosis: a study of 1942-1978 birth cohorts in The Netherlands. Psychol Med 1998; 28:871..879.
129. Wessely S, Castle D, Der G, Murray R. Schizophrenia and Afro-Caribbeans. A case-control study. Br J Psychiatry 1991; 159:795..801.
130. Eaton WW, Mortensen PB, Frydenberg M. Obstetric factors, urbanization and psychosis. Schizophr Res 2000; 43:117..123.
131. Marcelis M, Takei N, van Os J. Urbanization and risk for schizophrenia: does the effect operate before or at the time of illness onset? Schizophr Res 1999; 36:48..49.
132. van Os J, Selten JP. Prenatal exposure to maternal stress and subsequent schizophrenia   The May 1940 invasion of The Netherlands. Br J Psychiatry 1998; 172:324..326.

133. Selten JP, van der Graaf Y, van Duursen R, Gispen-de Wied CC, Kahn RS. Psychotic illness after prenatal exposure to the 1953 Dutch Flood Disaster. Schizophr Res 1999; 35:243..245.
134. Odegaard. Emigration and Insanity: a study of mental disease among Norwegian-born population in Minnesota. Acta Psychiatr Neurol Scand 1932; 7:1..206.
135. Harrison G, Glazebrook C, Brewin J, et al. Increased incidence of psychotic disorders in migrants from the Caribbean to the United Kingdom. Psychol Med 1997; 27:799..806.
136. Selten JP, Slaets JP, Kahn RS. Schizophrenia in Surinamese and Dutch Antillean immigrants to The Netherlands: evidence of an increased incidence. Psychol Med 1997; 27:807..811.
137. Selten JP, Veen N, Feller W, et al. Incidence of psychotic disorders in immigrant groups to The Netherlands. Br J Psychiatry 2001; 178:367..372.
138. Mortensen PB, CantorGraae E, McNeil TF. Increased rates of schizophrenia among immigrants: some methodological concerns raised by Danish findings. Psychol Med 1997; 27: 813..820.
139. Weyerer S, Hafner H. The high incidence of psychiatrically treated disorders in the inner city of Mannheim. Susceptibility of German and foreign residents. Soc Psychiatry Psychiatr Epidemiol 1992; 27:142..146.
140. McDonald C, Murray RM. Early and late environmental risk factors for schizophrenia. Brain Res Brain Res Rev 2000; 31:130..137.
141. Lipska BK, Weinberger DR. Subchronic treatment with haloperidol and clozapine in rats with neonatal excitotoxic hippocampal damage. Neuropsychopharmacology 1994; 10:199..205.
142. Lipska BK, Swerdlow NR, Geyer MA, Jaskiw GE, Braff DL, Weinberger DR. Neonatal excitotoxic hippocampal damage in rats causes post-pubertal changes in prepulse inhibition of startle and its disruption by apomorphine. Psychopharmacology (Berl) 1995; 122:35..43.
143. Lipska BK, Weinberger DR. To model a psychiatric disorder in animals: schizophrenia as a reality test. Neuropsychopharmacology 2000; 23:223..239.
144. Lipska BK, Jaskiw GE, Weinberger DR. Postpubertal emergence of hyperresponsiveness to stress and to amphetamine after neonatal excitotoxic hippocampal damage: a potential animal model of schizophrenia. Neuropsychopharmacology 1993; 9:67..75.
145. Saunders RC, Kolachana BS, Bachevalier J, Weinberger DR. Neonatal lesions of the medial temporal lobe disrupt prefrontal cortical regulation of striatal dopamine. Nature 1998; 393: 169..171.
146. Bertolino A, Knable MB, Saunders RC, et al. The relationship between dorsolateral prefrontal N-acetylaspartate measures and striatal dopamine activity in schizophrenia. Biol Psychiatry 1999; 45:660..667.
147. Suddath RL, Christison GW, Torrey EF, Casanova MF, Weinberger DR. Anatomical abnormalities in the brains of monozygotic twins discordant for schizophrenia. N Engl J Med 1990; 322:789..794.
148. Weinberger DR. Cell biology of the hippocampal formation in schizophrenia. Biol Psychiatry 1999; 45:395..402.
149. Heckers S, Rauch SL, Goff D, et al. Impaired recruitment of the hippocampus during conscious recollection in schizophrenia. Nat Neurosci 1998; 1:318..323.
150. Sapolsky RM. Glucocorticoids and hippocampal atrophy in neuropsychiatric disorders. Arch Gen Psychiatry 2000; 57:925..935.
151. Brown AS, Susser ES, Butler PD, Richardson Andrews R, Kaufmann CA, Gorman JM. Neurobiological plausibility of prenatal nutritional deprivation as a risk factor for schizophrenia. J Nerv Ment Dis 1996; 184:71..85.
152. Brake WG, Boksa P, Gratton A. Effects of perinatal anoxia on the acute locomotor response to repeated amphetamine administration in adult rats. Psychopharmacology 1997; 133: 389..395.

153. El-Khodor BF, Boksa P. Birth insult increases amphetamine-induced behavioral responses in the adult rat. Neuroscience 1998; 87:893..904.
154. Moore H, Ghajarnia M, Grace AA. Anatomy and function of prefrontal and limbic cortico-striatal circuits in a rodent model of schizophrenia. American College of Neuropsychopharmacology (ACNP), 1998, vol. 37.
155. Rakic P. Experimental Deletion of Specific Cortical Neurons: Relevance to Schizophrenia, American College of Neuropsychopharmacology (ACNP), 1996, vol. 35.
156. Johnston MV, Barks J, Greenamyre T, Silverstein F. Use of toxins to disrupt neurotransmitter circuitry in the developing brain. Prog Brain Res 1988; 73:425..446.
157. Black MD, Selk DE, Hitchcock JM, Wettstein JG, Sorensen SM. On the effect of neonatal nitric oxide synthase inhibition in rats: a potential neurodevelopmental model of schizophrenia. Neuropharmacology 1999; 38:1299..1306.
158. Weinstock M. Does prenatal stress impair coping and regulation of hypothalamic-pituitary-adrenal axis? Neurosci Biobehav Rev 1997; 21:1..10.
159. Hayashi A, Nagaoka M, Yamada K, Ichitani Y, Miake Y, Okado N. Maternal stress induces synaptic loss and developmental disabilities of offspring. Int J Dev Neurosci 1998; 16:209..216.
160. Vallee M, MacCari S, Dellu F, Simon H, Le Moal M, Mayo W. Long-term effects of prenatal stress and postnatal handling on age-related glucocorticoid secretion and cognitive performance: a longitudinal study in the rat. Eur J Neurosci 1999; 11:2906..2916.
161. Erlenmeyer-Kimling L, Rock D, Roberts SA, et al. Attention, memory, and motor skills as childhood predictors of schizophrenia-related psychoses: the New York High-Risk Project. Am J Psychiatry 2000; 157:1416..1422.
162. David AS, Malmberg A, Brandt L, Allebeck P, Lewis G. IQ and risk for schizophrenia: a population-based cohort study. Psychol Med 1997; 27:1311..1323.
163. Davidson M, Reichenberg A, Rabinowitz J, Weiser M, Kaplan Z, Mark M. Behavioral and intellectual markers for schizophrenia in apparently healthy male adolescents. Am J Psychiatry 1999; 156:1328..1335.
164. Done DJ, Crow TJ, Johnstone EC, Sacker A. Childhood antecedents of schizophrenia and affective illness   social adjustment at ages 7 and 11. BMJ 1994; 309:699..703.
165. Jones P, Rodgers B, Murray R, Marmot M. Child developmental risk factors for adult schizophrenia in the British 1946 birth cohort. Lancet 1994; 344:1398..1402.
166. Goldstein JM, Seidman LJ, Buka SL, et al. Impact of genetic vulnerability and hypoxia on overall intelligence by age 7 in offspring at high risk for schizophrenia compared with affective psychoses. Schizophr Bull 2000; 26:323..334.
167. Cannon TD, Huttunen MO, Lonnqvist J, et al. The inheritance of neuropsychological dysfunction in twins discordant for schizophrenia. Am J Hum Genet 2000; 67:369..382.
168. Lemaire V, Koehl M, Le Moal M, Abrous DN. Prenatal stress produces learning deficits associated with an inhibition of neurogenesis in the hippocampus. Proc Natl Acad Sci USA 2000; 97:11032..11037.
169. Poland RE, Cloak C, Lutchmansingh PJ, McCracken JT, Chang L, Ernst T. Brain N-acetyl aspartate concentrations measured by H MRS are reduced in adult male rats subjected to perinatal stress: preliminary observations and hypothetical implications for neurodevelopmental disorders. J Psychiatr Res 1999; 33:41..51.
170. Stohr T, Schulte Wermeling D, Szuran T, et al. Differential effects of prenatal stress in two inbred strains of rats. Pharmacol Biochem Behav 1998; 59:799..805.
171. Lipska BK, Weinberger DR. Genetic variation in vulnerability to the behavioral effects of neonatal hippocampal damage in rats. Proc Natl Acad Sci USA 1995; 92:8906..8910.

172. Sternberg EM, Glowa JR, Smith MA, et al. Corticotropin releasing hormone related behavioral and neuroendocrine responses to stress in Lewis and Fischer rats. Brain Res 1992; 570:54..60.
173. Berger N, Vaillancourt C, Boksa P. Genetic factors modulate effects of C-section birth on dopaminergic function in the rat. Neuroreport 2000; 11:639..643.
174. Wilcox JA, Nasrallah HA. Childhood head trauma and psychosis. Psychiatry Res 1987; 21: 303..306.
175. Malaspina D, Goetz RR, Friedman JH, et al. Traumatic brain injury and schizophrenia in members of schizophrenia and bipolar disorder pedigrees. Am J Psychiatry 2001; 158:440..446.
176. Rantakallio P, Jones P, Moring J, VonWendt L. Association between central nervous system infections during childhood and adult onset schizophrenia and other psychoses: a 28-year follow-up. Int J Epidemiol 1997; 26:837..843.
177. Lewis G, David AS, Malmberg A, Allebeck P. Non-psychotic psychiatric disorder and subsequent risk of schizophrenia. Cohort study. Br J Psychiatry 2000; 177:416..420.
178. Andreasson S, Allebeck P, Engstrom A, Rydberg U. Cannabis and schizophrenia. A longitudinal study of Swedish conscripts. Lancet 1987; 2:1483..1486.
179. Egan MF, Goldberg TE, Kolachana BS, et al. Effect of COMT Val108/158 Met genotype on frontal lobe function and risk for schizophrenia. Proc Natl Acad Sci USA 2001; 98: 6917..6922.

II THE VULNERABILITY TO SCHIZOPHRENIA

4 The Nature of the Prodrome in Schizophrenia

Jaak Rakfeldt, PhD
and Thomas H. McGlashan, MD

INTRODUCTION

In 1927, Harry Stack Sullivan *(1)* wrote about the onset of schizophrenia stating the following:

> The psychiatrist sees too many end states and deals professionally with too few of the pre-psychotic . With this in mind, it would seem as if we should lay great stress on the prompt investigation of failing adjustment, rather than, as is so often the case, wait and see what happens . I feel certain that many incipient cases might be arrested before the efficient contact with reality is completely suspended, and a long stay in institutions made necessary. (p. 135)

This chapter provides an overview of current thinking as well as ongoing research dealing with the "incipient" stages of schizophrenia.

Longitudinal studies indicate that the clinical chronicity of schizophrenia occurs in the early phase of the illness, predominantly within the first 5 years from the time of onset *(2)*. These and related findings have suggested that the earliest episodes of psychosis may reflect an active pathophysiologic process that, if sustained, can produce enduring impairment in patients and may reduce their capacity to respond to treatment *(3–5)*. Thus, therapeutic interventions in this early phase of the illness may be of critical importance *(4)*. Furthermore, it has been hypothesized that the morbidity of the illness may be limited by providing effective treatment at the onset or in the early phase of the illness *(6,7)*. In short, a critical need exists to identify persons better who are on the pathway of experiencing the early signs and symptoms of schizophrenia (i.e., in the symptomatic prodromal phase of illness).

From: *Early Clinical Intervention and Prevention in Schizophrenia*
Edited by: W. S. Stone, S. V. Faraone, and M. T. Tsuang © Humana Press Inc., Totowa, NJ

This chapter outlines the nature of the prodrome in schizophrenia and places it in the context of the overall etiology and development of the disorder in its earliest stages. Much has been written about the pathogenesis and phenomenological evolution of schizophrenia, but this chapter does not aim to be an exhaustive review of this literature. Instead, we selectively present contributions from the past generation and especially from the past decade that we consider pivotal to our picture and understanding of the prodrome.

DEFINITIONS

Prodrome As a Term

The word *prodrome* comes from the Greek word *prodromos*, which means the forerunner of an event. A prodrome refers to the early signs and symptoms preceding the full acute onset of illness. The prodrome usually refers to a period of prepsychotic disturbance that distinctly deviates from a person's typical, usual, and previous experiences and behaviors.

Prodrome to Relapse vs Prodrome to Onset

The term *prodrome* has also been used to denote both the preonset period as well as the period before relapse in those persons who already have psychotic illnesses. The relapse prodrome should be distinguished, however, from the prepsychotic phase that precedes the very first onset of a psychotic illness, or what might be termed the initial prodrome. This chapter focuses primarily on the initial prepsychotic phase, reflecting the interval from the first changes in a person's experiences and behaviors until development of the first frank psychotic symptoms.

Related Theories of Pathophysiology

The vulnerability stress model of schizophrenia was first clearly proposed by Meehl *(8)*, who stated that a defect in neural integration was inherited, which ultimately became the schizophrenia phenotype. Specific genetic factors were considered by Meehl to be necessary etiologically. The possibility, however, could not be excluded that some unknown environmental factor may also have some direct etiological significance. Genetic and environmental factors combined to build up vulnerability, which was regarded as a certain susceptibility of the central nervous system. Meehl designated this as *schizotaxia*, and postulated that schizotaxia involved a lack of selectivity of synaptic functioning and could be associated with subtle phenotypic manifestations.

This genetic vulnerability combined with environmental stressors led to behavioral abnormalities such as cognitive slippage, anhedonia, ambivalence, and an

aversion to intimate human relationships. Meehl termed this *schizotypy*. A person described as a schizotype, when confronted with cumulative and/or severe mental stress or environmental challenges, could decompensate into schizophrenia.

The vulnerability to schizophrenia is viewed as an enduring trait. This means that it exists before the onset of any symptomatology, and it may continue through to remission. The trait is not static or fixed, however, but it is shaped by transactions with the world. Some aspects of this may be a genetic vulnerability, whereas others may be acquired through faulty coping strategies. At the same time, strengths and other supports may buffer against these stressors and may help to minimize or even prevent the full expression of the vulnerability in clinical terms. Intrauterine circumstances, birth complications, season-of-birth issues, and perhaps socioeconomic factors may play a role as well. Because stressors and triggering mechanisms can be internal or external, or both, they may evoke a broad range of coping strategies required for adaptation. These coping styles may, in turn, exacerbate or minimize the impact of the stress and the effect of the neurodevelopmental vulnerability.

Tienari et al. *(9)* reported the findings from a nationwide Finnish sample of offspring of schizophrenic mothers who were adopted away and were raised by nonrelatives ($N = 155$). This group was compared in a blindly rated protocol with matched controls of adopted away offspring of nonschizophrenia parents. A broad range of psychological tests as well as a intensive interviews suggested that the adopted away offspring of schizophrenic mothers had a significantly higher frequency of psychoses and other severe forms of mental illness. These findings certainly support a genetic hypothesis. The authors caution, however, that these differences between the groups emerged only in the context of families who were rated by the interviewers as being markedly disturbed. The authors conclude by suggesting that genetic factors only become manifest in the presence of specific environmental circumstances, i.e., disturbed family contexts. They point to the additional fact that not only are individuals influenced by their environments, but they also influence their environments, meaning that disturbed behavior of these genetically at-risk prepsychotic persons may have helped to foster the disturbed family environments, which then were associated with greater disturbed behavior.

EXPRESSION OF SCHIZOPHRENIA PREMORBIDLY

Early and Mid-Premorbid Phase
(Usually Childhood Through Adolescence)

Olin and Mednick *(10)* consider premorbid indicators of psychosis that may be relevant to primary intervention. They review a substantial literature on risk factors for schizophrenia and conclude that several premorbid characteristics

have been identified to be risk markers for future psychosis. These premorbid characteristics fall into two categories. The first contains precursors related to early etiological factors, including a family history of schizophrenia, birth and delivery complications, maternal exposure to influenza during pregnancy, neurobehavioral deficits, early parental separation (usually) during the first year of life, institutional rearing, and stress related to poor family functioning. The second group involves social and behavioral precursors of mental illness usually identified during childhood or early adolescence by teachers and clinicians. These are personality variables identified during interviews and through the use of questionnaires.

The authors report that teachers are frequently able to judge accurately children and adolescents who later become diagnosed with schizophrenia. Such children are reported to be more emotionally labile and more susceptible to emotional and psychological breakdown. Teachers consistently rated males who later became psychotic as being more disruptive, as having disciplinary problems, and being more anxious, lonely and rejected by peers, and as more likely to have repeated a grade. In contrast, teachers rated females as being more nervous and withdrawn.

The authors conclude that these findings underscore the importance of the interaction between genetic vulnerability, environmental attributes, and individual traits. They point out that aside from very early parental separation, institutionalization, and neurobehavioral deficits, these characteristics have also been identified as risk factors in individuals who are not at genetic risk for schizophrenia, suggesting that such characteristics can be generalized to individuals in the general population.

Protective factors may also become more clear from these studies such as maternal mental health being a buffer against genetic vulnerability. Studies report that women diagnosed with schizophrenia and other psychiatric disorders suffer from more stress during pregnancy and engage in more risk-related behaviors during pregnancy such as using medications and alcohol, smoking, and not seeking prenatal care until very late in their pregnancies (11). Such behaviors, of course, may also increase the risk of perinatal and obstetric complications, which in turn increase the risk for future psychosis in persons who are already genetically more vulnerable. On the other hand, parents who have adequate social supports, and who are mentally and emotionally healthy are more likely to provide stable home environments, and to provide the essential emotional support for healthy child development.

All of this evidence, the authors conclude, supports the hypothesis that schizophrenia is a developmental disorder. It follows, therefore, that teachers may be a particularly helpful resource in identifying adolescents at risk for future psychosis. Certainly, teachers spend a great deal of time with adolescents and are, there-

fore, in a unique position to assess how students cope with social and cognitive demands as compared to their peers in classroom and other school-based situations.

Jones et al. *(12)* studied the associations between adult-onset schizophrenia and childhood sociodemographic, neurodevelopmental, cognitive, and behavioral factors among the British 1946 birth cohort. This was a prospective study that explored the association between various developmental domains and adult-onset schizophrenia. The cohort included 5362 members, of whom 30 developed schizophrenia between the ages of 16 and 43 years of age. For this subset, milestones of motor development were reached later than by cohort members who did not develop schizophrenia. The authors note that, for example, there was a 1- to 2-month delay in learning how to walk. In addition, up to the age of 15, persons who later developed schizophrenia had significantly more speech problems. Lower educational tests scores at ages 8, 11, and 15 also marked those who became ill. Solitary play preferences at ages 4 and 6 also predicted those who would later develop schizophrenia, as did lower ratings of social confidence at age 13. At age 15, those who later became ill were rated by teachers as being more anxious in social situations. And finally, home health aides rated mothers of the group destined to develop schizophrenia as having lower mothering skills and as being less able to understand their children when the child was 4 years old. The authors conclude that clear differences between people who later develop schizophrenia and the others in the 1946 birth cohort were found across a range of developmental domains, leading to the possibility that the origins of schizophrenia may be found early in life.

These studies point out that personal and behavioral attributes present in childhood and adolescence well before the onset of psychosis are frequently associated with the illness. It is important to realize, however, that these associations have been determined retrospectively, and the characteristics described are associated with some but not all cases of schizophrenia. From the prospective perspective, these personal and behavioral attributes have little power and accuracy in identifying children and adolescents who are likely to become psychotic later on. Their "predictive" power in the asymptomatic premorbid phase of illness in childhood and adolescence is small *(13)*. Teacher ratings of childhood classroom behavior in the British birth cohort study, for example, predicted schizophrenia in only 5% of students *(14)*.

Late Premorbid Phase

Davidson et al. *(15)* noted that often the diagnosis of schizophrenia is made at the time of the onset of dramatic psychotic symptoms. Mounting evidence, however, suggests that subtle behavioral and intellectual abnormalities often precede psychotic episodes by many years. In fact, apparently healthy children and

adolescents who later developed schizophrenia frequently manifested lower intelligence, social withdrawal, conduct and adjustment disorders, and neurological deficits when compared to siblings, classmates, and population norms. Davidson and his colleagues used a follow-back or historical, prospective design. The strength of their study was that it included the entire national population. They merged the Israeli national psychiatric hospitalization case registry with the Israeli draft board registry. The latter contains scores of behavioral and intellectual functioning for males ages 16..17 years. The specific purpose of the study was to determine if psychiatric hospitalization for schizophrenia could be predicted from these Israeli draft board registry assessments.

The results suggest that individuals destined to be hospitalized for schizophrenia ($N = 509$) had statistically significantly worse scores on all measures as compared to matched nonpatients ($N = 9215$). The authors conclude that these results suggest that scores measuring social functioning, organizational ability, and intellectual functioning can be used to predict future hospitalization for schizophrenia with a positive predictive value of 71.6%. The authors note as well that behavioral attributes such as the ability to function independently in everyday life and organizational ability are lower in persons destined to be hospitalized. The authors also stress that these findings are consistent with earlier research that points to relatively poor premorbid behavioral and personality adjustment, especially in terms of impaired social relationships, among those who are later diagnosed with schizophrenia (15).

Davidson's findings relate to the late premorbid phase. The Israeli draftees were 16 and 17 years old. Those who were destined to develop schizophrenia were on average 5 years from onset. The impairments they displayed, if measured prospectively, would have considerably more predictive power than the impairments noted above from studies of the early premorbid phase. In Davidson's cohort, the intellectual and social deficits of the draftees had a positive predictive value (PPV) for developing schizophrenia 5 years later (on average) of 75%, as compared to 5% PPV of the teachers' reports of children in the British cohort study (14). This is still not sufficiently accurate prediction to justify intervention at this point, but it does indicate that illness activity is building silently but steadily, even though on the surface the situation is still "premorbid."

EXPRESSIONS OF SCHIZOPHRENIA PRODROMALLY

Retrospective Descriptions

In a trenchant article dealing with the onset of schizophrenia, Sullivan (1), stressed that the appearance of the disorder is late in a long series of subjectively felt experiences, and that objective manifestations of maladjustment often exists for years before the full psychotic break.

Yung and McGorry *(16)* review the prodrome for first-episode psychosis and conclude by proposing their own "Hybrid/Interactive" model for conceptualizing the prodrome. The authors define the initial prodrome as the time interval from the first changes people experience until development of the first frank psychotic symptoms. They also point to difficulties defining this prodromal interval. Based on retrospective data, people often first notice some change in themselves. These are not, however, usually psychotic symptoms. They may, for example, notice that they are not coping as well with stress, or they may notice vague feelings of uneasiness and depression. Uncharacteristic moments of disinhibition may occur. Although these experiences are becoming more and more noticeable to the persons themselves, these changes may be so subtle at first that others may not notice them at all. After this phase, as these early signs intensify, families and friends often begin to notice changes, described as the person becoming more irritable, anxious, or doing things that are clearly out of character. These changes are often normalized and minimized, particularly among adolescents, for whom such behaviors are often viewed as normal phases of growing up, or "typically" erratic teenage behavior.

Of course, making meaning out of such subtle experiences retrospectively is problematic. People are prone to identify almost any event as triggering. These may, however, not really be causally linked to the onset of the prodrome at all. Moreover, family members may feel guilty about not having noticed subtle changes in their loved ones, leading them later to deny that such changes had even occurred, at least not until a very clear psychotic episode has ensued. The degree of "sealing over" *(17)* may also influence recall. Patients may not want to remember such painful and turbulent experiences, and as pointed out, their family members may not wish to do so either. In short, the unique coping styles of both patients and their family members may diminish the accuracy of retrospective descriptions of the prodrome.

During this time, people tend to isolate themselves from others, resulting in greater destruction of social networks, and impairment of schoolwork and occupational functioning. There is heightened danger of potentially life-threatening crises such as increased aggressiveness and suicidal behavior, coupled with increased substance use and abuse. All of these factors may lead to a precipitous downward course in many domains for patients, which is also often accompanied by extreme social disruptions for friends and family members.

The authors call for a more accurate characterization of the prodrome. This would help to identify high-risk persons during their first manifestations of the subtle changes suggesting impending psychosis. The authors urge that such people be studied in order to investigate the pathogenesis of psychosis and to identify clear markers that predict onset. The presence and duration of prodromal symptoms may also have prognostic significance: longer duration of prodromal symptoms may

indicate poorer prognoses *(18)*. There may well be subtypes of schizophrenia such as the "process" and "reactive" types long discussed in the literature *(19,20)*.

Yung and McGorry *(16)* list prodromal symptoms in order from most to least frequently occurring. The list is as follows: reduced concentration and attention, reduced drive and motivation or anergia, depressed mood, sleep disturbances, anxiety, social withdrawal, suspiciousness, deterioration in role functioning, and irritability.

The authors caution, however, that the onset of the prodrome is not captured by simply a list of symptoms at one point in time, but involves a process that is unfolding and evolving. Regarding these changes, two schools of thought have emerged. The first group views these as nonspecific changes followed by specific prepsychotic symptoms that are then followed by psychosis. In fact, most authors in this camp consider the prodrome to consist of nonspecific "neurotic" symptoms that are then followed by more marked deviations leading to frank psychosis *(21–23)*. The subjective symptoms are usually accompanied by some deterioration of role functioning and some marked behavioral changes as well. They cite Cameron's (1938) *(24)* work that describes these nonspecific symptoms as lasting from a few weeks to several years before the specific symptoms emerge that herald the impending psychosis. The nonspecific symptoms include nervousness, restlessness, tenseness, unease, apprehension, and anxiety. In contrast, the "specific symptoms" are clearly and recognizably schizophrenic in quality, and consist of a sense that one's environment has lost the feeling of familiarity, combined with subjective feelings of being dazed or confused. These symptoms were viewed as being attenuated forms of frank psychotic experience.

In the second pattern, there are early specific changes in perception, attention, speech, or motility, followed by neurotic symptoms thought to be a reaction to these first changes, followed by psychosis *(25)*. The authors cite the work of Chapman (1966) *(25)* who suggested that specific subjective changes occur first, and are then followed by neurotic symptoms and behavioral changes.

"Outpost syndromes" *(26)* are clusters of symptoms and behaviors that crosssectionally appear to resemble prodromes but that often remit spontaneously. Huber described outpost syndromes as resembling a defect or a residual state in schizophrenia. He coined the term "basic symptoms," which consist of subjective complaints about impairment in cognitive, emotional, motor, and autonomic functioning, as well as in bodily sensation, energy, external perception, and tolerance to stress *(27)*.

Yung and McGorry suggest a "Hybrid/Interactive" model of the prodrome, which combines the patterns described earlier. In this conceptualization, people move in and out of symptomatic periods of both the nonspecific and the specific, attenuated psychotic, types. Both of these types may precede psychosis and may occur primarily. Reactive neurotic symptoms such as anxiety and depression can

occur in response to specific symptoms, and to the behavioral changes that may result from any of these symptoms.

McGorry suggests that a more accurate term for this period would be "at-risk mental states" *(28)*. This perspective has significant implications for clinical practice and for research. It allows for a sequential screening of persons who combine risk factors into prospectively designed research studies, recruiting people who are more likely to transition into psychosis. Thus, an at-risk mental state may be combined with other risk factors, such as family history, and persons can be followed along to see if they do, or do not convert to frank psychosis.

A major concern of such prospective studies is that psychiatric attention and intervention would be given to persons who never go on to develop the psychotic disorder, or false positives. Cross-sectionally, specific changes in mental state may resemble the prodrome but not result in psychosis. Such persons may have incipient major mood disorders, or an anxiety disorder, or may simply be reacting to an environmental or situational crisis. On the other hand, such changes in mental state may occur in people who are potentially prepsychotic, but factors such as effective coping, increased social support, and other ameliorative circumstances could prevent or delay the psychosis. These persons then might have what Huber describes as "outpost syndromes."

Häfner and colleagues *(29)* used a retrospective assessment approach to study the onset of schizophrenia. In a representative sample ($N = 232$) of first-admission persons from a regional population of 1.5 million, the authors investigated both positive and negative symptoms, age, gender, and social factors among first-admission patients. The authors developed a structured Interview for the Retrospective Assessment of the Onset of Schizophrenia (IRAOS). The IRAOS was used to interview patients and their closest reference persons. Additional medical records were also reviewed to gather more data. This sample was part of the authors' Age, Beginning, and Course (ABC) study and consisted of a sample of 276 patients (143 women and 133 men), who were between 12 and 59 years of age. The inclusion criteria involved patients who had had their first admission within the previous 2-year period, and who had a diagnosis of schizophrenia. Shortly following admission, after the acute symptoms had subsided, patients were given the Present State Exam and were interviewed using the IRAOS.

The authors assessed the early course of illness and recorded which symptoms were present before onset (*see* Fig. 1).

The results suggest that negative and nonspecific signs of mental disorder initiate the prodrome 2.3 years (median) prior to onset. Positive symptoms emerge later, 0.8 years (median) prior to onset. The year prior to onset in particular is marked by considerable symptomatic activity, particularly in the last 4.6 months, which sees an acceleration of positive symptoms. According to Häfner and colleagues, the prodrome is 1 year or longer in 68% of cases and less than 1 year in

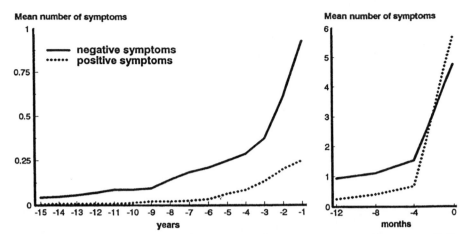

Fig. 1. Cumulative values of positive and negative symptoms over 15 years until first hospitalization for schizophrenia (*N* = 232). Reproduced with permission from ref. *30.*

32%, with only 18% appearing abruptly only 4 weeks prior to onset. The prodrome is initated by nonspecific negative symptoms in 73% of cases, positive and negative symptoms in 20% of cases, and positive symptoms exclusively in only 7% of cases *(29).* These findings are important in that they represent the first, and largest empirical study of the prodrome based on careful retrospective systematic assessment.

In a retrospective study, Møller and Husby *(31)* interviewed 19 first-episode schizophrenia patients, explored prodromal phenomena in depth, and described experiences and behaviors that appeared to be essential components of initial prodromes. From eight groups of experiences, they highlighted two as being tentative core dimensions: "disturbance of self" and "extreme preoccupation by and withdrawal to overvalued ideas." Four prodromal behaviors are also identified: (a) quit school, university, or job, or major school truancy, (b) marked and lasting observable shift of interests, (c) marked and lasting social passivity, withdrawal, or isolation, and (d) marked and lasting change in global appearance or behavior.

Using a combination of qualitative and quantitative research approaches Møller *(32)* interviewed the above sample of first-episode persons as well as their relatives in order to explore the phenomenology of the initial prodrome and the phase of untreated psychosis. The findings suggest that a later onset of the prodrome, an initial presence of grandiosity and disorganization, and a mild level of social withdrawal comprise a pattern that may reduce treatment delay and

shorten the duration of untreated psychosis (DUP). More blatant and bizarre behavior leads to earlier detection and treatment. In contrast, social withdrawal is likely to make identification of psychosis more difficult, and may therefore increase DUP.

Prospective Descriptions With Predictive Validity

Klosterkötter et al. *(33)* relate how during the 1960s Huber described subtle symptoms (often perceptible only to persons themselves) that often marked the earliest signs of illness, and he termed these "basic symptoms" *(34)*. The Bonn Scale of the Assessment of Basic Symptoms (BSABS) operationalized these pre-psychotic deviations in the form of a semistructured interview.

Klosterkötter and his colleagues *(33)* report on the Cologne early-recognition project in which persons suspected of being in the initial prodromal phase were studied prospectively for the first time. The purpose of the study was to examine the prognostic accuracy of initial prodromal symptoms assessed by the BSABS to determine its ability to predict subsequent psychoses. The results suggest that about 50% had developed schizophrenia in the follow-up. The mean transition time to schizophrenia occurred at 4.3 years after the onset of the initial prodrome in women, and after 6.7 years in men. The positive predictive value of the BSABS was 70% for predicting schizophrenia with certain symptoms such as thought interference, disturbances of receptive language, and visual distortions being most predictive.

Yung et al. *(35)* describe how in the 1990s young people were referred to their first-episode program who were not psychotic but at risk for becoming psychotic in the near future. They set up a separate clinic called the Personal Assessment and Crisis Evaluation (PACE) Clinic for these people and found that a significant number did indeed become psychotic.

Yung et al. *(35)* studied these symptomatic youth carefully over time and identified three types of prodromal constellations. Positive symptoms defined two out of the three prodromal states or groups. The first group consisted of persons with positive psychotic symptoms that are brief and do not meet the frequency or duration criteria specified by most diagnostic systems of psychosis. Such patients may meet criteria for *DSM–IV* Brief Psychosis or Psychosis NOS (not otherwise specified), but they do not meet criteria for *DSM–IV* Schizophreniform Disorder. The second group was defined by the onset within the past year of nonpsychotic, attenuated positive symptoms that occurred at least once a week in the past month. The third group was not characterized by positive symptoms but by genetic risk (i.e., first-degree relative with psychosis) and recent deterioration of functioning. The first group they called Brief Limited Intermittent Psychosis Prodromal State (BLIPS); the second they called Attenuated Positive Symptom Prodromal States (APSPS); and the third group they called Genetic Risk and Deterioration

(GRD). They assessed patients for these prodromal syndromes using a structured assessment instrument, the Comprehensive Assessment of At-Risk Mental States (CAARMS).

Miller et al. *(36)* and McGlashan et al. *(37)* describe a scale to characterize, quantify, and track prodromal symptoms and states, the Scale of Prodromal Symptoms (SOPS), and a structured interview, The Structured Interview for Prodromal Symptoms (SIPS). The SOPS and SIPS were developed to accomplish three tasks: (a) define the presence/absence of psychosis, (b) assess the presence/absence of one or more of the three prodromal states as defined by Yung et al. *(35)*, and (c) measure the severity of prodromal symptoms cross-sectionally and longitudinally. Miller et al. *(36)* tested the SIPS for interrater reliability for the prodromal vs not prodromal judgment, and agreement among raters was 93% ($\kappa = 0.82$, 95% CI 0.55-0.93). These data suggest that raters using the SIPS can make a diagnostic judgment regarding the presence of the prodrome with excellent interrater reliability.

The diagnostic criteria for the prodrome developed by Yung, McGorry, and colleagues identified a group of prodromal patients, approx 40% of whom converted to an actively psychotic state within 1 year *(16)*. These pivotal findings demonstrate that their prodromal criteria have robust predictive validity. Miller et al. (36) tested the predictive validity of the SIPS on a sample of patients assessed for the prodrome and followed for 1 year without treatment. Among patients diagnosed as prodromal at baseline, 46% developed schizophrenic psychosis by 6 months and 64% by 12 months, thus replicating the findings of Yung and McGorry (1996) et al. *(16)*.

PRODROMAL INTERVENTION:
EARLIEST CLINICAL TRIALS

Falloon et al. *(38)* described a preliminary uncontrolled study of an intensive early intervention with persons who displayed signs and symptoms of schizophrenia. The intervention was carried out in a semirural area in England that previously had lacked established mental health services. This allowed Falloon and his colleagues to develop an early-intervention project from scratch. He situated this intervention within the already established network of family practice physicians in the area.

Falloon's early-detection procedures involved a two-stage approach that entailed training family practitioners to recognize prodromal symptoms and without delay to refer such persons for immediate specialized mental health assessment. The second phase involved mental health assessment. Falloon established a multidisciplinary team of mental health professionals that ensured assessment within a few hours of a request. The assessment included the patient and significant

caregivers who completed an instrument that tapped features of the prodrome in schizophrenia.

The early-intervention procedures included education about the nature of the illness, a comprehensive stress management program, and neuroleptic medication when necessary. The specific mix of these components was always targeted and tailored to the individual needs of the patients. Within 24 hours of detection of symptoms, patients and their primary caregivers were provided with educational seminars that stressed the rationale for early intervention. They were told that these symptoms could possibly be early signs of an impending schizophrenia, and that the application of treatment strategies could be effective in preventing a major psychiatric decompensation. People were also told that these features might be found in a range of other disorders as well. It was stressed that recovery was very possible with application of effective treatment methods, as well as from continued support for family and friends, backed up by around-the-clock services from well-trained mental health specialists. Questions and concerns were discussed in an open and frank manner that fostered treatment alliance, and that minimized fears. After the education, informed consent to participate in the intervention was sought and in every case it was granted.

Falloon also incorporated a home-based stress management effort, which occurred at the conclusion of the initial educational phase. This included a brief assessment of the major stressors that may have triggered the onset of symptoms. The participants, as well as their caregivers, were then helped to cope better with these situations, and were aided in strategies to resolve any continuing stress related to these events. Daily sessions usually included significant others as well as participants and focused on problem-solving techniques. Intensive residential care was available if necessary, and was supported by a range of psychological, social work, and occupational therapy services.

The stress management techniques and drug therapy were combined with crisis-oriented supports and continued until the prodromal signs and symptoms remitted. Continued monitoring of stress and assessing of patients' ability to deal with stressors enabled treaters to define specific coping strategies still needed. This ongoing analysis allowed for targeting further training and for the use of specific problem-solving skills for all members of the household. Training was continued until proficiency with problem-solving efforts in all forms of stress management had been developed. In addition, a regular weekly household meeting was conducted to ensure sustained use of the skills. These meetings occurred at the patients' homes, and specifically addressed problematic issues for participants as well as for other household members.

Falloon described the procedure of monitoring for any reoccurrence of prodromal symptoms by having the participants and their significant others trained to recognize the specific early-warning signs. A wallet-size card was given to all

participants that listed the significant signs that were most likely to occur during prodromal episodes. These cards also contained detailed procedures as to how to contact the family practitioner immediately as well as the mental health specialists.

The most dramatic and encouraging outcome from this project was that Falloon had conducted a study using similar case definitions in the same region 10 years earlier. At that time, he had found an annual schizophrenia incidence of 7.4 persons per 100,000 population, which was consistent with that for the rest of England (about 8 per 100,000). During the course of Falloon's intervention project, however, the annual incidence rate for his region had fallen to only 0.75 per 100,000 total population. This reflects a dramatic and striking 10-fold reduction of the incidence of schizophrenia during the 4-year period of this study, leading to hope that such early intervention may really help. A major caveat, however, is power. It was a very small sample ($N = 16$) and treatments were preliminary, nonrandomized, and not controlled.

Phillips and McGorry *(39)* completed a randomized trail of early intervention with young people who are prodromal to schizophrenia (PACE). Their results are quite promising. The study design was nonblind and involved randomizing participants to either active treatment or follow-along for 6 months. The active-treatment condition consisted of risperidone 1.2 mg per day, which was augmented by anxiolytics or antidepressants as needed. The intervention also involved between 12 and 24 sessions of cognitive behavioral treatment. The control condition consisted of basic social support plus antidepressants and anxiolytics as needed. The sample size was 60 participants, all of whom completed the 6-month protocol. There were 32 participants in the treatment condition, and 28 in the control condition. At the end of the first 6-month phase, 10 persons in the control condition (36%) and 4 members of the active-treatment condition (12.5%) had converted to psychosis, a statistically significant finding. During the second 6-month interval, more of the treatment group members had converted to psychosis than did controls. These findings suggest that active treatment postponed the onset of psychosis but did not actually prevent it.

SUMMARY OF THE PRODROME
AS REVEALED IN THESE SELECTED STUDIES

This chapter has selectively reviewed what we regard as the pivotal literature related to the prodrome, or the symptomatic stage of illness prior to onset of diagnosable psychosis.

Meehl's *(8)* classic paper introduced the concept of vulnerability to schizophrenia. He proposed that the disorder is a result of neural deficits (schizotaxia) that when combined with unique life experiences and interpersonal contexts may lead to specific personality configurations (schizotypy) that confer greater vul-

nerability to schizophrenia. This was thought to be necessary but not sufficient since many people with schizotypy do not develop schizophrenia. These hypotheses are supported by Tienari et al. *(9)* whose work suggested that genetic vulnerability factors only became manifest in the presence of disturbed family contexts.

Premorbid characteristics that are related to later onset of psychosis include factors that may be regarded as etiologic or factors that reflect early neurodevelopmental deficits. Etiological factors include family history of schizophrenia, birth and delivery complications, maternal exposure to influenza, early parental separation, institutional rearing, and stress related to poor family functioning *(10)*. Phenomenologically, children who later become psychotic are reported by their teachers as being more emotionally labile, being more disruptive, having more disciplinary problems, being more anxious, lonely, and rejected by peers, and being more likely to have repeated a grade. During the late premorbid phase, individuals destined to be hospitalized for schizophrenia performed more poorly on measures of social functioning, organizational ability, and intellectual functioning *(15)*.

During the initial prodrome, persons often notice that they are not coping as well with stress; or they sense vague feelings of uneasiness and depression; and at times they may act out in uncharacteristically disinhibited ways *(16)*. The list of prodromal symptoms from most to least frequently occurring includes: reduced concentration and attention, reduced drive and motivation, depressed mood, sleep disturbances, anxiety, social withdrawal, suspiciousness, deterioration of role functioning, and irritability *(16)*. The work of Häfner and colleagues supports this list of prodromal symptoms in that negative and nonspecific signs of mental disorder occur first, and often years prior to onset. Positive symptoms emerge during the year prior to the first psychotic episode, particularly in the last 4. 6 months *(30)*. These nonspecific signs may, however, be prodromal to disorders other than schizophrenia.

Yung et al. *(35)* define three constellations of prodromal symptoms. The first consists of brief psychotic episodes that do not meet frequency and duration criteria for diagnosis. The second pattern involves attenuated positive symptoms of schizophrenia. The third type is characterized by genetic risk and recent deterioration of functioning. Miller et al. *(36)* and McGlashan *(37)* incorporated these types into a structured interview schedule, the SOPS, and a rating scale that quantifies and tracks prodromal symptoms, the SIPS.

Many people have contributed to the substantial and growing literature dealing with the prodrome in schizophrenia. Our aim in this chapter was to highlight the central themes, e.g., the prodrome as an early expression of psychosis with predictive validity for later schizophrenia, and the encouraging development of reliable and valid instruments to identify persons at risk, thus opening up possibilities for accurate early identification and timely intervention. Knowledge about the prodrome is important in that there may be only a narrow window of

opportunity during which vulnerable persons may be able to cope more effectively with the onset of illness, e.g., engaged in treatment while cognitive abilities are still relatively intact. It is also a time when social networks may still be together, when hopes and goals for the future are still alive, and where dramatic declines in volition and intentionality have not yet occurred.

By becoming better able to identify persons truly vulnerable for first-episode psychosis during this narrow window, we may help them marshal more effective coping strategies and, perhaps, lessen the severity and the collateral damage of their illnesses.

REFERENCES

1. Sullivan HS. The onset of schizophrenia. Am J Psychiatry 1994; 151(6):135..139.
2. McGlashan TH. A selective review of recent North American long-term follow-up studies of schizophrenia. Schizophr Bull 1988; 14(4):515.542.
3. Lieberman JA, Kinon BJ, Loebel AD. Dopaminergic mechanisms of idopathic and drug induced psychosis. Schizophr Bull 1990; 16(1):97..110.
4. Wyatt RJ. Early intervention for schizophrenia: can the course of the illness be altered? Biol Psychiatry 1995; 38(1):1..3.
5. Loebel AD, Lieberman JA, Alvir JMJ, Mayerhoff DI, Deisler SH, Szymanski SR. Duration of psychosis and outcome in first episode schizophrenia. Am J Psychiatry 1992; 149:1183..1188.
6. McGlashan TH, Johannessen JO. Early detection and intervention with schizophrenia: rationale. Schizophr Bull 1996; 22(2):201.222.
7. McGlashan, TH. Early detection and intervention in schizophrenia: editor's introduction. Schizophr Bull 1996; 22(2):197..199.
8. Meehl P. Schizotaxia, schizotypy, schizophrenia. Am Psychol 1962; 17:827.838.
9. Tiernari P, Wynne L, Moring J, et al. The Finnish adoptive family study of schizophrenia: implications for family research. Br J Psychiatry 1994; 164(Suppl 23):20.26.
10. Olin SS, Mednick SA. Risk factors of psychosis: identifying vulnerable populations premorbidly. Schizophr Bull 1996; 22(2):223.240.
11. Sameroff A, Seifer R, Zax M, Barocas R. Early indicators of developmental risk: Rochester Longitudinal Study. Schizophr Bull 1987; 13(3):383..394.
12. Jones P, Rodgeres B, Murray R, Marmot M. Child developmental risk factors for adult schizophrenia in the British 1946 birth cohort. Lancet 1994; 344:1398..1402.
13. Jones P, van Oss H. Predicting schizophrenia in teenagers pessimistic results from the British 1946 birth cohort. Conference on Schizophrenia Research, Colorado Springs, CO, April 1997.
14. Jones P, Croudace J. Predicting schizophrenia from teachers' reports of behaviour: results from a general population birth cohort. In: Miller T, et al., eds. Early Intervention in Psychotic Disorders. Dordrecht, Netherlands: Kluwer Academic, 2001:1..28.
15. Davidson M, Reichenberg MA, Rabinowitz J, Weiser M, Kaplan Z, Mark M. Behavioral and intellectual markers for schizophrenia in apparently healthy male adolescents. Am J Psychiatry 1999; 156(9):1328..1335.
16. Yung AR, McGorry PD. The prodromal phase of first-episode psychosis: past and current conceptualizations. Schizophr Bull 1996; 22(2):353.370.
17. McGlashan TH, Levy ST, Carpenter W. Integration and sealing over: clinically distinct recovery styles from schizophrenia. Arch Gen Psychiatry 1975; 32:1269..1272.

18. Johnstone EC, Crow TJ, Johnson AL, MacMillan JF. The Northwick Park Study of first episode schizophrenia: I. Presentation of the illness and problems relating to admission. Br J Psychiatry 1986; 148:115..120.

19. Chapman JP, Day D, Burstein A. The process-reactive distinction and prognosis in schizophrenia. J Nerv Ment Dis 1961; 133:383.391.

20. Fenton WS, McGlashan TH. The prognostic scale for chronic schizophrenia. Schizophr Bull 1987; 13(2):277..286.

21. Bowers MB. The onset of psychosis: a diary account. Psychiatry 1965; 28:346..358.

22. Bowers MB. Pathogenesis of acute schizophrenia. Arch Gen Psychiatry 1968; 19:348..355.

23. Henrichs DW, Carpenter WT. Prospective study of prodromal symptoms in schizophrenic relapse. Am J Psychiatry 1985; 142:371.373.

24. Cameron DE. Early schizophrenia. Am J Psychiatry 1938; 95:567..578.

25. Chapman JP. The early symptoms of schizophrenia. Br J Psychiatry 1966; 112:225..251.

26. Huber G, Gross G, Schüttler R, Linz M. Longitudinal studies of schizophrenic patients. Schizophr Bull 1980; 6(4):592..605.

27. Koehler K, Sauer H. Huber's basic symptoms: another approach to negative psychopathology in schizophrenia. Compr Psychiatry 1984; 25:174..182.

28. McGorry RD, Singh BS. Schizophrenia: risk and possibility of prevention. In: Raphael B, Burrows GD, eds. Handbook of Preventive Psychiatry. Amsterdam: Elsevier, 1995:492..514.

29. Häfner H, Maurer K. The prodromal phase of psychosis. In: Miller T, et al., eds. Early Intervention in Psychotic Disorders. Dordrecht, Netherlands: Kluwer Academic, 2001:71..100.

30. Maurer K, Häfner H. Methodological aspects of onset assessment in schizophrenia. Schizophr Res 1995; 15:265..276.

31. Møller P, Husby R. The initial prodrome in schizophrenia: searching for naturalistic core dimensions of experience and behavior. Schizophr Bull 2000; 26(1):217..232.

32. Møller P. First-episode schizophrenia: do grandiosity, disorganization, and acute initial development reduce duration of untreated psychosis? An exploratory naturalistic case study. Compr Psychiatry 2000; 41(3):184..190.

33. Klosterkötter J, Helmich M, Steinmeyer EM, Scultze-Lutter F. Diagnosing schizophrenia in the initial prodromal phase. Arch Gen Psychiatry 2001; 58(2):158..164.

34. Gross G. The "basic symptoms" of schizophrenia. Br J Psychiatry 1989; Suppl 7:21..25.

35. Yung AR, McGorry PD, McFarlane CA, Jackson HJ, Patton GC, Rakker A Monitoring and care of young people at incipient risk of psychosis. Schizophr Bull 1996; 22(2):283..303.

36. Miller TJ, McGlashan TH, Woods SW, et al. Symptom assessment in schizophrenic prodromal states. Psychiatr Q 1999; 70(4):273..287.

37. McGlashan TH, Miller TJ, Woods SW, Hoffman RE, Davidson L. Instrument for the assessment of prodromal symptoms and states. In: Miller T, et al., eds. Early Intervention in Psychotic Disorders. Dordrecht, Netherlands: Kluwer Academic, 2001:135..149.

38. Falloon IRH. Early intervention for first episodes of schizophrenia: a preliminary exploration. Psychiatry 1992; 55:4..15.

39. Philips L, McGorry PD. The development of preventive interventions for early psychosis. Paper presented at the Second International Conference on Early Psychosis, New York, April 2, 2000.

5   The Nature of Schizotaxia

Stephen V. Faraone, PhD,
Ming T. Tsuang, MD, PhD, DSc
and Sarah I. Tarbox, BA

SUMMARY

In this chapter, we show that (a) schizotaxia (Meehl's term for the predisposition to schizophrenia) is a clinically consequential condition and (b) that distinguishing it from schizotypal personality disorder (SPD) may be useful from both clinical and scientific perspectives. We review prior work indicating that some of the nonpsychotic and nonschizotypal relatives of schizophrenic patients have a psychiatric syndrome characterized by negative symptoms, neuropsychological impairment, and psychosocial dysfunction. Following Meehl, we call this constellation of clinical and neurobiologic features schizotaxia. The studies we review suggest it may be worthwhile to consider schizotaxia as a separate diagnostic class. Doing so would alert clinicians to a neurobehavioral syndrome not adequately covered by current diagnostic criteria and would motivate researchers to develop diagnostic and therapeutic approaches aimed at helping schizotaxic individuals and, perhaps, preventing the onset of schizophrenia.

INTRODUCTION

Neuroanatomical abnormalities, neuropsychological deficits, and psychosocial difficulties have been observed consistently in high-risk children and adolescents, and in nonpsychotic adult relatives of schizophrenic individuals [1]. These observations, in conjunction with the presence of similar, nonclinical (i.e., not psychosis) abnormalities in individuals with schizophrenia, support the idea that the liability to schizophrenia is a neurodevelopmental condition produced by a combination of genetic and environmental factors that exists prior to the onset of psychosis. Several lines of evidence support this view. For example, autopsy

From: *Early Clinical Intervention and Prevention in Schizophrenia*
Edited by: W. S. Stone, S. V. Faraone, and M. T. Tsuang © Humana Press Inc., Totowa, NJ

studies on brains of schizophrenic individuals show structural abnormalities consistent with malformations occurring during the second and third trimesters of pregnancy *(2,3)*. In addition, children at risk for developing schizophrenia show deficits in several areas including motor, intellectual, and social functioning (e.g., refs. *4,5*). Moreover, psychotic symptoms generally manifest after puberty, a time when ongoing brain development, hormonal changes, and environmental stressors all co-occur *(6)*. This type of evidence, considered in conjunction with elevated risks for schizophrenia in relatives of schizophrenic patients *(7)*, supports the conceptualization of the predisposition to schizophrenia as an interactive, neurodevelopmental process fashioned from genetic and environmental factors.

Based on this premise that the neurobiological basis for schizophrenia is formed by the combined effect of genes and adverse environmental risk factors, we proposed a modified view of Meehl's concept of "schizotaxia" to describe the neurodevelopmental condition underlying the predisposition to schizophrenia *(8)*. In this chapter, we present this conceptualization of schizotaxia as the liability for schizophrenia, by describing first Meehl's original hypothesis, and then our rationale for its reformulation. Evidence supporting the consideration of schizotaxia as a separate diagnostic category will then be reviewed in two ways: first, by considering its clinical features in the relatives of schizophrenic individuals, and second, by comparing features of schizotaxia with symptoms of SPD. We conclude by delineating recent steps taken to assess the validity of schizotaxia as a syndrome, and suggest directions for future research.

In 1962, Paul Meehl used the term *schizotaxia* to describe the genetic predisposition to schizophrenia *(9)*. Schizotaxic individuals, he surmised, would develop either schizotypy or schizophrenia, depending on environmental circumstances. In a reformulation of his theory, Meehl *(10)* conceded the possibility that some schizotaxic persons might not develop schizotypal personality, although he thought this outcome would require "a sufficiently well-managed prophylaxis" (p. 938). Subsequent data have shown that even without intervention many schizotaxic persons will become neither schizotypal nor schizophrenic.

Although, outside of Meehl's work, the term schizotaxia had not been widely used, several investigators began to document clinical or neurobiological defects among relatives of schizophrenic patients. For example, a program of research by Holzman's group found smooth pursuit eye movement dysfunction among schizophrenic patients and their relatives *(11–13)*. These researchers concluded that the pattern of dysfunction in patients and families was consistent with the presence of a genetically mediated latent trait, which could lead to schizophrenia in some relatives and smooth pursuit eye movement dysfunction in others *(14)*. Further early evidence for the existence of Meehl's schizotaxia came from the New York High-Risk (NYHRP) study, and showed attentional deviance among

the children of schizophrenic parents *(15,16)*. Likewise, the Jerusalem Infant Development Study (JIDS) began to document motor and sensorimotor abnormalities in high-risk infants *(17)*.

Likewise, much research since Meehl's original formulation suggests that schizotaxia may be a clinically consequential condition. Abnormalities in affect, cognition, and social functioning among the nonschizotypal and nonpsychotic relatives of schizophrenic patients show that schizotaxia is not merely a theoretical construct; it has psychiatric and neurobiological features that may justify further research about its nosologic validity.

Although our use of the term schizotaxia is consistent with Meehl's view of it as the underlying defect among people genetically predisposed to schizophrenia, we do not endorse other aspects of his theory unless expressly stated. For example, Meehl proposed a solely genetic etiology, whereas we consider the etiology of schizotaxia to stem from both genetic liability and environmental risk factors. Moreover, having written his theory prior to the availability of molecular genetic data, Meehl favored a single major gene theory of schizophrenia, which has since been falsified by genetic linkage studies. In addition, Meehl viewed schizotypy as the only clinical phenotype of schizotaxia. We suggest that, when not expressed as schizotypy (or schizophrenia), schizotaxia produces a stable syndrome of neuropsychological deficits and negative symptoms in many relatives of schizophrenic individuals.

There have already been comprehensive reviews of these schizotaxic features (*see*, e.g., ref. *18*). Our purpose here is not to reproduce that information but to highlight the clinical features of schizotaxia and to motivate researchers to develop diagnostic criteria and therapeutic approaches aimed at helping those with schizotaxia.

CHARACTERIZATION OF SCHIZOTAXIA

Typically, clinical descriptions of most psychiatric conditions are derived initially from reports of patients who present with a specified cluster of signs and symptoms. In contrast, clinical descriptions of schizotaxia originate from studies of people genetically predisposed to schizophrenia: the relatives of schizophrenic patients. Such studies infer a clinical or neurobiologic abnormality to be a potential feature of schizotaxia if it is present among these relatives and among schizophrenic patients. However, for schizotaxia to be established as a useful diagnostic category, it first requires the formulation of specific diagnostic criteria. Second, validation of the schizotaxia syndrome must be substantiated with converging evidence from multiple domains *(19)*. Moreover, the divergent validity of schizotaxia will need to be established. In this section, we begin by considering three areas of deficit (i.e., psychiatric symptoms, neuropsychological performance, and psychosocial functioning) that are observed consistently in relatives of schizophrenic patients, and that form the basis for working diagnostic criteria

for the syndrome of schizotaxia. We then address the most difficult differential diagnostic hurdle for schizotaxia: is it sufficiently different from schizotypal personality to warrant a separate category? Finally, we describe the initial steps that have been taken to validate schizotaxia as a syndrome, and some implications for future research.

Clinical Features of Schizotaxia

Psychiatric Signs and Symptoms

Family, adoption, and twin studies firmly support the idea that relatives of schizophrenic patients are at high risk for SPD (20–22). Several studies have attempted to determine which schizotypal symptoms are most common among the relatives of patients with schizophrenia. For example, Gunderson et al. (23) found that relatives of schizophrenic patients were at high risk for social isolation, interpersonal dysfunction, and impoverished affective experiences. In that study, mild psychotic-like symptoms such as recurrent illusions and magical thinking were more common in relatives who also were diagnosed with borderline personality disorder. Tsuang et al. (24) reported that negative symptoms (especially flat affect and avolition) were elevated significantly in the schizophrenia families, whereas positive symptoms were not. In the Roscommon family study, odd speech, social dysfunction, and negative symptoms strongly discriminated relatives of schizophrenic patients from controls. In contrast, positive symptoms, suspicious behavior, and avoidant symptoms were less discriminating (25).

Consistent with these studies, psychometric assessments of schizotypal symptoms among relatives of patients with schizophrenia find a predominance of negative rather than positive symptoms. For example, Grove et al. (26) showed that relatives of schizophrenic patients have greater deficits on the Physical Anhedonia Scale (which measures negative schizotypal features) than the Perceptual Aberration Scale (which measures positive schizotypal features). Despite the possibility that artifacts of self-report scales such as defensiveness might have led to these results, their consistency with direct-interview studies is compelling.

In summary, the literature to date provides firm support for the idea that nonpsychotic relatives of schizophrenic patients are at risk for schizotypal personality traits. The literature also shows that the relatives in schizophrenia families are more likely to express negative symptoms than positive symptoms, although, as the Roscommon study showed, positive schizotypal symptoms are also found among nonpsychotic relatives of schizophrenic patients.

Given that negative schizotypal symptoms are prominent among relatives of schizophrenic patients, we would expect these relatives to also show an excess of schizoid personality disorder. However, relevant data are mixed. In the Danish adoption study, the biological relatives of schizophrenic patients did not show an excess of schizoid personality (27). Similar results were reported in a family

study by Maier et al. *(28)* and a twin study by Torgersen et al. *(29)*. In contrast, two family studies found higher rates of schizoid personality among relatives of schizophrenic patients compared with parents of controls *(30,31)*. As there are no systematic differences between studies that do and do not find schizoid personality in schizophrenia families, further work is needed to clarify the nature of the negative symptoms of schizotaxia and to determine why these are expressed in negative schizotypal, but not schizoid traits.

NEUROPSYCHOLOGICAL PERFORMANCE

Several decades of research suggest that when the liability for schizophrenia does not lead to frank psychosis, it will nonetheless produce neurobiologic abnormalities and neuropsychological deficits *(32)*. Abnormalities found among relatives of schizophrenic patients include neurologic signs *(33)*, neuroimaging assessed brain abnormalities *(34)*, psychophysiological deficits *(35,36)*, and neuropsychological impairment *(37)*. Although each of these domains of research has provided valuable data about the neurobiologic features of schizotaxia, here we focus briefly on psychophysiological deficits and then concentrate on the neuropsychological findings because they describe deficits that have clinically meaningful implications for members of schizophrenia families.

Psychophysiological abnormalities observed in relatives of schizophrenic patients include difficulties in smooth pursuit eye tracking *(35,38)*, prepulse inhibition *(39)*, and suppression of auditory evoked potentials *(36,40)*. These deficits are similar to those observed in schizophrenic patients *(36,41–45)*. The likelihood of having such abnormalities increases with a greater degree of biological relatedness to a schizophrenic individual (e.g., ref. *45*) and worse performance in relatives is associated with worse performance of the schizophrenic proband *(46)*. Interestingly, these psychophysiological abnormalities are more prevalent in relatives who have schizophrenia spectrum personality symptoms (e.g., schizotypal personality) *(47–49)*.

Two research paradigms provide data about the neuropsychological features of schizotaxia: studies of children of schizophrenic patients and studies of adult relatives of schizophrenic patients. It is useful to distinguish studies of child and adult relatives because, unlike children, adults have lived through some, or all, of the risk period for schizophrenia. Thus, both types of relative groups will include some schizotaxic individuals but studies of children are more likely to include cases that eventually will become schizophrenic.

One neuropsychological function that differentiates child relatives is *motor ability*. Impaired motor ability presents in children as soft neurological signs such as disturbed gait, poor balance, incoordination, motor impersistence, and impaired mirror drawing *(50,51)*. Impaired motor ability in childhood has been shown to predict future schizophrenia-related psychopathology. For example, poor motor

coordination in elementary school, as evidenced by difficulties in athletics and craft-making, was shown to be a risk factor for later development of schizophrenia in Finnish schoolchildren *(52)*. These results are supported by recent findings from the NYHRP *(53)*. In contrast, motor functioning has been less consistently impaired among adult relatives of schizophrenic patients *(54–58)*.

Perceptual-motor speed tests assess the ability to perceive stimuli and react to them quickly in an appropriate manner. Among the children of schizophrenic patients, there is consistent evidence for deficits on such tests *(33,59)*. Similar results have also been found among adult relatives. For example, in studies from three different research groups, nonpsychotic relatives were significantly slower on the Trail Making test *(60–63)*. Similar findings were reported by others *(64,65)*.

Tests of *short-term memory* assess the ability to retain information in memory for a brief duration (e.g., recalling a phone number after finding it in the directory). In most *(66–68)* but not all *(69)* studies, children of schizophrenic patients showed poor short-term memory as measured by oral arithmetic scores (which require short-term memory to manipulate mathematical concepts). They are not impaired consistently when asked to recall a string of digits *(51,66,69,70)*, but do show deficits if distracted during digit recall *(70–73)*. Short-term digit recall has not been impaired in studies of adult relatives *(54,74)*, probably because of the lack of a distraction component in those studies.

Impaired *sustained attention* usually is measured with a continuous performance test (CPT), which presents a long series of stimuli and asks the subject to respond whenever a rare target stimulus appears. Cornblatt et al.'s *(75)* review of 40 studies using the CPT shows that sustained attention deficits are evident among both the adult and child relatives of schizophrenic patients.

There has been little neuropsychological evaluation of *verbal ability and language* among children of schizophrenic patients. However, in a recent study of early-onset schizophrenia (prior to age 12), premorbid impairments in speech and language were associated with measures of increased risk for schizophrenia (e.g., obstetrical complications and number of family members with schizophrenia-spectrum disorders) *(76)*. Most studies of adult relatives have not found differences in general verbal ability although there was some evidence for poorer vocabulary scores in one sample *(54)*. Notably, four studies found significant impairments in speed and ease of verbal production *(60–63,74)* and Cannon et al. *(55)* found deficits in language abilities.

Difficulties with language have also been documented in studies of *communication deviance*, which have found unclear, amorphous, disruptive, or fragmented communication among the parents of schizophrenic patients *(77–88)*. Moreover, Docherty et al. *(89)* showed that disordered communication, especially involving referential failures, is related to family history of psychosis and/or high schizotypy scores.

Given these communication problems, it is not surprising that adult relatives of schizophrenic patients also show signs of *thought disorder (77,78,90–98)*. Indeed, communication deviance and thought disorder usually are associated with one another *(79)*. The thought disorder observed among relatives is never as severe as that seen among schizophrenic patients, but it does share qualitatively similar characteristics such as looseness of associations, autistic logic, word-finding difficulties, perseveration, and conceptual disorganization.

Studies of children of schizophrenic patients have provided scant information about the *ability to learn and recall verbal material*. Adult relatives, however, have difficulties recalling the details of a short story *(54,55,74)* or using the semantic similarities of words to aid in their recall *(99)*. In contrast, deficits in simple *visual-spatial learning and memory* tasks are not usually found in schizotaxic adults *(54,55,59,100,101)*.

Executive functions are essential for planning, processing abstract concepts, and using retained information in other cognitive tasks. Children of schizophrenics do poorly on measures of concept formation *(102)*, but not on object-sorting tests that require them to abstract a rule from a series of stimulus presentations *(72)*. Adult relatives also do poorly on concept formation tests *(64,103)* and, although there is some contrary evidence *(61,62,64,74)*, most studies have found them to be impaired on sorting tests *(54,60,104,105)*. Consistent with these findings of executive dysfunction, adult relatives are impaired on tests of working memory that assess the ability to remember information over a short period of time so that it can be used in a subsequent task *(41,106)*.

Table 1 summarizes the neuropsychological studies of child and adult relatives. It renders a clear conclusion: in schizophrenia families, some relatives have neuropsychological deficits in multiple domains. The domains impaired in these relatives are consistent with the cognitive dysfunctions thought to be central to schizophrenic patients themselves. Also, these deficits are stable over a 4-year follow-up period *(106)*, and are more severe in persons with multiple first-degree schizophrenic relatives as compared to persons with only one affected relative *(107)*. Moreover, deficits in childhood (i.e., verbal memory, gross motor skills, and attention) predict schizophrenia-related psychosis in adulthood *(53)*. This evidence supports the idea that some relatives in schizophrenia families have a familially transmitted syndrome   schizotaxia, which manifests as abnormalities in neuropsychological performance.

PSYCHOSOCIAL FUNCTIONING

If schizotaxia is a clinically significant condition, it should be associated with disability at work, in school, or with interpersonal relationships. For adult relatives, one might infer such disability from their profile of neuropsychological impairments. For example, at work and in school impaired executive functions

Table 1
Neuropsychological Functions Impaired in Child and Adult Relatives

	Type of Relative	
Neuropsychological Domain	Children/Adolescents	Adults
Motor Ability	+	+/–
Perceptual-Motor Speed	+	+
Short-Term Memory	+/–	–
Sustained Attention	+	+
Verbal Ability and Language	?	+/–
Verbal Learning and Memory	?	+
Visual-Spatial Memory	?	+/–
Executive Functions	+	+/–

Note: +, Impaired; –, Not Impaired; +/–, Variable Results; ?, Not sufficiently studied.

From ref. 8. Clinical Implications and New Directions for Research. Schizophr Bull 27:1..18.

will jeopardize successful achievement, which requires planning and organizational skills and the ability to process abstract concepts. Moreover, impairments in vigilance will make it difficult for schizotaxic people to succeed in settings that require concentration over long periods of time. One might also infer interpersonal dysfunction from the subtle thought disorder and communication associated with schizotaxia.

Although these neuropsychological inferences are compelling, few studies of adult relatives have directly examined psychosocial functioning. One exception is the work of Toomey et al. *(108)*, which showed that compared with controls, adult relatives demonstrated deficits in perception on nonverbal social cues as assessed using the Profile of Nonverbal Sensitivity (PONS) test. Moreover, these deficits correlated significantly with slower reaction times on vigilance tasks *(108)*, supporting previous results linking social deficits with poor attention. We also know that schizotaxia leads to negative symptoms, which include indices of psychosocial failure such as impersistence at school or work, recreational interests and activities, sexual activity, and relationships with friends and peers.

In contrast to the dearth of psychosocial information about adult relatives, psychosocial dysfunction has been documented among the adolescent relatives and children of schizophrenic patients ("child relatives" for short). For example, data from JIDS demonstrated poor social adjustment in adolescents with a schizophrenic parent including immaturity, unpopularity with peers, and difficulty relating with peers (especially members of the opposite sex). Poor social adjustment was not related to concurrent onset of schizophrenia or other disorders *(109)*.

Notably, Asarnow's review *(110)* determined that all studies of adolescent relatives have found them to have significant social dysfunction.

Results from the NYHRP found child relatives to have poorer social functioning and more restricted interests than psychiatric or normal controls *(111)*. Social competence decreased between childhood and early adolescence, but remained stable from early to late adolescence *(5)*. In the Israeli high-risk study, Auerbach et al. *(112)* found boys of schizophrenic parents to be more withdrawn than boys of nonschizophrenic parents. The boys who developed schizophrenia-related disorders had been shy and withdrawn or aggressive and antisocial *(113)*. In the Danish high-risk study, child relatives were described by teachers as passive and socially isolated, and by mothers as both passive and aggressive. When compared with controls, teachers described child relatives as less socially competent and more aggressive; peers described them as more aggressive, withdrawn, and unlikable *(114)*.

Thus, like neuropsychological impairment, there is consistent evidence for psychosocial dysfunction among children at risk for schizophrenia. Moreover, studies of children link these two domains of dysfunction. For example, in Auerbach et al.'s *(112)* study, the socially withdrawn children also had motor abnormalities. Walker and Lewine *(4)* rated videotapes of children who subsequently became schizophrenic. These children had neuropsychological impairments (poor fine and gross motor coordination) and evidence of social dysfunction (poor eye contact, more negative affect and low social responsiveness). In the NYHRP, attentional problems in childhood predicted social dysfunction in adolescence and social isolation in adulthood *(115)*. Notably, an association between neuropsychological performance and functional impairment is also seen for schizophrenic patients *(116)*.

Because neuropsychological impairment is evident at an early age (e.g., ref. *117*) and typically emerges prior to social dysfunction *(115)*, it is intriguing to speculate about a causal link between these two features of schizotaxia. As suggested by Cornblatt and Keilp *(75)*, an early attentional deficit could impair the processing of interpersonal information and lead to failure in social interactions.

Cornblatt and Keilp's model predicts that interpersonal interactions will frequently fail, leading to increased stress and a repeated cycle of increased psychosocial difficulties and stress. We would extend this model to include other neuropsychological deficits as potential causes of psychosocial dysfunction. Future confirmation of these causal links would suggest that treatment of neuropsychological deficits might improve the psychosocial functioning of schizotaxic people.

Relationship of Schizotaxia to Schizotypal Personality Disorder

RATIONAL FOR DIFFERENTIATING SCHIZOTAXIA FROM SPD

In a reformulation of his theory, Meehl *(10)* conceded the possibility that some schizotaxic persons might not develop schizotypal personality, although

he thought this outcome would require "a sufficiently well-managed prophy-laxis" (p. 938). Subsequent data have shown that   even without intervention many schizotaxic persons will become neither schizotypal nor schizophrenic. Two lines of evidence support the differentiation of schizotaxia from SPD. First, the core features of schizotaxia (negative symptoms and neuropsychological impairments) occur in 20. 50% of such relatives *(54,118)* as compared with only about 10% of relatives who will become psychotic and less than 10% who will be diagnosed with SPD *(21,119)*. Thus, unlike schizotypal personality, schizotaxia appears to be common among relatives of schizophrenic patients. Since schizotypal personality should be evident by adulthood, finding that many schizotaxic adults are not schizotypal shows that the former condition does not always evolve into the latter.

A second line of support for separating schizotaxia from schizotypal personality is that the latter is a heterogeneous disorder. Four types of studies provide evidence in support of this assertion. First, factor analytic studies find evidence for two to four dimensions of schizotypal personality (e.g., refs. *120,121–125*). The three dimensions that have been identified most consistently include: a cognitive-perceptual factor, an introversion-anhedonia factor, and a disorganization-social impairment factor. Of those, the first two receive the strongest support: the cognitive-perceptual factor, which comprises symptoms similar to the "positive" symptoms of schizophrenia, and the introversion-anhedonia factor, which encompasses schizophrenia-like "negative" symptoms *(126)*.

Second, biological studies also find evidence for two types of schizotypal personality. An early review by Siever *(127)* concluded that a subgroup of schizotypal subjects exhibited biological abnormalities that were similar to those seen in schizophrenic patients. This subgroup manifested negative symptoms and neuropsychological impairment (two features of schizotaxia), but rarely exhibited positive symptoms. Moreover, Condray and Steinhauer *(64)* found impaired language comprehension among schizotypal subjects with a family history of schizophrenia, but not among those without such a history. In addition, Kendler et al. *(128)* showed that among schizotypal subjects, negative symptoms predicted attentional and eye-tracking dysfunction (ETD) (likely features of schizotaxia), but the positive syndrome did not. Results consistent with these were reported by Thaker et al. *(129)*, who assessed eye tracking among subjects with paranoid, schizoid, and schizotypal personality. Eye-tracking abnormalities were associated with these disorders, but only for those subjects with a family history of schizophrenia.

Third, the two methods used to study schizotypal personality provide further evidence of this heterogeneity. The "clinical method" identifies personality-disordered patients who seem to exhibit a mild form of schizophrenic symptomatology, and results in an emphasis on positive symptoms. The "family research

method" identifies relatives of patients with schizophrenia who exhibit subtle schizophrenia-like psychopathology, and results in an emphasis on negative symptoms (130). Although the people recruited by these two methods show some clinical similarities, several studies suggest that "clinical" and "familial" schizotypal personality may be different disorders (130). For instance, among subjects diagnosed with schizotypal personality, Torgersen (20) reported that the negative symptoms of social withdrawal and impairment were genetically related to schizophrenia whereas positive, psychotic-like symptoms were not. Thaker et al. (131) found clinical schizotypal subjects to show more evidence of magical ideation and perceptual ideation than familial schizotypal subjects. The two groups, however, did not differ in either physical or social anhedonia. Recent work supports these findings, suggesting that measures of positive schizotypy (e.g., Magical Ideation) are associated with family environmental factors, whereas negative schizotypy measures are influenced by genetic as well as family variables (132).

Fourth, family studies provide additional support for the idea that schizotypal personality is a heterogeneous disorder. For example, Thaker et al.'s review (133) shows that most studies of clinically derived, schizotypal probands did not find elevated rates of schizophrenia among their relatives. Subsequent reports also have supported that assertion (119). These findings suggest that many clinically ascertained schizotypal patients do not carry the genetic predisposition to schizophrenia; i.e., they do not have schizotaxia.

DEFINING THE COMORBIDITY OF SCHIZOTAXIA AND SPD

Figure 1 illustrates our conceptualization of the overlap of schizotaxia and schizotypal personality disorder. Schizotaxia (the left circle) and schizotypal personality (the right circle) are shown as conditions that sometimes co-occur. The area of overlap between the circles corresponds to people showing both schizotaxic and schizotypal symptoms. These individuals have been described as having "familial" or "negative" schizotypal personality in the research literature. The lack of complete overlap between the two circles illustrates the notion that schizotaxia is a broader construct than the subset of schizotypal persons who have predominantly negative symptoms. The portion of the schizotypal personality circle not overlapping with the schizotaxia circle contains those patients described as having "clinical" or "positive" schizotypal personality. Thus, although negative schizotypal personality does not account for all of the relatives with schizotaxic symptoms, it more closely echoes the concept of schizotaxia than does positive schizotypal personality.

Future research now has the task of continuing to parse the comorbidity between schizotypal personality and schizotaxia. Because comorbidity is a common feature of psychiatric illness, recognizing both conditions and their comorbidity might be a reasonable solution. In contrast, it may be preferable to sharpen diagnostic

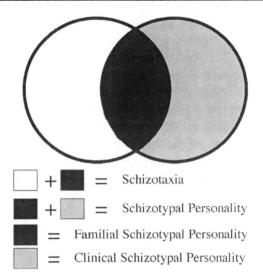

Fig. 1. Overlap between schizotaxia and schizotypal personality. Reproduced with permission from ref. *8.*

criteria with the goal of separating schizotaxia from schizotypal personality. This requires psychometric studies that would find diagnostic criterion sets that eliminate the extensive comorbidity between the two conditions.

If successful, such studies would designate schizotaxia as the syndrome of negative symptoms and neuropsychological dysfunction observed among relatives of schizophrenic patients (all of Fig. 1's schizotaxia circle) and SPD as the schizophrenia-like syndrome in which positive symptoms dominate the clinical picture (the portion of Fig. 1's schizotypal personality circle that does not overlap with the schizotaxia circle). Reformulating the diagnoses in this manner would increase the homogeneity of schizotypal personality and free researchers to define schizotaxia in a manner that might further validate it as a syndrome.

TOWARD DEFINING SCHIZOTAXIA AS A SYNDROME

As stated above, several steps must be taken for schizotaxia to become a useful diagnostic category. First, specific diagnostic criteria must be operationalized. Second, the validity of the schizotaxia syndrome must be assessed with converging evidence from multiple domains *(19).* Moreover, the divergent validity of schizotaxia will need to be substantiated to merit a separate category from other disorders (e.g., SPD).

Tsuang et al. *(134)* proposed preliminary research diagnostic criteria based on two of these core features: negative symptoms and neuropsychological deficits. These criteria included negative symptoms of moderate or greater severity as

assessed using the Scale for the Assessment of Negative Symptoms (SANS) *(135)*, and at least moderately impaired neuropsychological functioning in two of the three domains assessed: attention/working memory, long-term verbal declarative memory, and executive functioning. (*See* ref. *134* for complete criteria and details of specific tests.) It is worth noting that these criteria are preliminary, and we expect such criteria to evolve as future research continues to assess the concurrent and predictive validity of schizotaxia criterion sets.

Using these criteria, Stone et al. *(136)* took the first steps toward validating schizotaxia as a syndrome by comparing adult relatives who met criteria for schizotaxia with those who did not on independent measures of clinical function. These measures included the Social Adjustment Scale (SAS) *(137)*, the Quality of Life (QOL) Scale *(138)*, the Symptom Checklist-90. R (SCL-90. R) *(139)*, Chapman's Physical Anhedonia Scale (PAS) *(140)*, and the *DSM–IV* Global Assessment of Functioning Scale (GAF) *(141)*. Schizotaxic subjects demonstrated greater deficits on these measures of social and clinical functioning as compared with relatives who did not meet criteria. These differences were not attributable to age, gender, education, IQ, parental education, family genetic loading, or co-morbid psychiatric disorders.

Further support for the validity of schizotaxia comes from analyses of ratings of the schizotaxic and nonschizotaxic subjects using the Structured Interview for Schizotypy *(142)*. Based on evidence supporting the notion that schizotaxia is similar to negative schizotypy, Stone et al. (unpublished data) compared global ratings of negative symptoms (social isolation, introversion, and restricted emotion) with global ratings of positive symptoms (ideal of reference, magical thinking, illusions, and psychotic-like phenomena) for the schizotaxic and nonschizotaxic groups. The schizotaxic subjects demonstrated significantly higher ratings on two of the three negative symptoms. In contrast, there were no group differences on measures of positive symptoms.

These findings, in conjunction with the body of research reviewed above, further support the notion of schizotaxia as a meaningful clinical condition in the relatives of schizophrenic individuals and provide groundwork for validating schizotaxia as a syndrome. If the validity of schizotaxia is established, it will facilitate the diagnosis and treatment of people in schizophrenia families, broaden our understanding of the interrelationships between the various conditions in the schizophrenia spectrum, and lead to a greater understanding of the liability to schizophrenia.

CONCLUSIONS

To recap, schizotaxia is a subtle syndrome of brain dysfunction expressed, in part, as negative symptoms and neuropsychological deficits, but not as psychosis. This syndrome is qualitatively similar   yet less severe   than that observed

among schizophrenic patients. Our inquiry into schizotaxia yields clear conclusions from prior work and intriguing hypotheses for future study. Schizotaxia, we conclude, is not merely a theoretical construct describing the unknown neural substrate of schizophrenia. Four decades after Meehl first coined the term, an accumulation of research reveals schizotaxia to be a clinically consequential condition. Indeed, the negative symptoms, neuropsychological deficits, and psychosocial disabilities of the schizotaxic person constitute a chronic syndrome that may compromise quality of life and goal attainment.

Because some schizotaxic people meet criteria for SPD, one might argue for incorporating the former into the latter. But that would blur the meaning of schizotypal personality, which is already a heterogeneous diagnosis. Moreover, cleaving schizotypal personality into groups with and without a family history of schizophrenia creates subgroups that differ on etiological, neurobiologic, and clinical features.

Thus, we propose to join schizophrenia-related "negative" SPD with other cases of schizotaxia. This leaves future research the goal of refining diagnostic criteria to accent the distinction between schizotaxia and SPD. In particular, although negative symptoms and neuropsychological impairments appear to be hallmarks of schizotaxia, some positive symptoms such as mild thought disorder might also be considered as diagnostic criteria as well as neurologic signs, neuroimaging-assessed brain abnormalities, and psychophysiological deficits. The validity of proposed diagnostic criteria could be examined in family studies of schizophrenia, but family studies of schizotaxia would also be needed to fully clarify the familial relationship between the two conditions.

If future work refines definitions of schizotaxia and schizotypal personality, it will also need to clarify how these conditions are related to schizophrenia, which is itself clinically and genetically heterogeneous (143). Such work would need to consider alternative theoretical models. For example, there may be several dimensions of schizotaxia and schizotypal personality. Predisposing to each of these may be different sets of genes that, in combination, predispose to schizophrenia. It is also possible that the genes predisposing to schizotaxia and schizotypal personality may be related to different forms of schizophrenia. Moreover, it is not clear if schizotaxia is a discrete entity or a quantitative trait that varies in severity from subclinical to clinically meaningful manifestations. Addressing such issues could facilitate genetic studies, and might clarify the treatment implications of schizotaxia for people in schizophrenia families.

Our reformulation of schizotaxia has several clinical implications. In conducting family interventions for schizophrenia, knowledge of schizotaxic deficits should help clinicians refine their clinical approach to relatives of schizophrenic patients. Likewise, the psychotherapy of schizotaxia would benefit from the clinical insights of those who work with other neuropsychological disorders (144).

Finally, the idea of psychopharmacologic intervention in schizotaxic adults *(134)* and the implication of potential treatment of schizotaxic adolescents at risk for schizophrenia, is intriguing *(8)*.

Our conclusions are limited in several ways. Because there are no agreed upon diagnostic criteria for schizotaxia, studies that have examined this construct among relatives of schizophrenic patients have not used comparable samples. Many of these studies have examined putative indicators of schizotaxia in samples that include subjects with personality disorders. This obscures the relative contributions of schizotaxia and known clinical conditions to the expression of schizotaxic traits. Moreover, we have also drawn inferences from studies of schizotypal personality disorder, which as we have discussed in this chapter, is itself heterogeneous. Finally, we view our thoughts on the treatment of schizotaxia and the possibilities of preventing schizophrenia as clinical hypotheses rooted in a nascent scientific literature. They call for further studies of schizotaxia: to describe its genetic roots, to delineate its risk factors, to detail its pathophysiology, and to determine why its outcome is not solely schizophrenia.

ACKNOWLEDGMENTS

Preparation of this chapter was supported in part by the National Institute of Mental Health Grants 1 R01MH41874-01, 5 UO1MH46318, and 1 R37MH43518 to Dr. Ming T. Tsuang.

REFERENCES

1. Erlenmeyer-Kimling L. Neurobehavioral deficits in offspring of schizophrenic parents: liability indicators and predictors of illness. Am J Med Genet (Neuropsychiatric Genetics) 2000; 97:65..71.
2. Bogerts B. Recent advances in the neuropathology of schizophrenia. Schizophr Bull 1993; 19(2):431..445.
3. Shenton ME, Wible CG, McCarley RW. A review of magnetic resonance imaging studies of brain abnormalities in schizophrenia. In: Krishnan KRR, Doraiswamy PM, eds. Brain Imaging in Clinical Psychiatry. New York: Marcel Dekker, 1997.
4. Walker E, Lewine RJ. Prediction of adult-onset schizophrenia from childhood home movies of the parents. Am J Psychiatry 1990; 147(8):1052..1056.
5. Dworkin R, Lewis J, Cornblatt B, Erlenmeyer-Kimling L. Social competence deficits in adolescents at risk for schizophrenia. J Nerv Ment Dis1994; 182(2):103..108.
6. Weinberger DR. Neurodevelopmental perspectives on schizophrenia. In: Bloom FE, Kupfer DJ, eds. Psychopharmacology: the Fourth Generation of Progress. New York: Raven, 1995: 1171..1183.
7. Gottesman II. Schizophrenia Genesis: The Origin of Madness. New York: Freeman, 1991.
8. Faraone SV, Green AI, Seidman LJ, Tsuang MT. "Schizotaxia": clinical implications and new directions for research. Schizophr Bull 2001; 27:1..18.
9. Meehl PE. Schizotaxia, schizotypy, schizophrenia. Am Psychol 1962; 17:827..838.
10. Meehl PE. Schizotaxia revisited. Arch Gen Psychiatry 1989; 46:935..944.

11. Holzman PS, Proctor LR, Hughes DW. Eye-tracking patterns in schizophrenia. Science 1973; 181(95):179..181.

12. Holzman PS, Kringlen E, Levy DL, Proctor LR, Haberman SJ, Yasillo NJ. Abnormal-pursuit eye movements in schizophrenia. Evidence for a genetic indicator. Arch Gen Psychiatry 1977; 34(7):802..805.

13. Holzman P, Proctor L, Levy D, Yasillo N, Meltzer H, Hurt S. Eye tracking dysfunctions in schizophrenic patients and their relatives. Arch Gen Psychiatry 1974; 31:136..139.

14. Matthysse S, Holzman PS, Lange K. The genetic transmission of schizophrenia: application of Mendelian latent structure analysis to eye tracking dysfunctions in schizophrenia and affective disorder. J Psychiatr Res 1986; 20:57..76.

15. Erlenmeyer-Kimling L. A prospective study of children at risk for schizophrenia: methodological considerations and some preliminary findings. In: Wirt R, Winokur G, Ross M, eds. Life History Research in Psychopathology. Minneapolis: University of Minnesota Press, 1975: 22..46.

16. Rutschmann J, Cornblatt B, Erlenmeyer-Kimling L. Sustained attention in children at risk for schizophrenia. Report on a continuous performance test. Arch Gen Psychiatry 1977; 34(5): 571..575.

17. Marcus J, Auerbach J, Wilkinson L, Burack CM. Infants at risk for schizophrenia. The Jerusalem Infant Development Study. Arch Gen Psychiatry 1981; 38(6):703..713.

18. Moldin SO, Erlenmeyer-Kimling L. Measuring liability to schizophrenia: progress report 1994: editor's introduction. Schizophr Bull 1994; 20(1):25..30.

19. Robins E, Guze SB. Establishment of diagnostic validity in psychiatric illness: its application to schizophrenia. Am J Psychiatry 1970; 126:983..987.

20. Torgersen S. Relationship of schizotypal personality disorder to schizophrenia: genetics. Schizophr Bull 1985; 11:554..563.

21. Battaglia M, Torgersen S. Schizotypal disorder: at the crossroads of genetics and nosology. Acta Psychiatr Scand 1996; 94:303..310.

22. McGuffin P, Thapar A. The genetics of personality disorder. Br J Psychiatry 1992; 160: 12..23.

23. Gunderson JG, Siever LJ, Spaulding E. The search for a schizotype: crossing the border again. Arch Gen Psychiatry 1983; 40:15..22.

24. Tsuang MT, Gilbertson MW, Faraone SV. Genetic transmission of negative and positive symptoms in the biological relatives of schizophrenics. In: Marneros A, Tsuang MT, Andreasen N, eds. Positive vs. Negative Schizophrenia. New York: Springer-Verlag, 1991:265..291.

25. Kendler KS, McGuire M, Gruenberg AM, Walsh D. Schizotypal symptoms and signs in the Roscommon family study. Arch Gen Psychiatry 1995; 52:296..303.

26. Grove WM, Lebow BS, Clementz BA, Cerri A, Medus C, Iacono WG. Familial prevalence and coaggregation of schizotypy indicators: a multitrait family study. J Abnorm Psychol 1991; 100(2):115..121.

27. Kety SS, Wender PH, Jacobsen B, et al. Mental illness in the biological and adoptive relatives of schizophrenic adoptees. Replication of the Copenhagen study in the rest of Denmark. Arch Gen Psychiatry 1994; 51:442..455.

28. Maier W, Lichtermann D, Minges J, Heun R. Personality disorders among the relatives of schizophrenia patients. Schizophr Bull 1994; 20(3):481..493.

29. Torgersen S, Onstad S, Skre I, Edvardsen J, Kringlen E. "True" schizotypal personality disorder: a study of co-twins and relatives of schizophrenic probands. Am J Psychiatry 1993; 150(11):1661..1667.

30. Dorfman A, Shields G, DeLisi LE. *DSM-III-R* personality disorders in parents of schizophrenic patients. Am J Med Genet (Neuropsychiatric Genetics) 1993; 48(1):60..62.
31. Kendler KS, McGuire M, Gruenberg AM, O'Hare A, Spellman M, Walsh D. The Roscommon family study. III. Schizophrenia-related personality disorders in relatives. Arch Gen Psychiatry 1993; 50:781..788.
32. Seidman LJ. Clinical neuroscience and epidemiology in schizophrenia. Harv Rev Psychiatry 1997; 3:338..342.
33. Erlenmeyer-Kimling L, Cornblatt B, Friedman D, et al. Neurological, electrophysiological, and attentional deviations in children at risk for schizophrenia. In: Henn FA, Nasrallah HA, eds. Schizophrenia as a Brain Disease. New York: Oxford University Press, 1982:61..98.
34. Seidman LJ, Faraone SV, Goldstein JM, et al. Reduced subcortical brain volumes in nonpsychotic siblings of schizophrenic patients: a pilot MRI Study. Am J Med Genet (Neuropsychiatric Genetics) 1997; 74:507..514.
35. Levy DL, Holzman PS, Matthysse S, Mendell NR. Eye tracking and schizophrenia: a selective review. Schizophr Bull 1994; 20(1):47..62.
36. Friedman D, Squires-Wheeler E. Event-related potentials (ERPs) as indicators of risk for schizophrenia. Schizophr Bull 1994; 20(1):63..74.
37. Kremen WS, Seidman LJ, Pepple JR, Lyons MJ, Tsuang MT, Faraone SV. Neuropsychological risk indicators for schizophrenia: a review of family studies. Schizophr Bull 1994; 20: 103..119.
38. McDowell JE, Brenner CA, Myles-Worsley M, Coon H, Byerley W, Clementz BA. Ocular motor delayed-response task perfomance among patients with schizophrenia and their biological relatives. Psychophysiology 2001; 38(1):153..156.
39. Braff DL, Swerdlow NR, Geyer MA. Symptom correlates of prepulse inhibition deficits in male schizophrenic patients. Am J Psychiatry 1999; 156:596..602.
40. Adler LE, Olincy A, Waldo M, et al. Schizophrenia, sensory gating, and nicotinic receptors. Schizophr Bull 1998; 24:189..202.
41. Park S, Holzman PS, Goldman-Rakic PS. Spatial working memory deficits in the relatives of schizophrenic patients. Arch Gen Psychiatry 1995; 52:821..828.
42. Ross RG, Harris JG, Olincy A, Radant A, Adler LE, Freedman R. Familial transmission of two independent saccadic abnormalities in schizophrenia. Schizophr Res 1998; 30:59..70.
43. Ross RG, Olincy A, Harris JG, Radant A, Adler LE, Freedman R. Anticipatory saccades during smooth pursuit eye movements and familial transmission of schizophrenia. Biol Psychiatry 1998; 44:690..697.
44. Clementz BA, Geyer MA, Braff DL. Poor P50 suppression among schizophrenia patients and their first-degree biological relatives. Am J Psychiatry 1998; 155:1691..1694.
45. Waldo MC, Carey G, Myles-Worsley M, et al. Codistribution of a sensory gating deficit and schizophrenia in multi-affected families. Psychiatry Res 1991; 39:257..268.
46. Curtis CE, Calkins ME, Grove WM, Feil KJ, Iacono WG. Saccadic disinhibition in patients with acute and remitted schizophrenia and their first-degree biological relatives. Am J Psychiatry 2001; 158(1):100..106.
47. Thaker GK, Ross DE, Cassady SL, Adami HM, Medoff DR, Sherr J. Saccadic eye movement abnormalities in relatives of patients with schizophrenia. Schizophr Res 2000; 45(3):235..244.
48. Cadenhead KS, Swerdlow NR, Shafer KM, Diaz M, Braff DL. Modulation of the startle response and startle laterality in relatives of schizophrenic patients and in subjects with schizotypal personality disorder: evidence of inhibitory deficits. Am J Psychiatry 2000; 157(10): 1660..1668.

49. Cadenhead KS, Light GA, Geyer MA, Braff DL. Sensory gating deficits assessed by the P50 event-related potential in subjects with schizotypal personality disorder. Am J Psychiatry 2000; 157:55..59.

50. Asarnow JR, Goldstein MJ. Schizophrenia during adolescence and early adulthood: a developmental perspective on risk research. Clin Psychol Rev 1986; 6:211..235.

51. Lifshitz M, Kugelmass S, Karov M. Perceptual-motor and memory performance of high-risk children. Schizophr Bull 1985; 11:74..84.

52. Cannon M, Jones P, Huttunen MO, et al. School performance in Finnish children and later development of schizophrenia: a population-based longitudinal study. Arch Gen Psychiatry 1999; 56(5):457..463.

53. Erlenmeyer-Kimling L, Rock D, Roberts SA, et al. Attention, memory, and motor skills as childhood predictors of schizophrenia-related psychoses: the New York High-Risk Project. Am J Psychiatry 2000; 157(9):1416..1422.

54. Faraone SV, Seidman LJ, Kremen WS, Pepple JR, Lyons MJ, Tsuang MT. Neuropsychological functioning among the nonpsychotic relatives of schizophrenic patients: a diagnostic efficiency analysis. J Abnorm Psychol 1995; 104:286..304.

55. Cannon TD, Zorrilla LE, Shtasel D, et al. Neuropsychological functioning in siblings discordant for schizophrenia and healthy volunteers. Arch Gen Psychiatry 1994; 51(8):651..661.

56. Rosen AJ, Lockhart JJ, Gants ES, Westergaard CK. Maintenance of grip-induced muscle tension: a behavioral marker for schizophrenia. J Abnorm Psychol 1991; 100:583..593.

57. Kinney DK, Yurgelun-Todd DA, Woods BT. Hard neurologic signs and psychopathology in relatives of schizophrenic patients. Psychiatry Res 1991; 39:45..53.

58. Kinncy DK, Woods BT, Yurgelun-Todd DM. Neurological abnormalities in schizophrenic patients and their families: II. Neurologic and psychiatric findings in relatives. Arch Gen Psychiatry 1986; 43:665..668.

59. Neuchterlein KH, Dawson ME. Information processing and attentional functioning in the developmental course of schizoprenic disorders. Schizophr Bull 1984; 10:160..203.

60. Pogue-Geile MF, Garrett AH, Brunke JJ, Hall JK. Neuropsychological impairments are increased in siblings of schizophrenic patients. Schizophr Res 1991; 4:390.

61. Keefe RSE, Silverman JM, Amin F, et al. Frontal functioning and plasma HVA in the relatives of schizophrenic patients. Schizophr Res 1992; 6:158.

62. Keefe RSE, Silverman JM, Roitman SEL, et al. Performance of nonpsychotic relatives of schizophrenic patients on cognitive tests. Psychiatry Res 1994; 53:1..12.

63. Laurent A, Biloa-Tang M, Bougerol T, et al. Executive/ attentional performance and measures of schizotypy in patients with schizophrenia and in their nonpsychotic first-degree relatives. Schizophr Res 2000; 46(2..3):269..283.

64. Condray R, Steinhauer SR. Schizotypal personality disorder in individuals with and without schizophrenic relatives: similarities and contrasts in neurocognitive and clinical functioning. Schizophr Res 1992; 7:33..41.

65. Goldberg TE, Ragland D, Torrey EF, Gold JM, Bigelow LB, Weinberger DR. Neuropsychological assessment of monozygotic twins discordant for schizophrenia. Arch Gen Psychiatry 1990; 47:1066..1072.

66. Mednick SA, Schulsinger F. Some premorbid characteristics related to breakdown in children with schizophenic mothers. In: Rosenthal D, Kety SS, eds. The Transmission of Schizophrenia. Oxford, England: Pergamon, 1968:267..291.

67. Landau R, Harth P, Othnay N, Scharfhertz C. The influence of psychotic parents on their children's development. Am J Psychiatry 1989; 129:70..75.

68. Sohlberg SC. Personality and neuropsychological performance of high-risk children. Schizophr Bull 1985; 11:48..60.
69. Worland J, Hesselbrock V. The intelligence of children and their parents with schizophrenia and affective illness. J Child Psychol Psychiatry 1980; 21:191..201.
70. Cornblatt B, Erlenmeyer-Kimling L. Global attentional deviance as a marker of risk for schizophrenia: specificity and predictive validity. J Abnorm Psychol 1985; 94:470..486.
71. Harvey P, Winters K, Weintraub S, Neale JM. Distractibility in children vulnerable to psychopathology. J Abnorm Psychol 1981; 90:298..304.
72. Winters KC, Stone AA, Weintraub S, Neale JM. Cognitive and attentional deficits in children vulnerable to psychopathology. J Abnorm Child Psychol 1981; 9:435..453.
73. Spring B. Distractibility as a marker of vulnerability to schizophrenia. Psychopharmacol Bull 1985; 21:509..512.
74. Roxborough H, Muir WJ, Blackwood DHR, Walker MT, Blackburn IM. Neuropsychological and P300 abnormalities in schizophrenics and their relatives. Psychol Med 1993; 23: 305..314.
75. Cornblatt BA, Keilp JG. Impaired attention, genetics, and the pathophysiology of schizophrenia. Schizophr Bull 1994; 20:31..46.
76. Nicolson R, Lenane M, Singaracharlu S, et al. Premorbid speech and language impairments in childhood-onset schizophrenia: association with risk factors. Am J Psychiatry 2000; 157(5): 794..800.
77. Wynne L, Singer M. Thought disorder and family relations of schizophrenics: I. A research strategy. Arch Gen Psychiatry 1963; 9:191..198.
78. Singer MT, Wynne LC. Thought disorder and family relations of schizophrenics. III: Methodology using projective techniques. Arch Gen Psychiatry 1965; 12:187..212.
79. Docherty NM. Cognitive characteristics of the parents of schizophrenic patients. J Nerv Ment Dis 1994; 182(8):443..451.
80. Miklowitz DJ. Family risk indicators in schizophrenia. Schizophr Bull 1994; 20(1):137..150.
81. Docherty NM, Grosh ES, Wexler BE. Affective reactivity of cognitive functioning and family history in schizophrenia. Biol Psychiatry 1996; 39:59..64.
82. Rund BR. Communication deviance in parental schizophrenics. Fam Process 1986; 25: 133..147.
83. Rund BR. The relationship between psychosocial and cognitive functioning in schizophrenic patients and expressed emotion and communication deviance in their parents. Acta Psychiatr Scand 1994; 90:133..140.
84. Docherty N. Communication deviance, attention, and schizotypy in parents of schizophrenic patients. J Nerv Ment Dis 1993; 181:750..756.
85. Doane J, West K, Goldstein M, Rodnick E, Jones J. Parental communication deviance and affective style: predictors of subsequent schizophrenia-spectrum disorders in vulnerable adolescents. Arch Gen Psychiatry 1981; 38:679..685.
86. Velligan D, Goldstein M, Nuechterlein K, Miklowitz D, Ranlett G. Can communication deviance be measured in a family problem-solving interaction? Fam Process 1990; 29: 213..226.
87. Velligan D, Funderburg L, Giesecke S, Miller A. Longitudinal analysis of communication deviance in the families of schizophrenic patients. Psychiatry 1995; 58(February 1995):6..19.
88. Velligan D, Miller A, Eckert S, et al. The relationship between parental communication deviance and relapse in schizophrenic patients in the 1-year period after hospital discharge A pilot study. J Nerv Ment Dis 1996; 184(8):490..496.

89. Docherty NM, Rhinewine JP, Labhart RP, Gordinier SW. Communication disturbances and family psychiatric history in parents of schizophrenic patients. J Nerv Ment Dis 1998; 186(12): 761..768.
90. Shenton ME, Solovay MR, Holzman PS, Coleman M, Gale HJ. Thought disorder in the relatives of psychotic patients. Arch Gen Psychiatry 1989; 46:897..901.
91. Saccuzzo DP, Callahan LA, Madsen J. Thought disorder and associative cognitive dysfunction in the first-degree relatives of adult schizophrenics. A reply to Romney. J Nerv Ment Dis 1988; 176(6):368..371.
92. McConaghy N. Thought disorder or allusive thinking in the relatives of schizophrenics? A response to Callahan, Madsen, Saccuzzo, and Romney. J Nerv Ment Dis 1989; 177(12):729..734.
93. Romney DM. Thought disorder in the relatives of schizophrenics. A meta-analytic review of selected published studies. J Nerv Ment Dis 1990; 178(8):481..486.
94. Arboleda C, Holzman P. Thought disorder in children at risk for psychosis. Arch Gen Psychiatry 1985; 42:1004..1013.
95. Lidz T, Wild C, Schafer S, Rosman B, Fleck S. Thought disorders in the parents of schizophrenic patients: a study utilizing the Object Sorting Test. J Psychiatric Res 1962; 1:193..200.
96. Rosman B, Wild C, Ricci J, Fleck S, Lidz T. Thought disorders in the parents of schizophrenic patients: a further study using the object sorting test. J Psychiatric Res 1964; 2:211..221.
97. Schopler E, Loftin J. Thought disorders in parents of psychotic children. Arch Gen Psychiatry 1969; 20:174..181.
98. Wynne L, Singer M. Thought disorder and family relations of schizophrenics. II. A classification of forms of thinking. Arch Gen Psychiatry 1963; 9:191..206.
99. Lyons MJ, Toomey R, Seidman LJ, Kremen WS, Faraone SV, Tsuang MT. Verbal learning and memory in relatives of schizophrenics: preliminary findings. Biol Psychiatry 1995; 37: 750..753.
100. Driscoll RM. Intentional and incidental learning in children vulnerable to psychopathology. In: Watt NF, Anthony EJ, Wynne LC, Rolf JE, eds. Children at Risk for Schizophrenia: a Longitudinal Perspective. New York: Cambridge University Press, 1984:320..325.
101. Orvaschel H, Mednick S, Schulsinger F, Rock D. The children of psychiatrically disturbed parents: differences as a function of the sex of the sick parent. Arch Gen Psychiatry 1979; 36:691..695.
102. Asarnow JR, Steffy RA, Mac Crimmon DJ, Cleghorn JM. An attentional assessment of foster children at risk for schizophrenia. In: Wynne LC, Cromwell RL, Matthysse S, eds. The Nature of Schizophrenia: New Approaches to Research and Treatment. New York: Wiley, 1978:339..358.
103. Pogue-Geile MF, Watson JR, Steinhauer SR, Goldstein G. Neuropsychological impairments among siblings of schizophrenic probands. Schizophr Res 1989; 2(1,2):70.
104. Franke P, Maier W, Hain C, Klingler T. Wisconsin Card Sorting Test: an indicator of vulnerability to schizophrenia? Schizophr Res 1992; 6:243..249.
105. Mirsky AF, Lochhead SJ, Jones BP, Kugelmass S, Walsh D, Kendler KS. On familial factors in the attentional deficit in schizophrenia: a review and report of two new subject samples. J Psychiatric Res 1992; 26:383..403.
106. Faraone SV, Seidman LJ, Kremen WS, Toomey R, Pepple JR, Tsuang MT. Neuropsychological functioning among the nonpsychotic relatives of schizophrenic patients: a four-year follow-up study. J Abnorm Psychol 1999; 108:176..181.
107. Faraone SV, Seidman LJ, Kremen WS, Toomey R, Pepple JR, Tsuang MT. Neuropsychological functioning among the nonpsychotic relatives of schizophrenic patients: the effect of genetic loading. Biol Psychiatry 2000; 48:120..126.

108. Toomey R, Seidman LJ, Lyons MJ, Faraone SV, Tsuang MT. Poor perception of nonverbal social-emotional cues in relatives of schizophrenic patients. Schizophr Res 1999; 40:121..130.
109. Hans SL, Auerbach JG, Asarnow JR, Styr B, Marcus J. Social adjustment of adolescents at risk for schizophrenia: the Jerusalem Infant Development Study. J Am Acad Child Adolesc Psychiatry 2000; 39(11):1406..1414.
110. Asarnow J. Children at risk for schizophrenia: converging lines of evidence. Schizophr Bull 1988; 14(4):613..631.
111. Small NE. Positive and negative symptoms and children at-risk for schizophrenia. Dissertation Abstracts International 1990; 51(2-B):1005.
112. Auerbach J, Hans S, Marcus J. Neurobehavioral functioning and social behavior of children at risk for schizophrenia. Isr J Psychiatry Relat Sci 1993; 30(1):40..49.
113. Hans SL, Marcus J, Henson L, Auerbach JG, Mirsky AF. Interpersonal behavior of children at risk for schizophrenia. Psychiatry 1992; 55:314..335.
114. Ledingham J. Recent developments in high risk research. In: Lahey BB, Kazdin AE, eds. Advances in Clinical Child Psychology. New York: Plenum, 1990:91..137.
115. Dworkin RH, Cornblatt BA, Friedmann R, et al. Childhood precursors of affective vs. social deficits in adolescents at risk for schizophrenia. Schizophr Bull 1993; 19:563..577.
116. Green MF. What are the functional consequences of neurocognitive deficits in schizophrenia. Am J Psychiatry 1996; 153:321..330.
117. Fish B, Hagin R. Visual-motor disorders in infants at risk for schizophrenia. Arch Gen Psychiatry 1973; 28:900..904.
118. Faraone SV, Kremen WS, Lyons MJ, Pepple JR, Seidman LJ, Tsuang MT. Diagnostic accuracy and linkage analysis: how useful are schizophrenia spectrum phenotypes? Am J Psychiatry 1995; 152:1286..1290.
119. Battaglia M, Bernardeschi L, Franchini L, Bellodi L, Smeraldi E. A family study of schizotypal disorder. Schizophr Bull 1995; 21:33..45.
120. Muntaner C, Garcia-Sevilla L, Fernandez A, Torrubia R. Personality dimensions, schizotypal and borderline personality traits and psychosis proneness. Personality and Individual Differences 1988; 9:257..268.
121. Raine A, Allbutt J. Factors of schizoid personality. Br J Clin Psychol 1989; 28:31..40.
122. Bentall RP, Claridge GS, Slade PD. The multidimensional nature of schizotypal traits: a factor analytic study with normal subjects. Br J Clin Psychol 1989; 28:363..375.
123. Kendler KS, Hewitt J. The structure of self-report schizotypy in twins. J Personal Disord 1992; 6:1..17.
124. Kelley MP, Coursey RD. Lateral preference and neuropsychological correlates of schizotypy. Psychiatry Res 1992; 41:115..135.
125. Chen WJ, Hsiao CK, Lin CCH. Schizotypy in community samples: the three-factor structure and correlation with sustained attention. J Abnorm Psychol 1997; 106:649..654.
126. Venables PH. Schizotypal status as a developmental stage in studies of risk for schizophrenia. In: Raine A, Lencz T, Mednick SA, eds. Schizotypal Personality. Cambridge, England: Cambridge University Press, 1995:107..131.
127. Siever LJ. Biological markers in schizotypal personality disorder. Schizophr Bull 1985; 11(4):564..575.
128. Kendler KS, Ochs AL, Gorman AM, Hewitt JK, Ross DE, Mirsky AF. The structure of schizotypy: a pilot multitrait twin study. Psychiatry Res 1991; 36:19..36.
129. Thaker GK, Cassady S, Adami H, Moran M, Ross DE. Eye movements in spectrum personality disorders: comparison of community subjects and relatives of schizophrenic patients. Am J Psychiatry 1996; 153:362..368.

130. Kendler KS. Diagnostic approaches to schizotypal personality disorder: a historical perspective. Schizophr Bull 1985; 11(4):538..553.
131. Thaker G, Moran M, Adami H, Cassady S. Psychosis proneness scales in schizophrenia spectrum personality disorders: familial vs. nonfamilial samples. Psychiatry Res 1993; 46(1): 47..57.
132. MacDonald AWR, Pogue-Geile MF, Debski TT, Manuck S. Genetic and environmental influences on schizotypy: a community-based twin study. Schizophr Bull 2001; 27(1):47..58.
133. Thaker G, Adami H, Moran M, Lahti A, Cassady S. Psychiatric illnesses in families of subjects with schizophrenia-spectrum personality disorders: high morbidity risks for unspecified functional psychoses and schizophrenia. Am J Psychiatry 1993; 150(1):66..71.
134. Tsuang MT, Stone WS, Seidman LJ, et al. Treatment of nonpsychotic relatives of patients with schizophrenia: four case studies. Biol Psychiatry 1999; 41:1412..1418.
135. Andreasen NC. The Scale for the Assessment of Negative Symptoms (SANS). Iowa City: University of Iowa, 1983.
136. Stone WS, Faraone SV, Seidman LJ, Green AI, Wojcik J, Tsuang MT. Concurrent validation of schizotaxia: a pilot study. Biol Psychiatry 2001; 50:434..440.
137. Weissman MM, Bothwell S. Assessment of social adjustment by patient self-report. Arch Gen Psychiatry 1976; 33:1111..1115.
138. Heinrichs DW, Hanlon ET, Carpenter WT. The quality of life scale: an instrument for rating the schizophrenic deficit syndrome. Schizophr Bull 1984; 10:388..398.
139. Derogatis LR. Symptom Checklist-90-R (SCL-90-R). Minneapolis, MN: Computer Systems, 1993.
140. Chapman LJ, Chapman JP, Miller EN. Reliabilities and intercorrelations of eight measures of proneness to psychosis. J Consult Clin Psychol 1982; 50(2):187..195.
141. American Psychiatric Association. Diagnostic and Statistical Manual of Mental Disorders, 4th ed. Washington, DC: American Psychiatric Association, 1994.
142. Kendler KS, Lieberman JA, Walsh D. The structured interview for schizotypy (SIS): a preliminary report. Schizophr Bull 1989; 15(4):559..571.
143. Tsuang MT, Faraone SV. The case for heterogeneity in the etiology of schizophrenia. Schizophr Res 1995; 17:161..175.
144. Seidman LJ. Listening, meaning, and empathy in neuropsychological disorders: case examples of assessment and treatment. In: Ellison JM, Weinstein CS, Hodel-Malinofsky T, eds. The Psychotherapist's Guide to Neuropsychiatry. Washington, DC: American Psychiatric Press, 1994.

6

A Neuropsychological Perspective on Vulnerability to Schizophrenia

Lessons From High-Risk Studies

Allan F. Mirsky, PhD
and Connie C. Duncan, PhD

INTRODUCTION

Dateline, Washington, DC: February 2, 2053. The Secretary of Health and Human Services has announced that scientists have positively identified all of the genes (26 in number) that confer vulnerability to schizophrenia.

March 25, 2053. The Associated Press quotes a report in *Nature Genetics* that five individuals have been genotyped who possess every one of the 26 schizophrenogenic alleles, but are not suffering from any major mental disorder, as defined by the *DSM–X*. The report goes on to state that all of these individuals were raised in suburban middle-class homes, received excellent medical care during their lives (including during their mothers' pregnancy), have had relatively stress-free lives, and have loving and supportive families.

These fictitious accounts of future research on the etiology of schizophrenia are meant to draw attention to the issues of risk and vulnerability in the disorder. Fifty years from now, we will likely not understand fully the nature of the risk in high-risk populations, nor the factors that account for the variability of outcomes in vulnerable persons. At present, we know that the risk of developing schizophrenia if one has a parent with the disorder is approx 10% and that the chances are roughly 50% if one's identical twin has the disorder *(1)*. Which variables account for the bad luck of certain vulnerable individuals? In this chapter, we review several factors in the etiology of schizophrenia, as illuminated in high-risk research. These factors include pernicious environmental influences and stressful

From: *Early Clinical Intervention and Prevention in Schizophrenia*
Edited by: W. S. Stone, S. V. Faraone, and M. T. Tsuang © Humana Press Inc., Totowa, NJ

115

familial and social factors. We then propose a modification of the diathesis. stress model in the development of schizophrenia that implicates brainstem function.

The central thesis of our model is that a major component of the schizophrenic diathesis is an abnormality in brainstem function, stemming from genetic and/or perinatal alterations in brainstem neuronal tissue. As the brainstem is a fundamental component of the brain's attention system, we maintain that the most salient manifestation of the schizophrenic diathesis is impaired attention. This impairment of attention may be exacerbated by exposure to neurodevelopmental and psychosocial stressors, which further compromise brainstem function. The attentional dysfunction is in itself a source of stress in that it distorts and degrades the quality of social interactions of the vulnerable individual. Compromised brainstem function is thus posited as underlying the impairment in sustained attention, a key component in the pathogenesis of schizophrenia-spectrum disorder.

We begin with a brief review of two of the earlier, single-factor theories of the development of schizophrenia, bad parenting and bad genes. Although simplistic, they helped to illuminate factors that contribute to the complex vulnerability of persons to schizophrenia-spectrum disorders.

EARLY VIEWS ON THE ROLE OF PARENTING IN THE DEVELOPMENT OF SCHIZOPHRENIA

Between 1940 and 1970, theories about the etiology of schizophrenia tended to focus on poor, inadequate, or harsh parenting as a causal factor. The concepts of the "schizophrenogenic life experience" and, especially, the "schizophrenogenic mother," were proposed initially by Fromm-Reichmann (2). This was later elaborated into the concept of the "schizophrenogenic family" (3,4). The concept of the schizophrenogenic family implicated confusing communication patterns and contradictory messages ("double bind"), leading to impaired ego development, disturbed social interactions, thought disorder, and, ultimately, to the development of schizophrenia.

EVIDENCE FOR A GENETIC DIATHESIS IN SCHIZOPHRENIA

Overlapping the era of "blame the parents" was the era, beginning in the mid-1960s, of "blame the genes." That is, convincing data supporting a genetic diathesis in schizophrenia were beginning to emerge. Earlier investigations had reported that the likelihood of a schizophrenic parent having a child with schizophrenia was far higher than what would be expected in the general population (5). In fact, Kraepelin had noted as early as 1907 in his textbook of psychiatry that "defective heredity is a very prominent factor (in dementia praecox)... in about

70% of the cases" (as cited in DeLisi, ref. 6). In his review of the epidemiology of schizophrenia, Jablensky *(7)* cited an earlier case-control study by Koller in 1895 of the aggregation of psychiatric disorders in a large number of probands and healthy controls. According to Jablensky, Koller concluded that the psychoses have a strong genetic loading.

Despite these early findings, many clinicians still believed that the disorder was passed from generation to generation by bad parenting. Needed were data from studies in which the parenting variable was separated, to the greatest extent possible, from the genetic variable. Information that would partially resolve this dilemma was provided by Heston *(8)*, who studied offspring of individuals with schizophrenia who were being raised, not by their biological parents, but in foster homes. At about the same time, Rosenthal and his coworkers used data provided by adoption registers in Denmark to conduct follow-up studies of adopted-away offspring of schizophrenic patients *(9)*. In both studies, the incidence of schizophrenia or schizophrenia-like disorders ("schizophrenia-spectrum disorders") was significantly higher in the offspring of patients with schizophrenia than in those of healthy parents. These data, as well as other analyses from Rosenthal's group, led to the current view that there is a substantial genetic component in the transmission of schizophrenia from generation to generation.

THE DIATHESIS STRESS MODEL

Genetic data have continued to accumulate: For example, a significantly greater incidence of schizophrenia was observed among the relatives of the Danish adoptees studied initially by Rosenthal than among the relatives of matched healthy controls *(10)*. In addition, a number of candidate schizophrenogenic genes have been identified (*see* Chapter 1, this volume). Nevertheless, the genetic hypothesis does not account for all of the data. Current information on the etiology of schizophrenia supports a diathesis. stress model. That is, the behavioral expression of the biological vulnerability for schizophrenia is influenced by exposure to stress. Figure 1 illustrates the diathesis. stress hypothesis that we proposed in 1986 *(11)*.

The schematic diagram summarizes our hypothesis that there is an interaction between "schizophrenogenic brain abnormalities" (including genetic loading as well as prenatal and perinatal biological insults) and psychosocial stressors. According to our model, the development of a schizophrenic disorder depends on the level of each of these factors. The phenotypic expression of schizophrenia must include schizophrenogenic brain abnormalities as a key element. However, the level of psychosocial stress affects the expression of the disorder. Thus, at high levels of stress, lower levels of schizophrenogenic brain abnormalities may be

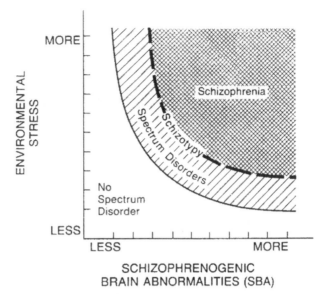

Fig. 1. Relation between schizophrenogenic brain abnormalities (SBAs) and environmental stress in the development of schizophrenic disorders. The model proposes that there is no phenotypic expression of schizophrenia that does not include SBA as a key element. At high levels of SBA, less environmental stress is needed to produce a schizophrenic disorder. Low levels of SBA or stress result in less severe outcomes. Adapted from ref. *11*.

sufficient to produce a disorder. In contrast, at low levels of psychosocial stress, a person with a low biological endowment for schizophrenia might show no disorder or a milder form of the disorder. We believe, as well, that schizophrenogenic brain abnormalities may intensify responsivity to stressors. Next, we consider sources of psychosocial and environmental stress in the etiology of schizophrenia.

SOURCES OF STRESS
IN THE DIATHESIS STRESS MODEL

Stressful Familial Influences

Although the concept of the schizophrenogenic mother is now largely rejected, research has shown that a chronically stressful rearing environment may interact with the effects of a schizophrenic diathesis to produce disorder, to enhance its severity, and/or to increase the risk of relapse. The findings supporting this view stem from four groups of studies that have implicated related psychosocial variables in the etiology of schizophrenic disorder.

COMMUNICATION DEVIANCE

"Communication deviance" refers to a form of communication in which the family group cannot maintain a clear focus of attention and meaning. This form of communication, observed in some families in which there is a proband with schizophrenia, was first described by Singer and Wynne *(12,13)*. They suggested that these deviant patterns of communication could influence the cognitive development of the offspring and lead to thought disorder in high-risk individuals.

We speculated previously on the possible schizophrenogenic effect of the interaction between impaired attention in individuals with, or at risk for, schizophrenia, and the communication deviance observed in families of patients with schizophrenia *(11)*. It seems reasonable to suggest that such pernicious familial experiences could have profound and persistent effects on the capacity for interpersonal communication, both inside and outside the family, thereby leading to feelings of alienation and social isolation.

EXPRESSED EMOTION AND AFFECTIVE STYLE

These two closely related characteristics of verbal behavior, observed in a group of families with a child referred for treatment, have been implicated in a series of investigations *(14)*. "Expressed emotion" involves critical, hostile comments and/or intense, emotion-laden statements directed to a specific person in the family *(15–19)*. "Affective style" comprises verbal behavior that is critical, guilt inducing, or intrusive *(20)*.

In a longitudinal study of children referred to an outpatient mental health clinic, it was observed that psychiatric outcome was significantly related to communication deviance, expressed emotion, and affective style *(14)*. In general, the more pathological the parental rating on these measures, the higher the likelihood of a schizophrenia-spectrum disorder in the offspring at age 30. This outcome was amplified considerably if there was a family history of psychiatric disorder. A similar result was reported in a follow-up study of adopted-away children of mothers with schizophrenia *(21,22)*. Adoptive families rated as "healthy" had a 7% rate of adopted children with a psychiatric disorder. In contrast, in adoptive families rated as "disturbed," 52% of the adopted, high-risk children had a disorder.

HARSH AND PUNITIVE TREATMENT

There is evidence for the role of harsh and punitive parental treatment in the exacerbation of the effects of a schizophrenic diathesis. The Genain quadruplets (Nora, Iris, Myra, and Hester) are a group of genetically identical women, all of whom developed schizophrenia by their mid-20s *(23,24)*. Despite their genetic identity, they developed schizophrenia to varying degrees of severity. Myra and Nora spent less time in mental hospitals than Iris and Hester, and were generally

adjudged to be healthier than their sisters. Myra married, had two sons, and worked for many years as a secretary. Nora worked for a time as a secretary, ran the household where three of the sisters lived, and managed most of their affairs. In contrast, Iris worked only briefly, and was institutionalized for many years with a dementing illness. Hester developed schizophrenia before any of her sisters and was never able to achieve an existence outside the family home.

In trying to account for the better life course of Myra and Nora, in comparison to their genetically identical siblings, one factor stands out, namely, the effects of the preferential treatment by their parents. In many of the accounts of their early life, carefully documented by Rosenthal (25), the impression is conveyed that their parents treated the quadruplets as two sets of twins, the "good twins" (Myra and Nora) and the "bad twins" (Iris and Hester). "From the beginning, it was clearly not possible to handle the four at once.... [the group of four was divided into] two sets of twins, Nora. Myra and Iris. Hester.... In this dichotomy, the Nora... Myra pair occupied the favored position. They were thought of as bigger, smarter, stronger, taller, more friendly, and more attractive than Iris and Hester" (26). Myra and Nora thus received higher expectations and more positive attention than Iris and Hester. Moreover, Hester, who developed the disorder earliest, and had probably the most severe form, was considered by both parents to be mentally retarded. The IQs reported by Bayley (27) indicate, however, that Hester's intelligence was in the normal range until age 14, when her IQ score dropped precipitously. This was about the time that she began to develop prodromal symptoms of schizophrenia. Rosenthal's (25) account of the quadruplets thus suggests a major contribution of parental mistreatment to the severity of schizophrenic disorder.

Another example of the noxious effects of parental behavior on a genetically vulnerable child is provided by a study by Lowing et al. (28), who reanalyzed the interview data obtained from Rosenthal's original Danish adoptees. The outcome data led to conclusions concerning the heritability of schizophrenia (9). Lowing et al. contrasted the incidence of reported stressors in individuals who developed "hard-spectrum" disorders (schizophrenia, schizotypal personality) with those of individuals who developed "soft-spectrum" disorders (schizoid personality, borderline personality, mixed-spectrum disorders). The number of stressors reported by the hard-spectrum group was significantly higher than that reported by the soft-spectrum group. Moreover, a particular set of stressors seemed to account for this difference: intrusive parents who denied the child decision-making power, coupled with alienation from the parent of the same sex, and generally harsh treatment by the parents.

Rosenfarb et al. (29) recently provided data of another negative effect on patients with schizophrenia following critical comments by family members   an

increase in "unusual" thoughts. They reported a significant positive correlation between the occurrence of critical remarks and evidence of odd thinking in a subgroup of patients who performed poorly on a memory-load version of the continuous performance test (CPT), a sensitive measure of sustained attention (e.g., Rosvold et al., ref. *30*). They interpreted this result as evidence of the interaction of neurocognitive vulnerability and psychosocial stressors.

These studies provide examples of the powerful interaction between stressful familial influences and a schizophrenic diathesis in the etiology of the disorder.

Stressful Community Influences

COMMUNITY REJECTION/DISAPPROVAL

This factor should probably be considered as a subset of harsh and punitive treatment observed under special circumstances. The identification of this stressor stems from a long-term follow-up study of a group of Israeli children with one schizophrenic parent (the National Institute of Mental Health [NIMH]-Israeli High-Risk Study) *(31)*. Half of the high-risk children were raised in kibbutzim throughout Israel; the other half were raised by their own parents in the nuclear family setting. There were matched healthy controls for both of the high-risk groups.

In the early, utopian days of the kibbutz movement in Israel, children were raised in groups, in relative isolation from their parents. Part of the motivation for this was to free the mother from child-care activities, so that she could participate more fully in the life of the kibbutz. Children were raised by a "metapelet," or professional child-care worker, and were visited by their parents for only a brief period during the day.

The goal of this investigation was to determine whether being raised on a kibbutz, with reduced exposure to a parent with schizophrenia, would yield better outcomes than being raised by one's own parents in a nuclear family *(32)*. The results indicated that, contrary to expectation, high-risk children on the kibbutzim were more than twice as likely as their nuclear-family-raised peers to develop psychiatric disorders by age 25. A total of 70% of the kibbutz-raised vs 30% of the parent-raised offspring had *DSM–III* diagnoses *(31)*.

The possibility of these results had been anticipated by Nagler *(32)*: he considered that there could be a pernicious effect of a kibbutz upbringing related to the level of scrutiny on the kibbutz. As a small, closed community (with residents numbering in the hundreds, at most), there are few secrets and even fewer opportunities for privacy. Psychopathology in one's parents is known by all; and expectations, stereotypes, and prejudices about the behavior of the parent could be readily transferred to the offspring. Nagler *(32)* noted that the chief support

provided by most kibbutzim to members is fiscal and not emotional, and that the kibbutz would not provide the ideal setting for a vulnerable child:

> In such a small closely-knit community it might be more difficult than in a city or town to keep knowledge of mental illness in the family [a secret]; parents' bizarre behavior in public might induce feelings of embarrassment and shame in children. Group life itself from earliest childhood on, with its clash of interests and friction, might be an unbearable burden to the kibbutz child. Unlike the child in town, the kibbutz child has to stay with his classmates day and night without any possibility of escape. (p. 25)

A later evaluation of the Israeli cohort, when the participants were on the average in their early 30s, found that the high-risk kibbutz group still had a significantly higher incidence of Axis I disorders than the other groups. Whereas 44% of the kibbutz-raised high-risk group had such a disorder, only 16% of the parent-raised high-risk group had an Axis I disorder. A combined total of 8% of the two groups of control children were diagnosed with an Axis I disorder *(33)*.

It should be noted that in the NIMH-Israeli High-Risk Study, the parents with a diagnosis of schizophrenia had all married, had children, and were part of an intact household. This suggests that they may have had a milder and/or later-onset form of the disorder.

It may appear that there is a contradiction between the results of the NIMH-Israeli High-Risk Study and the results cited in the immediately preceding sections on communication deviance, expressed emotion and affective style, and harsh and punitive treatment. In contrast to the "unbearable burden" presumably carried by the kibbutz-raised high-risk children, the parent-raised high-risk children may have had a relatively benign and protected family environment, provided by caring, albeit disordered, parents. This contrasts with the deleterious effects of high levels of family tension described earlier. In the studies of familial stressors, the parents had not been diagnosed as having a schizophrenic disorder; rather, the emphasis was on the harsh and punitive intrafamilial interactions and the effects on offspring.

There may not, therefore, be a contradiction. The actual contrast in these two bodies of research may be between the effects on a high-risk child of parents who are critical and hostile and those who are not. Genetics aside, whether or not the parent has a schizophrenic disorder appears to be less important than parental behavior in its effects on exacerbating the development of schizophrenia in a vulnerable child.

URBAN POVERTY

Urban. rural differences in the prevalence of schizophrenia were described first by Faris and Dunham in a landmark book published more than 60 years ago

Table 1
Deleterious Environmental
Effects Associated With Poverty

Environmental effect	Representative references
Fetal alcohol syndrome/effect	Streissguth et al. *(36)*
	Connor et al. *(37)*
Pregnancy/birth complications	Chamberlain et al. *(38,39)*
Malnutrition	Levav et al. *(40,41)*
Lead intoxication	Needleman et al. *(42)*
	Mirsky et al. *(43)*
Parasitic infections	Levav et al. *(44)*
	Cruz et al. *(45)*
	Marmor et al. *(46)*
Lack of intellectual stimulation	Bahrudin and Luster *(47)*
	Mirsky et al. *(48)*
	Mirsky *(49)*

Adapted from ref. *50.*

(34). These authors described the higher rate of schizophrenia among city dwellers than among persons living in rural areas. Researchers in other countries have reported similar findings. For example, Eaton et al. *(35)* reported recently that the risk of hospitalization for schizophrenia for individuals residing in the city of Copenhagen is 4.20 times higher than for those in rural areas of Denmark.

In view of these findings, we propose that there are factors associated with urban life, namely poverty, that may act as biopsychosocial stressors. There is evidence supporting the view that certain conditions of poverty, interacting with a schizophrenic diathesis, may facilitate the development of a schizophrenia-spectrum disorder in vulnerable persons.

Some of the deleterious factors associated with poverty are summarized in Table 1. It has been argued that a number of conditions associated with poverty (e.g., maternal drinking, pregnancy and birth complications, malnutrition, toxic substances in the environment, infections, reduced intellectual stimulation) have profoundly adverse effects on attentional capacities *(49)*. The research studies evaluating these environmental effects are also listed in Table 1. It is unclear why urban, as opposed to rural poverty, is more likely to be associated with a higher incidence of schizophrenia. This is possibly related, in part, to conditions of crowding in cities   which foster the spread of infection   and to poorer nutrition and greater concentrations of toxic substances, such as lead, in urban environments.

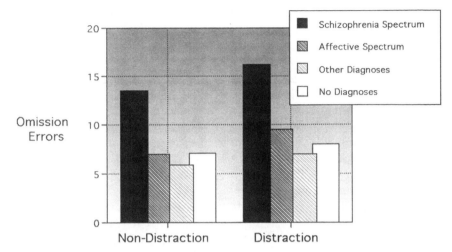

Fig. 2. The relationship between scores on a digit cancellation task at age 11 and *DSM–III* diagnoses at age 26. Scores on the left were obtained under nondistraction conditions (*p* < .04); those on the right, under auditory distraction (*p* < .03). The sample sizes for the respective groups at age 26 were as follows: schizophrenia spectrum = 9; affective spectrum = 11; other diagnoses = 7; no diagnosis = 63. Adapted from ref. *33*.

COMPONENTS OF DIATHESIS IN THE DIATHESIS STRESS MODEL

Identifying Characteristics of High-Risk Children

In addition to the issue of what we have referred to as *Community Rejection/ Disapproval*, there were a number of other lessons to be learned from the NIMH-Israeli High-Risk Study. There was a set of characteristics that differentiated the high-risk subjects from the controls in evaluations conducted at ages 11 and 17. Consistent with the findings of previous research (*see* reviews by Mirsky et al., refs. *33,51*), high-risk children were impaired in a variety of skills that could be subsumed under the heading of attention (e.g., arithmetic proficiency, arithmetic achievement, concentration, perceptual and especially visuomotor functioning).

An example of impaired attention in a subgroup of the high-risk children is illustrated in Fig. 2. Shown is performance at age 11 on a cancellation test under two conditions, nondistraction and distraction. The error rates of those children who would be diagnosed 15 years later with a schizophrenia-spectrum disorder were significantly elevated, and this difference was greater in the distraction condition.

The issue of distraction and its effect on performance in this group of vulnerable children deserves further comment. We know that in adults with schizophre-

nia, there is reduced capacity to overcome the effects of distraction in the performance of a sustained attention task *(52)*. This effect was also seen in patients whose symptoms were in remission *(53)*. That is, when required to perform the CPT in the presence of intermittent intrusive visual or auditory stimuli, patients with schizophrenia either active or in remission are more affected by the distraction than are comparison groups of healthy persons. Moreover, the effects of the distractor stimuli in the patients carry over into subsequent nondistraction portions of the task *(52)*. Related studies have shown that patients with schizophrenia are more impaired than healthy participants on attention tasks in which the stimulus quality is degraded, thereby making the task more demanding *(48, 54)*. This effect was also seen in first-degree relatives of patients *(48,54)*.

These data indicate that the attentional performance of patients with schizophrenia is more susceptible to the effects of distraction and task demands than is that of healthy persons. If distraction and increased task demands are viewed as forms of stress, these findings lend some support to the proposition that vulnerable children may be more affected by stressful events than healthy children.

In addition to impaired attention, the Israeli high-risk children also had inadequate psychosocial and interpersonal relations, a variety of "soft" neurological signs, and poor communication skills *(51)*. There were thus three major identifying characteristics of the high-risk children: (1) impaired attention/concentration; (2) poor motor function and/or perceptual-motor integration; and (3) deficits in social adaptation and low self-esteem. With respect to the latter, Mirsky et al. *(51)* summarized the social adaptation and self-esteem profile of the high-risk child who later developed a schizophrenia-spectrum disorder:

> He or she was an antisocial person; did not get along well with parents, teachers, or peers; was rated low in social desirability by peers; had a poor opinion of himself or herself; was suspicious and withdrawn; and had poor communication skills. In addition, the child was hypochondriacal, accident prone, and a daydreamer... the affective cases... in contrast, were seen as friendly, bright, engaging, eager to please both teachers and examiners, and in some ways more appealing and engaging than the children who developed no disorder. The future affective disorder cases in fact had the highest IQ scores of any of the groups... *higher IQ scores (may) serve to some extent as a protective factor in the development of an affective rather than a schizophrenia spectrum disorder.* (italics added; pp. 234.235)

Cognitive strengths may indeed provide protection against the depredations of schizophrenic thought processes. We propose that the reverse may be true, as well; namely, environmental conditions that damage the brain and thereby impair cognitive skills may lower the resistance of vulnerable persons to the development of a schizophrenia spectrum disorder.

Impairment of Attention Exacerbates the Risk for Schizophrenia

A number of environmental risk factors for developing schizophrenia have been proposed. Among these factors are pregnancy and birth complications (*see* Chapter 2, this volume), winter or spring births *(55)*, viral infections *(56)*, urban residence *(34)*, and stressful psychosocial factors, including harsh and punitive parenting *(20)*. However, the evidence suggests that a high level of family tension plays a role in the development of schizophrenia largely, if not exclusively, in children who are vulnerable by virtue of their genetic endowment *(1)*.

DIATHESIS STRESS REVISITED: THE VULNERABLE-BRAINSTEM HYPOTHESIS

We propose that many of the conditions associated with increased vulnerability to a schizophrenia-spectrum disorder share common neurodevelopmental effects. Specifically, they may all serve to compromise brainstem systems that support sustained attention *(57–60)*.

Myers' studies of experimental asphyxia in monkeys have established that acute total asphyxia and prolonged partial asphyxia (corresponding to two types of difficult labor and delivery in humans) are accompanied by damage to brainstem structures *(61–63)*. The structures include the inferior colliculus, the superior olivary complex, and other regions of the mesencephalon. Myers' work presents a model for perinatal brain damage. In a vulnerable individual, such damage could foster the development of a schizophrenic disorder by compromising the integrity of the brainstem. The crucial role of the brainstem in supporting activation or sustained attention is explicated by many theorists, including Mesulam *(64)*, Posner and Petersen *(65)*, and Mirsky et al. *(57)*.

The British studies of perinatal mortality (cited in Table 1) provide convincing evidence that early damage to the brain is more prevalent in the offspring of women living in impoverished circumstances, presumably due to inadequate prenatal care and obstetrical services *(38,39)*. The question arises as to whether other factors associated with poverty, such as malnutrition, lead intoxication, maternal drinking during pregnancy, and parasitic infections of the brain, may also contribute to reduced attentional capacity via damage to the brainstem system supporting attention.

Aston-Jones *(59)* and Usher et al. *(60)* have emphasized the role of brainstem noradrenergic locus coeruleus neurons in attention. Their findings highlight the role of the neurotransmitter systems that underlie the relay of impulses from brainstem to thalamus and cortex. The interplay among transmitter systems is complex, involving interactions among levels of noradrenaline, dopamine, and stress hormones. The increased stress occasioned by an unremittingly harsh and punitive familial environment and/or repeated interpersonal failures may lead to sustained

increases in cortisol and catecholamine (including noradrenaline) secretion. These altered titers may upset the balance of neurotransmitters and lead, in a vulnerable person, to permanent changes in brainstem-related systems necessary for the maintenance of normal attention.

INTERVENTIONS

The vulnerable-brainstem hypothesis proposed here is admittedly speculative. Nevertheless, it has implications for prevention, in that alleviating the stressors that have been identified should reduce the likelihood of developing disorder. Among the stressors that could be targeted for intervention are aberrant intrauterine development, birth trauma, malnutrition, environmental toxins, and aversive family interactions. Thus, for example, the delivery of prenatal and obstetrical care to low-income women at risk for schizophrenia could lessen a source of neurodevelopmental stress   perinatal brain insult. Similarly, education programs targeted at improving patterns of interaction in families of vulnerable children could reduce a potent psychosocial stressor.

The vulnerable-brainstem hypothesis proposed here suggests another avenue of intervention, namely treating the attentional dysfunction exhibited by high-risk children. That is, pharmacologic and/or behavioral treatment of impaired attention could be administered to high-risk children. The issues of prevention and early intervention are discussed at length in a subsequent section of this volume. In terms of our model, enhancing attentional capacity would break the cycle of poor attention and disturbed social interactions posited as major risk factors in the development of schizophrenia-spectrum disorders.

SUMMARY

We have reviewed information on vulnerability to schizophrenia based on studies of individuals at genetic risk for the disorder. We believe that the data provide support for the view that schizophrenia is best understood as the product of an interaction between a neurobiological predisposition, or diathesis, and chronically stressful life events. This interaction is illuminated by the study of high-risk populations.

We have emphasized the role of impaired attention, which is not only an indicator of vulnerability to schizophrenia, but also plays a key role in the pathogenic process. We have highlighted the critical role of brainstem function and related neurochemical systems that support attention as factors in the development of schizophrenia. Our model is summarized in Fig. 3, which depicts in schematic form the interplay among genetic, neurodevelopmental, psychosocial, and attentional variables in the development of schizophrenia-spectrum disorders.

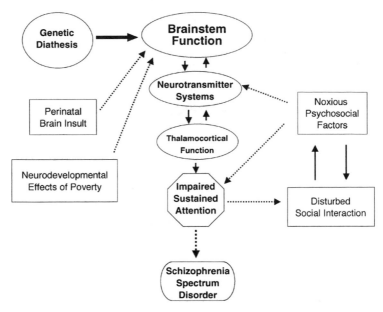

Fig. 3. The vulnerable brainstem hypothesis of the diathesis. stress model of schizophrenia. The diagram displays the influence of perinatal brain insult and neurodevelopmental effects of poverty on the brain-stem of an individual with a genetic diathesis for schizophrenia. Noxious psychosocial factors act on brainstem function via stress-related neurotransmitter systems. Compromised brain-stem function is posited as underlying an impairment in sustained attention, a key component in the development of schizophrenia-spectrum disorders. Dashed lines indicate influences that may be moderated by interventions, including delivery of prenatal and obstetrical care, reducing environmental hazards associated with poverty, and improving psychosocial milieu. Direct treatment of impaired attention may also reduce the risk of developing a schizophrenia-spectrum disorder.

According to our model, the impaired attention system associated with a schizophrenic diathesis may be exacerbated by pernicious neurodevelopmental and/or psychosocial factors. Factors often associated with impoverished living conditions act, via direct effects on brainstem function, to compromise attention. The impairment of attention in turn has a deleterious effect on the vulnerable individual's social transactions, and is itself a source of stress. Chronic stress caused by repeated interpersonal failures and/or a harsh and punitive family environment are thought to alter brainstem function via effects on neurotransmitter systems. The development of disorder, or the severity of its symptomatology, may reflect the presence and/or the magnitude of these stressors. The model also suggests the possibility of specific interventions that could reduce the likelihood of developing a schizophrenia-spectrum disorder. A diathesis. stress model under-

scores the importance for future research on schizophrenia and related spectrum disorders of focusing on the nature of stressful life experiences, and their effects on vulnerable persons, as well as on genetic and neurobiological factors.

REFERENCES

1. Gottesman II, Shields J. Schizophrenia, the Epigenetic Puzzle. Cambridge, England: Cambridge University Press, 1982.
2. Fromm-Reichmann F. Notes on the development of treatment of schizophrenics by psychoanalytic psychotherapy. Psychiatry 1948; 11:263..273.
3. Bateson GA, Jackson DD, Haley J, Weakland J. Toward a theory of schizophrenia. Behav Sci 1956; 1:251..264.
4. Bateson GA, ed. Perceval's Narrative: A Patient's Account of His Own Psychosis, 1830... 1832. Stanford, CA: Stanford University Press, 1961.
5. Kallman FJ, Rypins S. The Genetics of Schizophrenia: A Study of Heredity and Reproduction in the Families of 1,087 Schizophrenics. New York: Augustin, 1938.
6. DeLisi LE. The genetics of schizophrenia: past, present, and future concepts. Schizophr Res 1997; 28:163..175.
7. Jablensky A. The 100-year epidemiology of schizophrenia. Schizophr Res 1997; 28:111..125.
8. Heston LL. Psychiatric disorders in foster home reared children of schizophrenic mothers. Br J Psychiatry 1966; 112:819..825.
9. Rosenthal D, Wender PH, Kety SS, Welner J, Schulsinger F. The adopted-away offspring of schizophrenics. Am J Psychiatry 1971; 128:307..311.
10. Kety SS, Wender PH, Jacobsen B, et al. Mental illness in the biological and adoptive relatives of schizophrenic adoptees: replication of the Copenhagen study in the rest of Denmark. Arch Gen Psychiatry 1994; 51:442..455.
11. Mirsky AF, Duncan CC. Etiology and expression of schizophrenia: neurobiological and psychosocial factors. Annu Rev Psychol 1986; 37:291..319.
12. Singer MT, Wynne LC. Principles for scoring communication defects and deviances in parents of schizophrenics: Rorschach and TAT scoring manuals. Psychiatry 1966; 29:260..288.
13. Wynne LC, Singer M, Bartko J, Toohey M. Schizophrenics and their families: recent research on parental communication. In: Tanner JM, ed. Psychiatric Research: The Widening Perspective. New York: International Universities, 1976:254..286.
14. Goldstein MJ. The UCLA high-risk project. Schizophr Bull 1987; 13:505..514.
15. Brown GW, Monck EM, Carstairs GM, Wing JK. The influence of family life on the course of schizophrenic disorders. Br J Prev Soc Med 1962; 16:55..68.
16. Brown GW, Birely JL, Wing JK. Influence of family life on the course of schizophrenic disorders: a replication. Br J Psychiatry 1972; 121:241..258.
17. Barrelet L, Ferrero F, Szigethy L, Giddey C, Pellizzer G. Expressed emotion and first-admission schizophrenia: nine-month follow-up in a French cultural environment. Br J Psychiatry 1990; 156:357..362.
18. Nuechterlein KH, Snyder KS, Mintz J. Paths to relapse: possible transactional processes connecting patient illness onset, expressed emotion, and psychotic relapse. Br J Psychiatry 1992; 161(Suppl 18):88..96.
19. Vaughn CE, Snyder KS, Jones S, Freeman WB, Falloon IR. Family factors in schizophrenic relapse: replication in California of British research on expressed emotion. Arch Gen Psychiatry 1984; 41:1169..1177.

20. Doane JA, West KL, Goldstein MJ, Rodnick EH, Jones JE. Parental communication deviance and affective style: predictors of subsequent schizophrenia spectrum disorders in vulnerable adolescents. Arch Gen Psychiatry 1981; 38:679..685.
21. Tienari P, Sorri A, Lahti I, et al. Interaction of genetic and psychosocial factors in schizophrenia. Acta Psychiatr Scand Suppl 1985; 319:19..30.
22. Tienari P. Interaction between genetic vulnerability and family environment: the Finnish adoptive family study of schizophrenia. Acta Psychiatr Scand 1991; 5:460..465.
23. DeLisi LE, Mirsky AF, Buchsbaum MS, et al. The Genain quadruplets 25 years later: a diagnostic and biochemical followup. Psychiatry Res 1984; 13:59..76.
24. Mirsky AF, Bieliauskas LA, French LM, van Kammen DP, Jönsson E, Sedvall G. A 39-year followup of the Genain quadruplets. Schizophr Bull 2000; 26:699..708.
25. Rosenthal D, ed. The Genain Quadruplets. A Case Study and Theoretical Analysis of Heredity and Environment in Schizophrenia. New York: Basic Books, 1963.
26. Quinn O.W. The public image of the family. In: Rosenthal D, ed. The Genain Quadruplets. A Case Study and Theoretical Analysis of Heredity and Environment in Schizophrenia. New York: Basic Books, 1963:355..372.
27. Bayley N. Intellectual and physical development. In: Rosenthal D, ed. The Genain quadruplets. A Case Study and Theoretical Analysis of Heredity and Environment in Schizophrenia. New York: Basic Books, 1963:193..201.
28. Lowing PA, Mirsky AF, Pereira R. The inheritance of schizophrenia spectrum disorders: a reanalysis of the Danish adoptee study data. Am J Psychiatry 1983; 140:1167..1171.
29. Rosenfarb IS, Nuechterlein KH, Goldstein MJ, Subotnik KL. Neurocognitive vulnerability, interpersonal criticism, and the emergence of unusual thinking by schizophrenic patients during family transactions. Arch Gen Psychiatry 2000; 57:1174..1179.
30. Rosvold HE, Mirsky AF, Sarason I, Bransome ED, Beck LH. A continuous performance test of brain damage. J Consult Psychol 1956; 20:343..350.
31. Mirsky AF, Silberman EK, Latz A, Nagler S. Adult outcomes of high-risk children: differential effects of town and kibbutz rearing. Schizophr Bull 1985; 11:150..154.
32. Nagler S, Mirsky AF. Introduction: the Israeli high-risk study. Schizophr Bull 1985; 11:19..29.
33. Mirsky AF, Ingraham LJ, Kugelmass S. Neuropsychological assessment of attention and its pathology in the Israeli cohort. Schizophr Bull 1995; 21:193..204.
34. Faris REL, Dunham HW. Mental Disorders in Urban Areas: An Ecological Study of Schizophrenia and Other Psychoses. Chicago: Chicago University Press, 1939.
35. Eaton WW, Mortensen PB, Frydenberg, M. Obstetric factors, urbanization and psychosis. Schizophr Res 2000; 43:117..123.
36. Streissguth AP, Sampson PD, Olson HC, et al. Maternal drinking during pregnancy: attention and short-term memory in 14-year-old offspring   a longitudinal prospective study. Alcohol Clin Exp Res 1994; 18:202..218.
37. Connor PD, Streissguth AP, Sampson PD, Bookstein FL, Barr HM. Individual differences in auditory and visual attention among fetal alcohol-affected adults. Alcohol Clin Exp Res 1999; 23:1395..1402.
38. Chamberlin R, Chamberlin G, Howlett B, Claireaux A. British Births 1970: The First Weeks of Life. Vol 1. London: Heineman Medical Books, 1975.
39. Chamberlin R, Chamberlin G, Howlett B, Claireaux A. British Births 1970: obstetrical care. Vol. 2. London: Heineman Medical, 1978.
40. Levav M, Cruz ME, Mirsky AF. EEG abnormalities, malnutrition, parasitism and goitre: a study of schoolchildren in Ecuador. Acta Paediatr 1995; 84:197..202.

41. Levav M, Mirsky AF, Cruz ME, Cruz I. Neurocysticercosis and performance on neuropsychologic tests: a family study in Ecuador. Am J Trop Med Hyg 1995; 53:552..557.
42. Needleman HL, Reiss JA, Tobin MJ, Biesecker GE, Greenhouse JB. Bone lead levels and delinquent behavior. JAMA 1996; 275:363..369.
43. Mirsky AF, Kellam SG, Pascualvaca D, Petras H, Todd AC. Bone lead level and sustained attention   a longitudinal study. Poster presented at the annual meeting of the American Psychological Association; San Francisco, CA, August 2001.
44. Levav M, Mirsky AF, Schantz PM, Castro S, Cruz ME. Parasitic infection in malnourished school children: effects on behavior and EEG. Parasitology 1995; 110:103..111.
45. Cruz ME, Levav M, Ramirez I, et al. Niveles de nutricion y rendimiento en pruebas neuropsicologicas en niños escolares de una comunidad rural andina. Parasitos Cerebral e Intestinal Problemas de Salud Publica. Academia Ecuatoriana de Neurociencias. Ecuador: Quito, 1993.
46. Marmor M, Glickman L, Shofer F, et al. Toxocara canis infection of children: epidemiologic and neuropsychologic findings. Am J Public Health 1987; 77:554..559.
47. Baharudin R, Luster T. Factors related to the quality of the home environment and children's achievement. J Fam Issues 1998; 19:375..403.
48. Mirsky AF, Yardley SJ, Jones BP, Walsh D, Kendler, KS. Analysis of the attention deficit in schizophrenia: a study of patients and their relatives in Ireland. J Psychiatric Res 1995; 29: 23..42.
49. Mirsky AF. Perils and pitfalls on the path to normal potential: the role of impaired attention. Homage to Herbert G. Birch. J Clin Exp Neuropsychol 1995; 17:481..498.
50. Mirsky AF, Duncan CC. A nosology of disorders of attention. In: Wasserstein J, Wolf LE, Lefever FF, eds. Adult Attention Deficit Disorder: Brain Mechanisms and Life Outcomes, Ann NY Acad Sci 2001; 931:17..32.
51. Mirsky AF, Kugelmass S, Ingraham LJ, Frenkel E, Nathan M. Overview and summary: twenty-five year followup of high-risk children. Schizophr Bull 1995; 21:227..239.
52. Stammeyer EC. The effects of distraction on performance in schizophrenic, psychoneurotic, and normal individuals [dissertation]. Washington, DC: Catholic University, 1961.
53. Wohlberg GW, Kornetsky C. Sustained attention in remitted schizophrenics. Arch Gen Psychiatry 1973; 28:533..537.
54. Mirsky AF, Lochhead SJ, Jones BP, Kugelmass S, Walsh D, Kendler KS. On familial factors in the attentional deficit in schizophrenia: a review and report of two new subject samples. J Psychiatric Res 1992; 26:383..403.
55. Torrey EF, Miller J, Rawlings R, Yolken RH. Seasonality of births in schizophrenia and bipolar disorder: a review of the literature. Schizophr Res 1997; 28:1..38.
56. Karlsson H, Bachmann S, Schroder J, McArthur J, Torrey EF, Yolken RH. Retroviral RNA identified in the cerebrospinal fluids and brains of individuals with schizophrenia. Proc Natl Acad Sci USA 2001; 98:4634..4639.
57. Mirsky AF, Anthony BJ, Duncan CC, Ahearn MB, Kellam SG. Analysis of the elements of attention: a neuropsychological approach. Neuropsychol Rev 1991; 2:109..145.
58. Pragay EB, Mirsky AF, Ray CL, Turner DF, Mirsky CV. Neuronal activity in the brain stem reticular formation during performance of a "go-no go" visual attention task in the monkey. Exp Neurol 1978; 60:83..95.
59. Aston-Jones G, Rajkowski J, Kubiak P, Alexinsky T. Locus coeruleus neurons in monkey are selectively activated by attended cues in a vigilance task. J Neurosci 1994; 14:4467..4480.
60. Usher M, Cohen JD, Servan-Schreiber D, Rajkowski J, Aston-Jones G. The role of locus coeruleus in the regulation of cognitive performance. Science 1999; 283:549..554.

61. Myers RE. Models of asphyxia brain damage in the newborn monkey. Paper presented at meeting of Pan American Congress of Neurology; San Juan, Puerto Rico, 1967.

62. Myers RE. The clinical and pathological effects of asphyxiation in the fetal rhesus monkey. In: Adamsons K, ed. Diagnosis and Treatment of Fetal Disorders. New York: Springer-Verlag, 1969:226.249.

63. Myers RE. Brain damage induced by umbilical cord suppression at different gestational ages in monkeys. In Goldsmith EI, Moor-Jankowski J, eds. Second Conference on Experimental Medicine and Surgery in Primates. New York: Karger, 1971:394.425.

64. Mesulam MM. Principles of Behavioral Neurology. Philadelphia: Davis, 1987.

65. Posner MI, Petersen SE. The attention system of the human brain. Annu Rev Neurosci 1990; 13:25.42.

7

Neurocognitive Deficits in the Biological Relatives of Individuals With Schizophrenia

William S. Kremen, PhD
and Anne L. Hoff, PhD

In the 1970s and early 1980s, there was considerable skepticism about whether cognitive, neuropsychological function could be validly measured in schizophrenia because an intuitive or commonsense view led to the conclusion that cognitive deficits were most likely secondary to poor cooperation and motivation, preoccupation with delusions and hallucinations, institutionalization, or side effects of antipsychotic medication. Indeed, it was not uncommon for clinicians to think that patients with schizophrenia did not have any significant cognitive or neuropsychological impairment. Since that time, there has been an explosion of cognitive and neuropsychological research on schizophrenia, and the study of cognitive dysfunction is now solidly mainstream.

Actually, early schizophrenologists such as Kraepelin and Bleuler directly or indirectly expressed the idea that cognitive dysfunction was a fundamental problem underlying behavior abnormalities in schizophrenia. Kraepelin theorized that sustained or directed attention was deficient in schizophrenia, and that this deficiency resulted in insufficient control over the continuity of thinking and behavior *(1)*. Bleuler reasoned that much of the symptomatology of schizophrenia was attributable to a disconnecting of associative links between ideas *(2)*. Since the mid-1980s, the predominant position has swung back firmly toward the view that cognitive deficits are core features of schizophrenic illness. Studies of biological relatives of individuals with schizophrenia have been a key part of that shift.

The term "core features" is used here to indicate dysfunctional features that reflect underlying processes of the illness, as opposed to consequences of symptoms or treatment. Such features would thus be primary dysfunctions that should

From: *Early Clinical Intervention and Prevention in Schizophrenia*
Edited by: W. S. Stone, S. V. Faraone, and M. T. Tsuang © Humana Press Inc., Totowa, NJ

be present in anyone with the disorder. Evidence from several areas of research supports the notion that cognitive dysfunction is a core feature of schizophrenia. First, cognitive and neuropsychological abnormalities exist prior to and at the onset of illness *(3–6)*. Second, even in individuals with schizophrenia who are classified as neuropsychologically normal, there is evidence that their performance still reflects compromised function relative to their premorbid level of ability *(7)*. Third, individuals with schizophrenia manifest neuropsychological impairment even when compared to normal controls who are individually matched with them on IQ *(8)*. Fourth, these neuropsychological deficits are unlikely to be a result of medication effects or impaired motivation because they are present even in people with schizophrenia who are able to achieve above-average IQ scores *(8)*. Fifth, it is reasonable to postulate that a core dysfunctional feature would tend to be more treatment resistant than would other illness characteristics. Although neurocognitive performance may fluctuate with changes in clinical state, impairment still usually persists even when symptoms are relatively remitted *(9)*. Sixth, as shown in this chapter, compromised neurocognitive function similar to deficits found in patients (although milder) is found in nonpsychotic biological relatives of individuals with schizophrenia.

When testing individuals with schizophrenia, one can never be entirely certain about the extent to which at least some aspects of impaired neurocognitive performance may be caused by poor motivation, institutionalization, medication side effects, or neurotoxic effects of psychosis. This dilemma is a major reason why biological relatives provide a valuable complement to the study of individuals with schizophrenia. These relatives share genes with a person with schizophrenia, but they do not have the illness themselves. Given this strategy, it is important that these relatives do not have psychotic symptoms; otherwise some of the same factors noted for those with schizophrenia could confound neurocognitive performance in the relatives. If they are nonpsychotic and not receiving antipsychotic medication, compromised neurocognitive function in family members cannot, by definition, reflect the effects of illness or treatment. Taken together, this evidence is consistent with the notion that neurocognitive performance reflects a core dysfunctional feature of schizophrenia. That being the case, it is important to bear in mind that although some neuropsychological deficit is likely to be present, a unique set of pathonogmonic deficits that is the same in all cases has not been identified.

To qualify as a risk indicator, an abnormality should be (a) present and relatively stable in persons with the disorder, (b) present in individuals at risk for the disorder, and (c) less common or less severe in persons with other psychiatric conditions *(10–13)*. Cognitive risk indicators may, in turn, be referred to as endophenotypes because they have a plausible biological and genetic relationship to schizophrenia and they presumably represent phenomena that are intermediate between genes

and overt symptom expression *(14,15)*. Given the overwhelming evidence for a significant genetic component in schizophrenia, we infer that cognitive deficits in biological relatives of individuals with schizophrenia are likely to reflect genetically mediated risk indicators for the illness. In support of this inference, Faraone et al. showed that relatives from multiplex families displayed greater neurocognitive impairment than did relatives from simplex families *(16)*. This pattern is consistent with the idea that the severity of deficits in relatives varies as a function of their degree of genetic liability to schizophrenia. There is also strong evidence for brain abnormalities in schizophrenia. Cognitive function reflects brain function, thus making it a logical phenomenon to consider as a potential risk indicator for schizophrenia.

This chapter does not cover the entire literature on neurocognitive function in relatives of individuals with schizophrenia, and it is, therefore, important to acknowledge some of its omissions. We focus primarily (although not exclusively) on adult relatives. Fortunately, the types of neurocognitive abnormalities observed in children at risk (including those who develop schizophrenia-spectrum disorders) and adult relatives are very similar *(11)*. Thus, it appears that abnormalities in adult relatives are quite likely to have implications for both early intervention and prevention. If similar abnormalities are found in adult relatives, most of whom are through the peak risk period for developing schizophrenia, then these putative endophenotypes are probably vulnerability indicators. However, they are clearly not sufficient to cause schizophrenia by themselves. Rather, genes that are associated with particular neurocognitive deficits are each likely to account for a small proportion of variance in the factors that ultimately combine to result in schizophrenia.

We also focus primarily on measures that have been utilized within the neuropsychological paradigm. Thus, for example, two information-processing measures that are putative risk indicators for schizophrenia (backward masking and span of apprehension) are not covered. Because we are interested in potential risk indicators, we also focus on nonpsychotic relatives. Indeed, all references to relatives in this chapter refer to those without psychotic symptoms. Finally, although we do occasionally refer to unpublished data, we have, for the most part, restricted our tallies of results to those of published studies.

GENERAL INTELLECTUAL FUNCTION

Studies of children of parents with schizophrenia and prospective general-population studies suggest that low IQ is a risk factor for the development of schizophrenia or nonaffective psychotic symptoms *(4–6,17–20)*. In a prospective study of a National Collaborative Perinatal Project (NCPP) cohort, Kremen et al. found that low IQ at age 7, and particularly, a large IQ decline from age 4 to age 7 were

associated with a nearly sevenfold increase in the risk of psychotic, but not manic or depressive symptoms at age 23 *(4)*. In another NCPP cohort, Cannon et al. showed that developing schizophrenia and being a sibling of someone who developed schizophrenia were both significantly associated with low IQs at age 4 and at age 7 *(20)*. Low IQ is certainly not specific to schizophrenia, but it would appear that low IQ in children who are genetically at risk for schizophrenia constitutes a cognitive risk indicator. On the other hand, studies of adult relatives of individuals with schizophrenia generally exclude individuals with low IQ because the focus is usually on identifying deficits in particular cognitive domains. There may be disagreement as to whether IQ should be equated in these cognitive studies of relatives vs controls (i.e., the kinds of studies referred to in this chapter), but it is our view that adjusting for IQ in such cases may result in "overcontrolling" because lowered IQ may reflect the effects of genes that predispose for schizophrenia. In individuals with schizophrenia, this idea has been supported by the fact that whereas IQs are lower in those with schizophrenia than in controls, there is often no difference in oral reading recognition scores   the latter being a measure that appears relatively resistant to cognitive decline in schizophrenia *(21,22)*. A similar pattern was found in relatives of individuals with schizophrenia in that relatives had greater reading. IQ discrepancy scores than did controls *(23)*. Perhaps more important, results of the studies discussed below did not change substantially after controlling for IQ.

NEUROCOGNITIVE FUNCTIONS

Extensive reviews of cognitive function in children and adult relatives of individuals with schizophrenia have been conducted previously *(11,13,24,25)*. Much of the earlier work focused on the information-processing paradigm, but since the 1990s there has been an increase in neuropsychological studies   particularly in adult relatives. Neuropsychological assessment has the advantage of covering a more extensive range of cognitive functions, but its disadvantage may be that it generally does so with broader brush strokes. There is also a critical need for parsing cognition in order to discern the component processes that are responsible for deficits and to be able to link those processes to brain function *(26)*. It is perhaps worth noting that there is overlap between neuropsychological and information-processing approaches; for example, continuous performance tests (CPTs) have been widely used as measures of sustained attention-vigilance in both paradigms.

Based on a review of the literature, Kremen et al. noted that there was a good deal of consistency in the neurocognitive abnormalities that were most often found in relatives and in individuals with schizophrenia, as well as in the abnormalities most often found in children of parents with schizophrenia and adult relatives *(11)*.

These patterns strengthen the notion that cognitive deficits are indeed risk indicators for schizophrenia. At the time of that review, Kremen et al. concluded that the strongest evidence for neurocognitive risk indicators was in the areas of sustained attention, perceptual-motor speed, and abstraction-executive formation, with somewhat weaker evidence for mental control-encoding (particularly with distraction) *(11)*. Verbal declarative memory and verbal fluency were also thought to be promising leads for cognitive risk indicators, but there was too little study of these functions to draw conclusions. We evaluate here how these conclusions and predictions have held up on the basis of previous work as well as studies conducted in the ensuing years.

Sustained Attention-Vigilance

There is strong evidence of impairment in sustained attention-vigilance, which has been covered by other reviews *(25,27,28)*. These studies show that relatives of individuals with schizophrenia are not impaired on simple versions of the CPT, but they do show impairments on CPTs with either high working memory or early perceptual loads. Visual CPTs have been studied far more than auditory CPTs, although there is evidence that relatives are impaired on auditory versions as well *(29–31)*. Further study of auditory CPTs may be important given the abundant evidence of dysfunction in auditory-verbal processing in schizophrenia *(32)*. It should be noted that although the phrase "sustained attention" is still typically applied to the CPT, the aforementioned studies also show that there is virtually no evidence for a vigilance decrement over time during the test in schizophrenia. There is also some evidence from family studies for the heritability of perceptual and working memory load CPTs *(33–35)*.

Abstraction-Executive Function

By far, the most widely used measure of abstraction-executive function was the Wisconsin Card Sorting Test (WCST) *(36,37)*. Eight studies found significant deficits in relatives compared with controls in terms of categories achieved or perseverations *(29,38–44)*. Seven studies did not find significant differences *(45–51)*. Cannon et al. found significant deficits in an abstraction function that included the WCST as well as other measures *(52)*; it was not possible to determine which of the individual tests were significantly different in relatives and controls. Some studies had small sample sizes, but lack of power did not appear to be a problem because those with negative results tended to have small effect sizes as well. Thus, abstraction-executive function *as measured by the WCST* has only mixed support as a cognitive risk indicator for schizophrenia.

The WCST has been of great interest in schizophrenia research because of its working memory component and evidence for its association with activation of

prefrontal neural circuitry *(53–55)*. One of its potential shortcoming in studies of relatives may be that it tends to have a ceiling effect in populations that may be only subtly impaired. As such, working memory tasks that tend to produce greater performance variability may be more likely to be consistent risk indicators.

Park et al. found deficits in relatives of individuals with schizophrenia on a test of spatial working memory *(56,57)*. Deficits among relatives on working memory load CPTs provide further support for working memory deficits as neurocognitive vulnerability indicators. It remains unclear as to whether these working memory deficits are specific to particular modalities. Park et al. suggested that individuals with schizophrenia have spatial, but not auditory-verbal working memory deficits because they did not find digit span deficits in patients with schizophrenia *(58)*. Stevens et al. found that patients with schizophrenia performed poorly on a verbal, but not a tones working memory task *(59)*. It would be useful to pursue this issue in relatives in order to shed light on which components of working memory may be vulnerability indicators.

Perceptual-Motor Speed

Tests used to measure this function have been primarily the Trail Making Test *(60)* or the Wechsler Digit Symbol subtest *(61)*. Factor analytic studies have shown that these tests tend to have high loadings on the same factor *(62,63)*. Relatives manifested significant deficits in at least one version of these measures in eight studies *(29,39–41,43,45,49,51)*. There were only two studies with negative results *(48,64)*, one of which was at a trend level of significance $p < .07$ *(64)*. In two studies Trails B, but not Trails A, was significant; in these two studies, it was also noted that Trails B remained significant after adjusting for Trails A *(43,49)*. This result suggests that deficits are due to the set shifting/executive component of the test, but the differences on Trails A in the other studies suggest that relatives have processing speed deficits even without this additional cognitive component. The evidence, thus, strongly supports perceptual-motor speed as a cognitive risk indicator.

Mental Control-Encoding

This function, derived from factor analytic studies of attention, comprises tests such as Digit Span and Arithmetic *(62,63)*. These measures are not well supported as risk indicators for schizophrenia. Seven studies found no differences between relatives and controls on individual or composite measures *(29,40,41, 51,64–66)*, whereas only three found significant deficits in relatives *(42,67,68)*. Docherty and Gordinier found no differential deficit on Digit Span with distraction *(66)*, a task that was previously found to be selectively impaired in children at risk *(69)*.

Most studies did not separate scores for digits forward and backward. This is a potentially important distinction in that it attempts to tease apart two components of working memory: maintenance and manipulation. These may be thought of as reflecting mnemonic and executive processes in working memory, respectively. Conklin et al. found that relatives performed significantly worse than controls on digits backward only, suggesting differential impairment in the executive-manipulation component of verbal working memory *(68)*. Chen et al. included digits forward and backward in a composite verbal memory measure *(42)*; individual measures were not statistically tested, but effect sizes based on Cohen's *(70) d* for relatives vs controls were .36 for digits forward and .71 for digits backward. This pattern is consistent with that of Conklin et al. *(68)*. However, other studies that separated digits forward and backward did not find impairment on digits backward *(64,65)*. The data are, thus, equivocal as to whether digits backward is a useful cognitive risk indicator for schizophrenia.

In any case, we believe that further examination of working memory measures in relatives that require internal manipulation of information is likely to be useful. Gold et al. found that letter-number span and WCST performance were correlated in patients with schizophrenia, consistent with the notion that the ability to manipulate information in working memory underlies some aspects of WCST performance *(71)*. Given the importance of executive-working memory deficits in schizophrenia, the Wechsler Letter-Number Sequencing subtest or other measures with more intensive working memory manipulation demands may ultimately prove to be useful cognitive risk indicators for schizophrenia.

Declarative Memory

Most, but not all, studies have utilized story recall or list-learning measures of verbal declarative memory, and figural design recall as a measure of visual-spatial declarative memory. Six studies reported that verbal memory was significantly impaired in relatives *(41,46,51,52,64,72)*, and three studies reported nonsignificant differences *(42,65,73)*. However, two of the three negative studies included scores in their composite verbal memory indices that might be likely to reduce differences. Staal et al. *(73)* included both free and cued recall scores from the California Verbal Learning Test *(74)*. Individuals with schizophrenia tend to perform better in cued recall or recognition conditions as compared with free recall *(32,75)*, and it, thus, seems reasonable to assume that relatives would manifest little difference from controls on such measures. Even with the cued recall scores included, the composite index of Staal et al. had a moderate effect size of .44 for relatives vs controls *(73)*. Without a significant difference on their composite verbal memory index, Chen et al. *(42)* did not conduct a separate test for their Wechsler *(76)* story recall measure. The effect size for the story recall measure in relatives

vs controls was .56, which would have constituted a significant difference in that study. Thus, we conclude that results of eight of nine studies were actually consistent with a verbal declarative memory deficit in relatives, making it a strong cognitive risk indicator for schizophrenia. In addition, Faraone et al. found that verbal declarative memory was the only function in which relatives from both simplex and multiplex families performed significantly worse than controls, and in which relatives from mulitplex families performed significantly worse than relatives from simplex families *(16)*. These results strengthen the idea that verbal declarative memory impairments indicate genetic liability to schizophrenia.

Findings for visual-spatial memory have not been nearly as strong as those for verbal memory. Two studies found significant deficits in relatives vs controls *(41,64)*, but five did not *(46,52,65,72,73)*. Faraone et al. found that simplex and multiplex families were significantly worse than controls in visual-spatial declarative memory, but the two subgroups of relatives did not differ significantly from one another *(16)*. The stronger evidence for deficits in verbal, but not visual-spatial, declarative memory could reflect greater left- than right-hemisphere dysfunction in relatives of individuals with schizophrenia. Recent findings by Seidman et al. are consistent with this notion; relatives had hippocampal volumes reductions compared with controls that were mainly in the left hemisphere, and hippocampal volume was positively correlated with verbal declarative memory performance in the relatives *(77)*.

Despite these impairments in immediate and/or delayed recall, we are unaware of any findings of abnormal rates of forgetting in relatives of individuals with schizophrenia. This pattern effectively rules out the possibility of deficits in retention. Further decomposition of declarative memory performance is still needed, however, in order to determine the extent to which impairment in encoding or retrieval accounts for the observed deficits.

Verbal Fluency

Verbal fluency deficits were found in relatives compared with controls in six published studies *(39,42,43,46,49,51)*, with the only negative study that found semantic fluency deficits at the .07 level *(64)*. Otherwise, the results were equally consistent for both phonemic (letter) and semantic (category) fluency. In a 4-year follow-up study of relatives, Kremen, Seidman, Faraone, Toomey, and Tsuang (unpublished data) found no differences in verbal fluency between relatives and controls. Verbal fluency measures were given for the first time in this follow-up study. Although it is possible that there was something different about the subset of subjects who participated in the follow-up study, these subjects remained impaired on declarative memory and abstraction measures as did the entire sample at the baseline assessment *(78)*. (See also Stability section below.) Nevertheless,

the overall findings strongly suggest that verbal fluency is a viable cognitive risk indicator for schizophrenia.

Inhibition

Inhibitory control refers to the ability to suppress inappropriate or irrelevant stimuli, whether external or internal. It is particularly important when inappropriate or irrelevant stimuli are primed or prepotent so that greater active effort is required to suppress a response. Inhibitory control is inextricably intertwined with selective attention when one must inhibit the tendency to respond to irrelevant stimuli presented simultaneously. It is intertwined with working memory functions when stimuli that were primed or were responded to appropriately on a previous trial must be inhibited on a current trial. Hasher and Zacks have suggested that inhibition in working memory can affect language discourse and comprehension and even long-term memory *(79)*. Neuroimaging studies have shown that different regions in prefrontal cortex are activated to greater or lesser degrees depending on the maintenance, manipulation, or inhibitory control demands of a working task *(80,81)*. An example of inhibitory deficits in early processing in relatives of individuals with schizophrenia is that of deficits on antisaccade tasks *(82–85)*.

Most neuropsychological studies have examined inhibition in later stages of information processing. In the study of Byrne et al. *(64)*, relatives made more errors on the Hayling Sentence Completion Test *(86)*, a measure with a strong response suppression component. A few studies have examined neuropsychological indices of cognitive inhibition using the Stroop test in relatives. In two published studies that reported specifically on the interference condition, one showed deficits in relatives at a trend level $p < .09$ *(64)*; and one had negative results *(87)*. Seidman, Kremen, Faraone, and Tsuang (unpublished data) did not find differences between relatives and controls on Stroop interference. Computerized versions of the Stroop test that allow for calculation of reaction times to congruent vs incongruent words have been utilized in patients with schizophrenia, and these more sensitive tests may prove useful in relatives as well *(88)*.

Cohen's AX-CPT is a task that assesses inhibitory control in working memory. It has been shown to elicit inhibitory deficits in individuals with schizophrenia *(89)*. In this version, subjects are primed to respond to X because there are many target AX sequences; however, patients with schizophrenia made more errors in responding to X when it followed a non-A cue. Seidman et al. developed an auditory CPT in which one responds to the target A when it is preceded by a Q appearing three letters before the target *(31)*. When the intervening letters include Qs or As, this task has a substantial inhibition/interference component. Unpublished results with these tasks show an excess of deficits in relatives of individuals with schizophrenia as well as differences from normal controls in terms of activation patterns during functional neuroimaging *(30,90)*.

These results suggest that these tests of cognitive inhibition are worthy of further study in relatives of individuals with schizophrenia. Cohen and colleagues integrated the functions of working memory and inhibition within the construct of context processing (89,91). In their model, the same processing mechanism is responsible for both functions, with deficits appearing to be manifestations of either function depending on task conditions. However, the work of D. Esposito and colleagues, as previously noted, does indicate differential change in regional brain activations for these two functions (80).

A common feature of CPTs studied in people with schizophrenia and their relatives is that examinees are typically asked to respond only to target stimuli. In contrast, the Conners' CPT, which is widely used in the assessment of attention deficit/hyperactivity disorders (ADHD), instructs the examinee to respond to all stimuli except the targets (92). Because the examinee is primed to respond to most of the stimuli presented and must hold back when confronted with target stimuli, it places greater demand on inhibitory control. To our knowledge, this type of CPT is virtually unstudied in schizophrenia. It would be of interest to see whether this type of CPT also appears to be a risk indicator for schizophrenia because inhibitory control deficits may be important in schizophrenia, but also because it would shed additional light on the question of specificity with regard another psychiatric disorder with prominent attentional deficits.

OVERVIEW OF RISK INDICATORS
IN SPECIFIC COGNITIVE DOMAINS

As noted, at the time of the previous review of Kremen et al., there were very few results reported for declarative memory and verbal fluency (11). The updated findings strongly support the notion that these are promising candidates for neurocognitive risk indicators for schizophrenia. No prediction was made regarding verbal vs declarative memory, but the data suggest that deficits are largely in verbal memory. Mental control deficits in relatives   assessed primarily by Digit Span

appear to be less consistent than they did in the previous review. Abstraction-executive function   assessed primarily by the WCST   was one of the stronger candidates for a risk indicator in the previous review, but the updated results were equivocal.

Digit Span and WCST are both tasks that involve working memory. The WCST is a complex task that also involves abstract reasoning and the ability to profit from feedback. Its working memory component involves the need to update information from trial to trial, but it does not necessarily place particularly great demands on working memory capacity per se. Moreover, the few findings of deficits on digits backward, but not forward, suggest that other measures that require more taxing manipulation of information in working memory may provide more

promising cognitive risk indicators. In order to elicit deficits in relatives, it may be necessary to increase the working memory load along with requirements for manipulation as well as maintenance functions. Another key factor might be whether or not working memory demands are combined with speed of processing demands. For example, the WCST appears to be less consistently impaired in relatives than are working memory load CPTs such as the identical-pairs CPT *(25)*. A key difference may be that the WCST is self-paced, whereas the CPT is experimenter paced. Furthermore, the results of several studies show that processing speed (i.e., perceptual-motor speed) continued to have strong support as a cognitive risk indicator for schizophrenia.

Finally, the pattern of declarative memory deficits in relatives in the absence of abnormal forgetting shares at least some similarities with the profile of memory deficits in patients with frontal lobe lesions *(93)*. It is, thus, possible that executive control or short-term working memory deficits account for many cognitive deficits   including long-term memory deficits   in relatives of individuals with schizophrenia. Similarly, the model of Cohen and colleagues posits that a single prefrontally mediated "module" is responsible for several types of cognitive deficits observed in schizophrenia *(89,91)*.

Consistent with the literature on schizophrenia itself, all of the measures that have been identified as putative cognitive risk indicators involve processes that implicate neural networks involving frontal, anterior cingulate, and/or temporal-limbic brain regions *(94–96)*. This shows a degree of consistency with neuroimaging findings in individuals with schizophrenia and their biological relatives. (*See* Chapter 9 of this volume for more detail.) It remains to be determined whether dysfunction in relatives is primarily in prefrontal cortex itself (as suggested by Cohen and colleagues) or in other components of these neural networks such as the thalamus or hippocampus. Indeed, one possibility is that relatives experience more dysfunction in subcortical or posterior cortical regions that are linked to prefrontal cortex than in prefrontal cortex itself. Such a pattern might be consistent with relatives having similar, but less severe, deficits than their family members with schizophrenia.

SPECIFICITY OF RISK INDICATORS

There is ample evidence that the kinds of neurocognitive abnormalities that we have described are very consistently present in individuals with schizophrenia. The findings described herein also indicate that some of these cognitive deficits are more common or more prominent in relatives of individuals with schizophrenia in comparison to normal controls. In this case, the controls may be thought of as a proxy for the general population. As such, the first two criteria for risk indicators have been met. Unfortunately, there are still few studies of the specificity of these deficits for risk for schizophrenia vs other psychiatric disorders.

In the New York High Risk Project, attention, working memory, and gross motor skill deficits at ages 7 to 12 were associated with increased risk for schizophrenia spectrum disorders in mid-adulthood in those who were genetically at risk for schizophrenia; associations were weak in those who were genetically at risk for affective disorder (97).

In a general-population sample, Cannon et al. found that low IQs at age 4 and at age 7 predicted adult diagnoses of both schizophrenia and affective disorder, but the pattern was familial only for schizophrenia. That is, low IQ was associated with being an unaffected sibling of someone with schizophrenia, but not someone with affective disorder. Kremen et al. found that when compared to adult relatives of individuals with bipolar disorder on an extensive neuropsychological battery, only relatives of individuals with schizophrenia manifested neuropsychological deficits compared with controls (98).

Both individuals with schizophrenia and those with major affective disorders frequently manifest cognitive deficits, but similar deficits appear to be found in relatives of those with schizophrenia only. One explanation for this set of findings would be that cognitive deficits reflect underlying genetically mediated dysfunction for schizophrenia, but are more a function of the effects of illness in major affective disorders (98). Unfortunately, the study of Kremen et al. included only female subjects (98); further work needs to be conducted to determine whether this pattern holds for men as well. Recent findings also suggest that unaffected siblings of individuals with ADHD   another condition that involves some overlap of cognitive deficits with schizophrenia   do not manifest neuropsychological deficits (99).

Perhaps because it is costly and requires very large numbers of subjects, there have been few direct comparisons of cognitive dysfunction in relatives (particularly adults) of individuals with schizophrenia and relatives of individuals with other psychiatric disorders. An unpublished report from one such study comparing relatives of individuals with schizophrenia and relatives of individuals with ADHD indicates that CPT and Span of Apprehension test deficits can differentiate these two groups of relatives (100). Thus far, the data suggest that certain neurocognitive deficits are schizophrenia endophenotypes, but they probably do not constitute affective disorder or ADHD endophenotypes. More extensive comparisons of this type will be important for confirming neurocognitive endophenotypes that are specific to schizophrenia.

IMPORTANCE OF MULTIPLE OR COMPOSITE INDICATORS

Faraone et al. showed that a composite cognitive measure was able to discriminate relatives of individuals with schizophrenia from controls better than many other symptom-based or psychophysiological measures (101). This work pro-

vided support for the idea that composite measures or single measures assessed across time are likely to have greater predictive power than individual measures based on a single time point *(101)*. This point had been emphasized by others as well *(102)*. Being impaired on several cognitive measures was a strong predictor of risk for developing schizophrenia-spectrum conditions in children of parents with schizophrenia *(103,104)*, and false positives were lowest when impairment was based on the combination of three different neurocognitive measures *(97)*. Being impaired across multiple time points is another type of composite measure that is useful *(97,105)*. Composite measures may also be of importance for identifying vulnerable subgroups (see Heterogeneity section below).

WHAT IS THE RELATIONSHIP
AMONG VULNERABILITY INDICATORS?

Thinking of cognitive or other vulnerability indicators as endophenotypes leads to the question of how they may be related to one another in relatives of individuals with schizophrenia and whether or not correlations reflect common underlying genetic influences. Toomey et al. found that putative cognitive vulnerability indicators (abstraction-executive function, verbal declarative memory, auditory attention) were correlated among relatives, but not among controls *(106)*. Correlations did not differ between groups for nonvulnerability indicator measures. In particular, the correlations of attention with each of the other two indicators were significantly higher among relatives than among controls. This finding suggests, but does not confirm, a common underlying mechanism in relatives. The auditory attention measure relied heavily on a dichotic digits task that involves a strong working memory component as well as demands on sustained and divided attention, and encoding. Thus, dysfunction in one or more of these processes could be the common underlying mechanism for all three vulnerability indicators.

In contrast, Yurgelun-Todd and Kinney found that WCST and Trail Making Test performance were positively correlated in patients with schizophrenia, but inversely correlated in their siblings *(48)*. This pattern fit with their hypothesis that these tests reflect independent factors that, in combination, significantly increase the risk of schizophrenia. According to this "two-hit" model, relatives who were impaired on one would be unlikely to be impaired on the other and remain unaffected.

Grove et al. found that CPT and eye-tracking performance were correlated in relatives *(34)*, whereas Keefe et al. found that the two were independent *(107)*. The CPT. eye tracking differences could be because of the fact that different abilities were being examined; the Grove et al. CPT had a high load on early perceptual processes, whereas the Keefe et al. CPT had a high working memory load. The differences in the Toomey and Yurgelun-Todd studies are more diffi-

cult to reconcile. The auditory attention tests of Toomey et al. load on a different attention-related factor than the Trail Making Test (62,63), but in a separate analysis Toomey et al. found that WCST and Trail Making performance in their sample of relatives was positively correlated (i.e., good performance on one associated with good performance on the other).

STABILITY

More stable or persistent deficits are consistent with being more traitlike, and are thus more likely to be valid endophenotypes (108). There is some evidence for stability of neurocognitive deficits in relatives of individuals with schizophrenia, but this is another area that calls for further study. Attention and working memory deficits persisted from childhood through early adulthood in the children of parents with schizophrenia, and the magnitude of impairment remained stable over time (97,105). The attentional and behavioral difficulties were relatively independent, and unlike the attentional deficits, behavioral difficulties were sensitive to environmental factors (105). This difference may be viewed as supporting the notion that attention deficits are valid endophenotypes. In a 4-year follow-up of adult relatives of individuals with schizophrenia, Faraone et al. found evidence of moderate stability for indices of deficit in verbal declarative memory and auditory attention (78). The auditory attention measure dichotic digits loaded heavily on a sustained attention factor, but it contains strong working memory and encoding demands as well (63). As noted above, support for the WCST as a cognitive vulnerability measure has been inconsistent. It is, thus, noteworthy that WCST scores in relatives were not stable over time in the study of Faraone et al., suggesting that it may not be a useful endophenotypic measure (78). On the other hand, relatives were impaired in other executive function tests (i.e., object alternation) that were given for the first time at the follow-up assessment. This pattern suggests that aspects of executive function or working memory may indeed constitute cognitive endophenotypes, but that the WCST may not be a particularly useful test for assessing cognitive endophenotypes in relatives. It seems worth emphasizing this specific test because it is one of the most widely used tests in schizophrenia research.

HETEROGENEITY

Identifying Vulnerable Subgroups

We have identified several neurocognitive measures that appear to be vulnerability indicators for schizophrenia. Ours was not intended to be a comprehensive review, and there are no doubt others as well. It is possible that a single under-

lying genetic mechanism accounts for all of these deficits, but it seems more likely that polygenic processes are involved *(109)*. This may also explain the heterogeneity in findings across studies of relatives. It should also be recalled that no single deficit has been found to be present even in all individuals with schizophrenia. Consequently, it is expected that only a subset of relatives would manifest any particular abnormality.

Failure to examine this heterogeneity could result in misinterpretation of findings, including failure to identify a meaningful vulnerability indicator. As noted above, composite measures composed of multiple indicators or single indicators that are stable across time may help to identify vulnerable subgroups. For example, Cornblatt et al. found that children of parents with schizophrenia had greater attention deficits than control children based on group-mean scores *(110)*. Mean performance did not differ in a second sample, but inspection of the data indicated that there were outliers at both the good- and poor-performing ends of the distribution among the high-risk children *(105)*. By classifying subjects in the bottom portion of the distribution as deviant, they found that a subgroup of high-risk, but no-control children was deviant in all three rounds of testing.

Similarly, Faraone et al. included two criteria in addition to group-mean differences that might identify vulnerability indicators *(41)*. One of these was a higher proportion of deviant responders based on some meaningful cutoff. The second was the presence of greater variability in relatives than in controls. The latter criterion was based on the notion that not all relatives are expected to carry the pathogenic gene(s) that might predispose to cognitive dysfunction. The presence of subgroups that presumably carry or do not carry the pathogenic gene(s) might increase variability among the relatives. Moreover, it is possible that different neurocognitive abnormalities are present in different subgroups of relatives, perhaps reflecting different sets of genes and different underlying brain regions.

Sex Differences

Sex differences represent another type of heterogeneity that may be of importance in the search for cognitive vulnerability indicators, although they have been rarely looked at in relatives of individuals with schizophrenia. Kremen et al. found significant or near-significant group × sex interactions in verbal declarative memory, auditory attention, and mental control-encoding such that only female relatives were impaired compared with female controls *(111)*. Male relatives were more impaired than male controls in motor function, but motor function has not received much support as a vulnerability indicator in adult relatives. The interaction for declarative memory was also present in a 4-year follow-up *(78)*. In addition, the interactions in declarative memory and auditory attention were extended in comparisons of relatives from simplex vs multiplex families. That is, female

relatives from multiplex families tended to be more impaired than female relatives from simplex families, whereas there was little difference between male relatives from simplex vs multiplex families *(16)*.

Some, but not all, epidemiological studies suggest that women may have a higher threshold than men for developing psychosis *(112,113)*. If so, male relatives with greater cognitive deficits would be more likely to develop psychosis and, thus, would be less likely to be in a sample that excluded relatives with psychotic symptoms in order to identify potential vulnerability indicators. Estrogen has been shown to be strongly correlated with cognitive performance in women with schizophrenia *(114)*. Another   not mutually exclusive   possibility is that these female relatives tend to have some sort of estrogen deficiency or dysfunction *(115)*.

Types of Relative Studied

As noted in the introduction, results have been largely consistent for adult relatives and children of parents with schizophrenia *(11)*. Nevertheless, it is possible that some findings may differ depending on whether one examines parents, siblings, or adult children. For some purposes, there are benefits to restricting one's sample to siblings; it is advantageous for study purposes that siblings shared the same familial environment as the person with the illness, and were not raised by a parent with schizophrenia. Fortunately, siblings represent the largest subgroup in most of the studies reviewed in this chapter. Different issues, such as age effects, may arise with the study of parents. In one study, elderly relatives who were mostly parents did not manifest cognitive impairments; it was suggested that parents may be "selected" for better functioning because they are, by definition, capable of marriage and reproduction *(116)*. On the other hand, recent unpublished findings indicated accelerated aging effects on cognition in relatives; if the older relatives were primarily parents, this finding would suggest greater worsening of cognitive function in parents *(117)*.

In an "obligate carrier" design, parents are classified on the basis of positive or negative family history of schizophrenia to determine who is presumably the carrier of the gene(s) that predispose to schizophrenia. Using this design, Harris et al. found that positive-history parents had similar attentional deficits (based on perceptual-motor speed, vigilance, and mental-control encoding tests), but better declarative memory performance compared with their offspring with schizophrenia *(118)*. They concluded that attentional deficits reflect a primary dysfunction and the memory deficits reflect a secondary disturbance that may be present in those who actually express the disorder of schizophrenia. This conclusion is difficult to reconcile with the majority of studies that found declarative memory deficits in nonpsychotic relatives. In any case, this strategy may provide a useful complement to the more traditional family study designs.

IMPLICATIONS FOR INTERVENTION AND PREVENTION

Genetic-Linkage Studies

Identifying the most promising cognitive risk indicators is important for applying these alternate phenotypes to genetic-linkage studies. Utilization of deficits in these neurocognitive functions as endophenotypes   such that individuals with any of these deficits are classified as affected cases (even if they do not manifest psychiatric symptoms)   may enhance the ability of genetic-linkage studies to identify genes that increase liability to schizophrenia. Such beneficial effects have, for example, been shown for the inclusion of eye-tracking dysfunction as an endophenotype in genetic-linkage studies of schizophrenia *(119)*. Applying neurocognitive phenotypes to genetic-linkage analysis is only in its infancy. With growing evidence that neurocognitive deficits are core deficits of schizophrenia, and that such deficits can effectively discriminate relatives from controls, we believe that the use of neurocognitive endophenotypes in genetic-linkage studies should be strongly encouraged. Ultimately, the identification of genes that increase risk for schizophrenia is what will serve as the springboard for early intervention and prevention.

As noted, Faraone et al. showed that a composite cognitive measure was better than most other measures at discriminating relatives of individuals with schizophrenia from controls *(101)*. Based on this work, it appears that cognitive risk indicators are among the more useful potential endophenotypes for genetic linkage analysis. Moreover, this cognitive index was able to discriminate a significant proportion of relatives at a level at which there were no false positives (i.e., no controls erroneously classified as relatives). This finding is important because false positives are a far more serious problem for linkage analysis than false negatives *(120)*.

It may be argued that cognitive and neuropsychological measures involve multiple cognitive processes, thus making it difficult to isolate the specific mechanisms underlying performance. Composite indices would make it even more difficult to identify such mechanisms. Utilizing this broader level of analysis is not necessarily a problem; rather, it depends on one's purpose. Isolating component processes is very important in order to delineate the particular brain regions or neural circuitry mediating performance, or a common cognitive ability that may underlie performance deficits on several tasks. It is unlikely that there is a one-to-one relationship between the number of component cognitive processes contained in a given measure and the number of genes that are linked to performance on that measure. Indeed, it is well known that single gene disorders can have far-reaching effects on cognitive and brain function. Utilizing multicomponent or composite cognitive measures may still be useful if the initial goal is to delineate alternate phenotypes that are useful in identifying individuals that are

likely to possess pathogenic gene(s) associated with risk for schizophrenia. Being less complex than the schizophrenia syndrome itself, these alternate phenotypes, or cognitive endophenotypes, might be associated with one or at least fewer genes than the full syndrome.

In addition to composite measures, we have noted that measures that display more stable deficits over time are likely to be better cognitive endophenotypes. Evidence of stability of deficits in relatives has been shown for sustained attention-vigilance (CPTs) and working memory (attention span, digit span) in children of parents with schizophrenia (97,105), and in verbal declarative memory (story recall) and auditory attention (dichotic digits) in adult relatives (78). As previously indicated, this dichotic listening test contained a strong working memory component. Several of these measures were also included in a successful composite measure (101). Thus, these measures, or other measures tapping these functions, are likely to be most the promising neurocognitive endophenotypes for use in genetic-linkage studies.

Another issue that may be considered is the finding of sex differences in cognitive function in relatives. Those results raise the interesting possibility that emphasizing the study of female relatives of individuals with schizophrenia may make it easier to identify potential cognitive endophenotypes. Finally, cognitive deficits were greater in relatives from multiplex families than in those from simplex families, consistent with the idea that these deficits reflect the degree of genetic predisposition (16). Thus, neurocognitive studies that may, in part, be a prelude to genetic-linkage studies may benefit from a focus on relatives that are specifically from multiplex families (as is typically done in linkage studies themselves).

Family Treatment

In one developmental model, early cognitive (attentional) deficits in at-risk individuals are hypothesized to lead to difficulties in processing complex interpersonal cues, which, in turn, increases risk for the development of social deficits and eventually symptoms (110). Studies of children of parents with schizophrenia have shown that attentional deficits tended to be present prior to the emergence of behavioral difficulties (121), and that neurocognitive, but not behavioral, deficits in childhood and adolescence were useful in screening individuals at greatest risk for developing schizophrenia-spectrum disorders (105). Also consistent with this model, adult relatives of individuals with schizophrenia manifested deficits in nonverbal social perception, and slower reaction times on sustained attention-vigilance tasks predicted these social perception deficits (122). The latter finding supports the notion that deficits in processing socioemotional cues in relatives are, in part, a result of underlying neurocognitive deficits.

The presence of cognitive deficits (including social cognition) in the relatives of individuals with schizophrenia not only has implications for understanding

the genetics of the illness, but may also be relevant in terms of family treatment strategies. Psychoeducational family treatment programs typically involve information about the illness, community resources, stress management, use of medication, and methods of communication or problem solving (123,124). Indeed, family members are often key people involved in the care and support of patients with schizophrenia. If some of those family members have deficits in attention, processing speed, or verbal declarative or working memory, then instructions provided in psychoeducational treatment models could be misinterpreted, misunderstood, or poorly recalled. Key information could be missed or distorted. Information may need to be broken down into more easily remembered and smaller chunks of information and presented in visual as well as auditory modes, such as in handouts. More repetition and clarification of information may be called for as well.

Several researchers have also suggested that disorders of language, thought, and communication in schizophrenia are, in part, manifestations of underlying cognitive and information-processing deficits (125). As such, communication deficits represent another phenomenon that may be influenced by neurocognitive impairments and may, in turn, negatively impact on family treatment. There has been very little study of language in relatives of individuals with schizophrenia from a neurocognitive perspective. Shedlack et al. found that well siblings were impaired on measures of linguistic complexity (degree of clausal embedding in free-speech samples) (65). This result is consistent with the notion that some aspects of language structure are abnormal in relatives. Only brothers with schizophrenia-spectrum disorders were impaired in language comprehension in the study of Condray et al. (126). Interestingly, the spectrum-disordered subgroup was more impaired than the brothers with schizophrenia.

In a study of communication disturbances (sometimes referred to as communication deviance), Docherty et al. found that parents of patients with schizophrenia had more communication failures in natural-speech samples than did normal controls (127). Examples of such failures were language structural breakdown and use of vague and overinclusive words and those with ambiguous meanings. Similarly, Shenton et al. found that relatives of individuals with schizophrenia had more thought disorder than controls (128).

In family therapy sessions, subtle thought disorder or communication deviance in family members may also need to be addressed in terms of teaching better receptive and expressive communication skills. Such difficulties in communication may be further compounded if relatives have deficits in the perception of socioemotional cues. These types of deficits may be particularly important during periods of heightened stress or discord, or during times of subtle exacerbation of symptoms in the patient with schizophrenia. Impaired communication or misreading of interpersonal cues could augment rather than attenuate worsening of the problems.

With regard to treatment implications, little systematic attention has been paid to the potential impact of such deficits in relatives. One could argue that it might be useful to cognitively evaluate relatives who are involved in family treatment with a patient. There are obvious dilemmas involved in addressing this issue. In most cases, these relatives do not come in seeking treatment for themselves, and many do not have any diagnosable psychiatric disorder. Nevertheless, the findings of neurocognitive deficits in relatives suggest that ignoring this issue could negatively impact treatment of the identified patient. Recent preliminary findings from Tsuang et al. even suggest that relatives without schizophrenia spectrum diagnoses who have subtle neurocognitive deficits could benefit from low-dose antipsychotic medication *(129)*. Although it cannot be risk-free, the thoughtful development of creative new approaches to this dilemma certainly appears to be something worthy of further study.

REFERENCES

1. Kraepelin E. Dementia Praecox and Paraphrenia. Chicago: Chicago Medical Books, 1919.
2. Bleuler E. Dementia Praecox or the Group of Schizophrenias. New York: International Universities, 1911/1950.
3. Hoff AL, Riordan H, O'Donnell DW, Morris L, DeLisi LE. Neuropsychological functioning of first-episode schizophreniform patients. Am J Psychiatry 1992; 149:898..903.
4. Kremen WS, Buka SL, Seidman LJ, Goldstein JM, Koren D, Tsuang MT. IQ decline during childhood and adult psychotic symptoms in a community sample: a 19-year longitudinal study. Am J Psychiatry 1998; 155:672..679.
5. Aylward E, Walker E, Bettes B. Intelligence in schizophrenia: meta-analysis of the research. Schizophr Bull 1984; 10:430..459.
6. Jones P, Rodgers B, Murray RM. Child developmental risk factors for adult schizophrenia in the British 1946 birth cohort. Lancet 1994; 344:1398..1402.
7. Kremen WS, Seidman LJ, Faraone SV, Toomey R, Tsuang MT. The paradox of normal neuropsychological function in schizophrenia. J Abnorm Psychol 2000; 109:743..752.
8. Kremen WS, Seidman LJ, Faraone SV, Tsuang MT. Intelligence quotient and neuropsychological profiles in patients with schizophrenia and normal volunteers. Biol Psychiatry 2001; 50:453..462.
9. Gold JM, Harvey PD. Cognitive deficits in schizophrenia. Psychiatr Clin North Am 1993; 16:295..312.
10. Kremen WS, Tsuang MT, Faraone SV, Lyons MJ. Using vulnerability indicators to compare conceptual models of genetic heterogeneity in schizophrenia. J Nerv Ment Dis 1992; 180:55..65.
11. Kremen WS, Seidman LJ, Pepple JR, Lyons MJ, Tsuang MT, Faraone SV. Neuropsychological risk indicators for schizophrenia: a review of family studies. Schizophr Bull 1994; 20:103..119.
12. Erlenmeyer-Kimling L. Biological markers for the liability to schizophrenia. In: Helmchen H, Henn FA, eds. Biological Perspectives of Schizophrenia. Chichester, England: Wiley, 1987: 33..56.
13. Nuechterlein KH, Dawson ME. Information processing and attentional functioning in the developmental course of schizophrenic disorders. Schizophr Bull 1984; 10:160..203.

14. John B, Lewis KR. Chromosome variability and geographic distribution in insects. Science 1966; 152:711..721.

15. Gottesman II, Shields J. Schizophrenia and Genetics: a Twin Study Vantage Point. New York: Academic, 1972.

16. Faraone SV, Seidman LJ, Kremen WS, Toomey R, Pepple JR, Tsuang MT. Neuropsychological functioning among the nonpsychotic relatives of schizophrenic patients: the effect of genetic loading. Biol Psychiatry 2000; 48:120..126.

17. Erlenmeyer-Kimling L, Rock D, Squires-Wheeler E, Roberts S, Yang J. Early life precursors of psychiatric outcomes in adulthood in subjects at risk for schizophrenia or affective disorders. Psychiatry Res 1991; 39:239..256.

18. Crow TJ, Done DJ, Sacker A. Childhood precursors of psychosis as clues to its evolutionary origins. Eur Arch Psychiatry Clin Neurosci 1995; 154:61..69.

19. Russell AJ, Munro JC, Jones PB, Hemsley DR, Murray RM. Schizophrenia and the myth of intellectual decline. Am J Psychiatry 1997; 154:635..639.

20. Cannon TD, Rosso IM, Bearden CE, Sanchez LE, Hadley T. A prospective cohort study of neurodevelopmental processes in the genesis and epigenesis of schizophrenia. Dev Psychopathol 1999; 11:467..485.

21. Dalby JT, Williams R. Preserved reading and spelling ability in psychotic disorders. Psychol Med 1986; 16:171..175.

22. Kremen WS, Seidman LJ, Faraone SV, Pepple JR, Lyons MJ, Tsuang MT. The "3 Rs" and neuropsychological function in schizophrenia: an empirical test of the matching fallacy. Neuropsychology 1996; 10:22..31.

23. Kremen WS, Seidman LJ, Faraone SV, Pepple JR, Lyons MJ, Tsuang MT. The "3 Rs" and neuropsychological function in schizophrenia: a test of the matching fallacy in biological relatives. Psychiatry Res 1995; 56:135..143.

24. Erlenmeyer-Kimling L, Cornblatt B, Friedman D, et al. Neurological, electrophysiological, and attentional deviations in children at risk for schizophrenia. In: Henn FA, Nasrallah HA, eds. Schizophrenia as a Brain Disease. New York: Oxford University Press, 1982:61..98.

25. Cornblatt BA, Keilp JG. Impaired attention, genetics, and the pathophysiology of schizophrenia. Schizophr Bull 1994; 20:31..46.

26. Holzman PS. Parsing cognition. The power of psychology paradigms. Arch Gen Psychiatry 1994; 51:952..954.

27. Nuechterlein KH. Vigilance in schizophrenia and related disorders. In: Steinhauer SR, Gruzelier JH, Zubin J, eds. Handbook of Schizophrenia, Vol. 5: Neuropsychology, Neurophysiology and Information Processing. Amsterdam: Elsevier, 1991:397..433.

28. Chen WJ, Faraone SV. Sustained attention deficits as markers of genetic susceptibility to schizophrenia. Am J Med Genet 2000; 97:52..57.

29. Mirsky AF, Lochhead SJ, Jones BP, Kugelmass S, Walsh D, Kendler KS. On familial factors in the attentional deficit in schizophrenia: a review and report of two new subject samples. J Psychiatric Res 1992; 26:383..403.

30. Seidman LJ, Goldstein JM, Breiter HC, et al. Functional MRI of attention in relatives of schizophrenic patients (abstract). Schizophr Res 1997; 24:172.

31. Seidman LJ, Breiter HC, Goodman JM, et al. A functional magnetic resonance imaging study of auditory vigilance with low and high information processing demands. Neuropsychology 1998; 12:505..518.

32. Seidman LJ, Cassens G, Kremen WS, Pepple JR. The neuropsychology of schizophrenia. In: White RF, ed. Clinical Syndromes in Adult Neuropsychology: The Practitioner's Handbook. Amsterdam: Elsevier, 1992:381..449.

33. Cornblatt BA, Risch NJ, Faris G, Friedman D, Erlenmeyer-Kimling L. The continuous performance test, identical pairs version (CPT-IP): I. New findings about sustained attention in normal families. Psychiatry Res 1988; 26:223..238.

34. Grove WM, Lebow BS, Clementz BA, Cerri A, Medus C, Iacono WG. Familial prevalence and coaggregation of schizotypy indicators: a multitrait family study. J Abnorm Psychol 1991; 100:115..121.

35. Chen WJ, Liu SK, Chang CJ, Lien YJ, Chang YH, Hwu HG. Sustained attention deficit and schizotypal personality features in nonpsychotic relatives of schizophrenic patients. Am J Psychiatry 1998; 155:1214..1220.

36. Grant DA, Berg EA. A behavioral analysis of degree of reinforcement and ease of shifting to new responses in a Weigl-type card sorting problem. J Exp Psychol 1948; 38:404..411.

37. Heaton RK. Wisconsin Card Sorting Test Manual. Odessa, FL: Psychological Assessment Resources, 1981.

38. Franke P, Maier W, Hain C, Klingler T. Wisconsin Card Sorting Test: an indicator of vulnerability to schizophrenia? Schizophr Res 1992; 6:243..249.

39. Franke P, Maier W, Hardt J, Hain C. Cognitive functioning and anhedonia in subjects at risk for schizophrenia. Schizophr Res 1993; 10:77..84.

40. Mirsky AF, Yardley SL, Jones BP, Walsh D, Kendler KS. Analysis of the attention deficit in schizophrenia: a study of patients and their relatives in Ireland. J Psychiatric Res 1995; 29: 23..42.

41. Faraone SV, Seidman LJ, Kremen WS, Pepple JR, Lyons MJ, Tsuang MT. Neuropsychological functioning among the nonpsychotic relatives of schizophrenic patients: a diagnostic efficiency analysis. J Abnorm Psychol 1995; 104:286..304.

42. Chen YLR, Eric UH, Chen, Felice M, Lieh. Semantic verbal fluency deficit as a familial trait marker in schizophrenia. Psychiatry Res 2000; 95:133..148.

43. Laurent A, Biloa-Tang M, Bougerol T, et al. Executive/attentional performance and measures of schizotypy in patients with schizophrenia and in their nonpsychotic first-degree relatives. Schizophr Res 2000; 46:269..283.

44. Saoud M, d'Amato T, Gutknecht C, et al. Neuropsychological deficit in siblings discordant for schizophrenia. Schizophr Bull 2000; 26(4):893..902.

45. Condray R, Steinhauer SR. Schizotypal personality disorder in individuals with and without schizophrenic relatives: similarities and contrasts in neurocognitive and clinical functioning. Schizophr Res 1992; 7:33..41.

46. Roxborough H, Muir WJ, Blackwood DHR, Walker MT, Blackburn IM. Neuropsychological and P300 abnormalities in schizophrenics and their relatives. Psychol Med 1993; 23:305..314.

47. Scarone S, Abbruzzese M, Gambini O. The Wisconsin Card Sorting Test discriminates schizophrenic patients and their siblings. Schizophr Res 1993:103..107.

48. Yurgelun-Todd DA, Kinney DK. Patterns of neuropsychological deficits that discriminate schizophrenic individuals from siblings and control subjects. J Neuropsychiatry Clin Neurosci 1993; 5:294..300.

49. Keefe RS, Silverman JM, Lees Roitman SE, et al. Performance of nonpsychotic relatives of schizophrenic patients on cognitive tests. Psychiatry Res 1994; 53:1..12.

50. Stratta P, Daneluzzo E, Mattei P, Bustini M, Casacchia M, Rossi A. No deficit in Wisconsin Card Sorting Test performance of schizophrenic patients' first-degree relatives. Schizophr Res 1997; 26:147..151.

51. Ismail B, Cantor-Graae E, McNeil TF. Minor physical anomalies in schizophrenia: cognitive, neurological and other clinical correlates. J Psychiatric Res 2000; 34:45..56.

52. Cannon TD, Zorrilla LE, Shtasel D, et al. Neuropsychological functioning in siblings discordant for schizophrenia and healthy volunteers. Arch Gen Psychiatry 1994; 51:651..661.

53. Weinberger DR, Berman KF, Zec RF. Physiological dysfunction of dorsolateral prefrontal cortex in schizophrenia. I. Regional cerebral blood flow evidence. Arch Gen Psychiatry 1986; 43:114..124.

54. Goldberg E, Seidman LJ. Higher cortical functions in normals and in schizophrenia: a selective review. In: Steinhauer SR, Gruzelier JH, Zubin J, eds. Handbook of Schizophrenia, Vol 5: Neuropsychology, Psychophysiology and Information Processing. Amsterdam: Elsevier, 1991:553..591.

55. Goldman-Rakic PS. Working memory dysfunction in schizophrenia. J Neuropsychiatry Clin Neurosci 1994; 6:348..357.

56. Park S, Holzman PS. Association of working memory and eye tracking dysfunction in schizophrenia. Schizophr Res 1993; 11:55..61.

57. Park S, Holzman PS, Goldman-Rakic PS. Spatial working memory deficits in the relatives of schizophrenic patients. Arch Gen Psychiatry 1995; 52:821..828.

58. Park S, Holzman PS. Schizophrenics show spatial working memory deficits. Arch Gen Psychiatry 1992; 49:975..982.

59. Stevens AA, Donegan NH, Anderson M, Goldman-Rakic PS, Wexler BE. Verbal processing deficits in schizophrenia. J Abnorm Psychol 2000; 109:461..471.

60. War Department AGsO. Army Individual Test Battery. Manual of directions and scoring. Washington, DC: War Department, Adjutant General's Office, 1944.

61. Wechsler D. Manual for the Wechsler Adult Intelligence Scale Revised. San Antonio, TX: Psychological Corporation, 1981.

62. Mirsky AF, Anthony BJ, Duncan CC, Ahearn MB, Kellam SG. Analysis of the elements of attention: a neuropsychological approach. Neuropsychol Rev 1991; 2:109..145.

63. Kremen WS, Seidman LJ, Faraone SV, Pepple JR, Tsuang MT. Attention/information-processing factors in psychotic disorders: replication and extension of recent neuropsychological findings. J Nerv Ment Dis 1992; 180:89..93.

64. Byrne M, Hodges A, Grant E, Owens DC, Johnstone EC. Neuropsychological assessment of young people at high genetic risk for developing schizophrenia compared with controls: preliminary findings of the Edinburgh High Risk Study (EHRS). Psychol Med 1999; 29:1161..1173.

65. Shedlack K, Lee G, Sakuma M, et al. Language processing and memory in ill and well siblings from multiplex families affected with schizophrenia. Schizophr Res 1997; 25:43..52.

66. Docherty NM, Gordinier SW. Immediate memory, attention and communication disturbances in schizophrenia patients and their relatives. Psychol Med 1999; 29:189..197.

67. Mirsky AF. The Israeli High-Risk Study. In: Dunner DL, Gershon ES, Barrett JE, eds. Relatives at Risk for Mental Disorder. New York: Raven, 1988:279..296.

68. Conklin HM, Curtis CE, Katsanis J, Iacono WG. Verbal working memory impairment in schizophrenia patients and their first-degree relatives: evidence from the digit span task. Am J Psychiatry 2000; 157:275..277.

69. Harvey P, Winters K, Weintraub S, Neale JM. Distractibility in children vulnerable to psychopathology. J Abnorm Psychol 1981; 90:298..304.

70. Cohen J. Statistical power analysis for the behavioral sciences. Hillsdale, NJ: Erlbaum, 1988.

71. Gold JM, Carpenter C, Randolph C, Goldberg TE, Weinberger DR. Auditory working memory and Wisconsin Card Sorting Test performance in schizophrenia. Arch Gen Psychiatry 1997:159..165.

72. Franke P, Gansicke M, Schmitz S, Falkai P, Maier W. Differential memory span abnormal lateralization pattern in schizophrenic patients and their siblings? Int J Psychophysiol 1999; 34:303..311.

73. Staal WG, Hijman R, Pol HEH, Kahn RS. Neuropsychological dysfunctions in siblings discordant for schizophrenia. Psychiatry Res 2000; 95:227..235.

74. Delis D, Kramer J, Kaplan E, Ober B. The California Verbal Learning Test. San Antonio: Psychological Corporation, 1987.
75. Gold JM, Randolph C, Carpenter CJ, Goldberg TE, Weinberger DR. Forms of memory failure in schizophrenia. J Abnorm Psychol 1992; 101:487..494.
76. Wechsler D. Manual for the Wechsler Memory Scale Revised. San Antonio, TX: Psychological Corporation, 1987.
77. Seidman LJ, Faraone SV, Goldstein JM, et al. Left hippocampal volume as a vulnerability indicator for schizophrenia. Arch Gen Psychiatry 2002; 59:839..849.
78. Faraone SV, Seidman LJ, Kremen WS, Toomey R, Pepple JR, Tsuang MT. Neuropsychological functioning among the nonpsychotic relatives of schizophrenic patients: a 4-year follow-up study. J Abnorm Psychol 1999; 108:176..181.
79. Hasher L, Zacks RT. Working memory, comprehension, and aging: a review and new view. In: Bower GH, ed. The Psychology of Learning and Motivation. Vol. 22. New York: Academic, 1988:193..225.
80. D'Esposito M, Postle BR, Ballard D, Lease J. Maintenance versus manipulation of information held in working memory: an event-related fMRI study. Brain Cogn 1999; 41:66..86.
81. D'Esposito M, Postle BR, Jonides J, Smith EE. The neural substrate and temporal dynamics of interference effects in working memory as revealed by event-related functional MRI. Proc Natl Acad Sci USA 1999; 96:7514..7519.
82. McDowell JE, Clementz BA. The effect of fixation condition manipulations on antisaccade performance in schizophrenia: studies of diagnostic specificity. Exp Brain Res 1997; 115: 333..344.
83. McDowell JE, Myles-Worsley M, Coon H, Byerley W, Clementz BA. Measuring liability for schizophrenia using optimized antisaccade stimulus parameters. Psychophysiology 1999; 36:138..141.
84. Crawford TJ, Sharma T, Puri BK, Murray RM, Berridge DM, Lewis SW. Saccadic eye movements in families multiply affected with schizophrenia: the Maudsley Family Study. Am J Psychiatry 1998; 155:1703..1710.
85. Curtis CE, Calkins ME, Grove WM, Feil KJ, Iacono WG. Saccadic disinhibition in patients with acute and remitted schizophrenia and their first-degree biological relatives. Am J Psychiatry 2001; 158:100..106.
86. Burgess PW, Shallice T. Response suppression, initiation and strategy use following frontal lobe lesions. Neuropsychologia 1996; 34:263..272.
87. Schreiber H, Rothmeier J, Becker W, et al. Comparative assessment of saccadic eye movements, psychomotor and cognitive performance in schizophrenics, their first-degree relatives and control subjects. Acta Psychiatr Scand 1995; 91:195..201.
88. Carter CS, Robertson LC, Nordahl TE. Abnormal processing of irrelevant information in chronic schizophrenia: selective enhancement of Stroop facilitation. Psychiatry Res 1992; 41: 137..146.
89. Servan-Schreiber D, Cohen JD, Steingard S. Schizophrenic deficits in the processing of context: a test of a theoretical model. Arch Gen Psychiatry 1996; 53:1105..1112.
90. MacDonald AW, Pogue-Geile MF, Carter C. Differential deficits in selective attention and working memory processes in the siblings of patients with schizophrenia (abstract). Schizophr Res 2001; 49:73.
91. Cohen JD, Servan-Schreiber D. Context, cortex and dopamine. Psychol Rev 1992; 99:45..77.
92. Conners K. Conners' Continuous Performance Test: Manual. New York: Multi-Health Systems, 1992.
93. Wheeler M, Stuss D, Tulving E. Frontal lobe damage produces episodic memory impairment. J Intl Neuropsychol Soc 1995; 1:525..537.

94. Alexander GE, DeLong MR, Strick PL. Parallel organization of functionally segregated circuits linking basal ganglia and cortex. Ann Rev Neurosci 1986; 9:357..381.
95. Goldman-Rakic PS. Circuitry of primate prefrontal cortex and regulation of behavior by representational memory. In: Plum F, Mountcastle V, eds. Handbook of Physiology The Nervous System, Vol. V: Higher Functions of the Brain. Bethesda, MD: American Physiological Society, 1987:373..417.
96. Fuster JM. Memory in the cerebral cortex: an empirical approach to neural networks in the human and nonhuman primate. Cambridge, MA: MIT Press, 1995.
97. Erlenmeyer-Kimling L, Rock D, Roberts SA, et al. Attention, memory, and motor skills as childhood predictors of schizophrenia-related psychoses: the New York high-risk PROJE project. Am J Psychiatry 2000; 157:1416..1422.
98. Kremen WS, Faraone SV, Seidman LJ, Pepple JR, Tsuang MT. Neuropsychological risk indicators for schizophrenia: a preliminary study of female relatives of schizophrenic and bipolar probands. Psychiatry Res 1998; 79:227..240.
99. Seidman LJ, Biederman J, Monuteaux MC, Weber W, Faraone SV. Neuropsychological functioning in nonreferred siblings of children with attention deficit/hyperactivity disorder. J Abnorm Psychol 2000; 109:252..265.
100. Asarnow RF, Nuechterlein KH, Subotnik KL, et al. Neurocognitive impairments in non-psychotic parents of children with schizophrenia and attention-deficit/hyperactivity disorder: the University of California Los Angeles Family Study. Arch Gen Psychiatry 2002; 59:1053..1060.
101. Faraone SV, Kremen WS, Lyons MJ, Pepple JR, Seidman LJ, Tsuang MT. Diagnostic accuracy and linkage analysis: how useful are schizophrenia spectrum phenotypes? Am J Psychiatry 1995; 152:1286..1290.
102. Gottesman II, McGuffin P, Farmer AE. Clinical genetics as clues to the "real" genetics of schizophrenia (a decade of modest gains while playing for time). Schizophr Bull 1987; 13: 23..47.
103. Cornblatt BA, Erlenmeyer-Kimling L. Global attentional deviance as a marker of risk for schizophrenia: specificity and predictive validity. J Abnorm Psychol 1985; 94:470..486.
104. Cornblatt B, Marcuse Y. Children at high risk for schizophrenia: predictions from childhood to adolescence. In: Erlenmeyer-Kimling L, Miller NE, eds. Life-Span Research on the Prediction of Psychopathology. Hillsdale, NJ: Erlbaum, 1986:101..117.
105. Cornblatt B, Obuchowski M, Roberts S, Pollack S, Erlenmeyer-Kimling L. Cognitive and behavioral precursors of schizophrenia. Dev Psychopathol 1999; 11:487..508.
106. Toomey R, Faraone SV, Seidman LJ, Kremen WS, Pepple JR, Tsuang MT. Association of neuropsychological vulnerability markers in relatives of schizophrenic patients. Schizophr Res 1998; 31:89..98.
107. Keefe RS, Silberman JM, Mohs RC, et al. Eye tracking, attention, and schizotypal symptoms in nonpsychotic relatives of patients with schizophrenia. Arch Gen Psychiatry 1997; 54:169..176.
108. Rice JP, McDonald-Scott P, Endicott J, et al. The stability of diagnosis with an application to bipolar II disorder. Psychiatry Res 1986; 19:285..296.
109. Gottesman II, Shields J. Schizophrenia: The Epigenetic Puzzle. Cambridge, England: Cambridge University Press, 1982.
110. Cornblatt BA, Lenzenweger MF, Dworkin RH, Erlenmeyer-Kimling L. Childhood attentional dysfunctions predict social deficits in unaffected adults at risk for schizophrenia. Br J Psychiatry 1992; 161:59..64.
111. Kremen WS, Goldstein JM, Seidman LJ, et al. Sex differences in neuropsychological function in non-psychotic relatives of schizophrenic probands. Psychiatry Res 1997; 66:131..144.

112. Goldstein JM. Gender and the familial transmission of schizophrenia. In: Seeman MV, ed. Gender and Psychopathology. Washington, DC: American Psychiatric, 1995:201..226.
113. Goldstein JM. The impact of gender on understanding the epidemiology of schizophrenia. In: Seeman MV, ed. Gender and Psychopathology. Washington, DC: American Psychiatric, 1995:159..199.
114. Hoff AL, Kremen WS, Wieneke M, et al. Estrogen levels are strongly associated with neuropsychological performance in women with schizophrenia. Am J Psychiatry 2001; 158:1134..1139.
115. Hoff AL, Kremen WS. Sex differences in neurocognitive function in schizophrenia. In: Lewis-Hall F, Williams TS, Panetta JA, Herrera JM, eds. Psychiatric Illness in Women: Emerging Treatments and Research. Washington, DC: American Psychiatric, 2002:215..238.
116. Faraone SV, Seidman LJ, Kremen WS, Toomey R, Lyons MJ, Tsuang MT. Neuropsychological functioning among the elderly nonpsychotic relatives of schizophrenic patients. Schizophr Res 1996; 21:27..31.
117. Nuechterlein KH, Asarnow AF, Jacobson KC, et al. Neurocognitive vulnerability factors in first-degree relatives of schizophrenic probands show accelerated aging effects (abstract). Schizophr Res 2001; 49:117.
118. Harris JG, Adler LE, Young DA, et al. Neuropsychological dysfunction in parents of schizophrenics. Schizophr Res 1996; 20:253..260.
119. Faraone SV, Tsuang D, Tsuang MT. Genetics of Mental Disorders: A Guide for Students, Clinicians, and Researchers. New York: Guilford, 1999.
120. Risch N. Genetic linkage and complex diseases, with special reference to psychiatric disorders. Genet Epidemiol 1990; 7:3..7.
121. Erlenmeyer-Kimling L, Cornblatt BA. A summary of attentional findings in the New York high-risk project. J Psychiatric Res 1992; 26:405..426.
122. Toomey R, Seidman LJ, Lyons MJ, Faraone SV, Tsuang MT. Poor perception of nonverbal social-emotional cues in relatives of schizophrenic patients. Schizophr Res 1999; 40:121..130.
123. Mueser KT, Gingerich SL, Rosenthal CK. Educational Family Therapy for schizophrenia: a new treatment model for clinical service and research. Schizophr Res 1994; 13:99..107.
124. Liberman RP, Kopelowicz A. Basic elements in biobehavioral treatment and rehabilitation of schizophrenia. Int Clin Psychopharmacol 1995; 9(Suppl 5):51..58.
125. Hoff AL. Neuropsychological function in schizophrenia. In: Shriqui CL, Nasrallah HA, eds. Contemporary Issues in the Treatment of Schizophrenia. Washington, DC: American Psychiatric, 1995:187..208.
126. Condray R, Steinhauer SR, Goldstein G. Language comprehension in schizophrenics and their brothers. Biol Psychiatry 1992; 32:790..802.
127. Docherty NM, Gordinier SW, Hall MJ, Cutting LP. Communication disturbances in relatives beyond the age of risk for schizophrenia and their associations with symptoms in patients. Schizophr Bull 1999; 25:851..862.
128. Shenton ME, Solovay MR, Holzman PS, Coleman M, Gale HJ. Thought disorder in the relatives of psychotic patients. Arch Gen Psychiatry 1989; 46:897..901.
129. Tsuang MR, Stone WS, Seidman LJ, et al. Treatment of nonpsychotic relatives of patients with schizophrenia: four case studies. Biol Psychiatry 1999; 45:1412..1418.

8   The Nature and Origin of Socioemotional Deficits in Schizophrenia

Elaine Walker, PhD
and Karen M. Hochman, MD

SUMMARY

Social and emotional behavior abnormalities are defining features of schizophrenia. They are also among the most debilitating symptoms of the illness, with implications for the patient's ability to form and maintain relationships. At the same time, socioemotional deficits may provide clues about the neuropathophysiology of schizophrenia, and aid in the identification of persons at heightened risk of succumbing to the illness. This chapter examines multiple facets of socioemotional deficits in schizophrenia, with an emphasis on the developmental course. There is now a large body of research documenting premorbid deficits in social behavior in schizophrenia patients. Present in subtle forms in early infancy, they are amplified as maturation proceeds, and become marked in adolescence. With the onset of the prodromal phase, socioemotional deficits worsen. Evidence from neuroimaging research, and other sources, indicates that abnormalities in limbic-cortical circuitry may subserve these deficits. Differences between males and females in the maturation of limbic-cortical brain circuits might play a role in the sex differences observed in the premorbid course of schizophrenia.

INTRODUCTION

One of the most consistent findings in the literature on schizophrenia is that the social networks of schizophrenia patients are significantly smaller than those of healthy individuals (1). Furthermore, as is the case with many other illnesses,

From: *Early Clinical Intervention and Prevention in Schizophrenia*
Edited by: W. S. Stone, S. V. Faraone, and M. T. Tsuang © Humana Press Inc., Totowa, NJ

the prognosis is better for patients with larger social networks. Schizophrenia inpatients who have regular contact with family and/or friends are less likely to be rehospitalized (1). For first-episode patients, the availability of social support predicts outcome 5 years later (2). But is the reduction in social networks a cause of the illness, a consequence of illness, or a component of the illness? A neuroimaging study found that patients with fewer social relationships tend to have larger brain ventricles (3). Other investigators have reported that enlarged ventricles are linked with poor social competence (4). These findings suggest that social deficits are linked with the biological vulnerability to schizophrenia.

For most people who succumb to schizophrenia, the clinical symptoms of the disorder are preceded by a variety of deficits. Impairments in socioemotional behavior are arguably the most pronounced and chronic of these. As early as infancy, many preschizophrenic children manifest subtle abnormalities in facial expressions of emotion. During adolescence, interpersonal problems are often reflected in a failure to form typical peer relationships and romantic attachments. Throughout adult life, social deficits persist, and few patients marry or establish their own nuclear families.

Researchers have been interested in socioemotional impairment in schizophrenia for several reasons. First, interpersonal deficits seem to be a key feature of the illness, and understanding the nature and origins of these deficits may help to elucidate the etiology of schizophrenia. Second, social deficits are often a major impediment to treatment, rehabilitation, and quality of life. Patients who are unable or unwilling to engage in interpersonal interactions have difficulty in family, educational, and work settings. Social-skills deficits also contribute to stigma and social rejection (5,6). Third, as interest in the prevention of schizophrenia has grown, investigators have begun to focus on social impairment as a key prodromal indicator of vulnerability.

In this chapter, we examine the nature and course of socioemotional deficits throughout the life span of schizophrenia patients. We review a range of such deficits, from abnormalities in the nonverbal expression of emotion to developmental changes in social behavior. Sex differences are apparent in many of these domains, and they are also described. We then turn briefly to the question of the origins of social deficits in schizophrenia. What is the source of these problems? Are they directly linked with congenital liability and/or brain dysfunction? It is also possible that social impairments in schizophrenia are secondary to other, more basic deficits. They may be a consequence of generalized cognitive deficits, such as attentional dysfunction or abnormalities in abstract thinking (e.g., deficits in "theory of mind"). Finally, they may simply be "epiphenomena" a side effect of treatment or a reflection of the patient's withdrawal from social interactions due to the illness. We revisit these alternatives following a review of the empirical literature.

NONVERBAL SOCIAL DEFICITS

Expressing Emotion

Abnormalities in the expression or *encoding* of emotion are a defining feature of schizophrenia. Flat or inappropriate facial expressions of emotion are considered major characteristic signs of the disorder. It is obvious that such deficits can have considerable implications for the individual's social experiences. Facial expressions of emotion convey important information in interactions among human beings. If an individual's social displays are aberrant, others may avoid them or misread their intentions. Researchers have systematically explored the extent and correlates of these expressive deficits in schizophrenia.

In general, the results of empirical research confirm that schizophrenia patients differ from controls in the encoding of facial emotion. When compared to controls, patients show fewer positive and more negative facial expressions of emotion *(7, 8)*. They also show less intense emotional expressions when compared to healthy controls and patients suffering from depression *(9,10)*. As would be expected, less intense facial expressions of emotion are linked with social-functioning impairments *(7)*.

However, a reduction in the intensity of facial emotion does not necessarily reflect less intense subjective experience on the part of patients. When schizophrenia patients are asked to produce facial expressions of specific emotions, such as sadness, fear, or happiness, they report subjective emotional experiences consistent with the facial emotion they are attempting to produce *(11)*. Furthermore, although they show less intense facial emotion than normals when viewing emotional films, they report subjective emotional experiences similar to normal controls, and they show *more pronounced* skin conductance responses to the films *(12)*. A recent study of facial muscle movement yielded further support for the assumption that there is no reduction in patients' subjective emotional experiences *(13)*. When normal subjects view facial expressions of emotion they manifest simultaneous movement in their own facial muscles, suggesting a subjective emotional reaction to the stimuli. Kring and colleagues found that schizophrenia patients actually show more pronounced facial muscle movement than normal subjects. Another intriguing aspect of nonverbal communication in schizophrenia is the dissociation between the various channels of emotional expression. For example, unlike normals and depressed patients, schizophrenia patients manifest inconsistencies between the facial and verbal aspects of their emotional expression *(14,15)*. Taken together, these findings suggest the associations among internal states and various external manifestations of emotion are weaker for schizophrenia patients. Again, given the pivotal role that nonverbal communication plays in social interaction, inconsistencies among channels of nonverbal expression would produce discomfort in interpersonal exchanges.

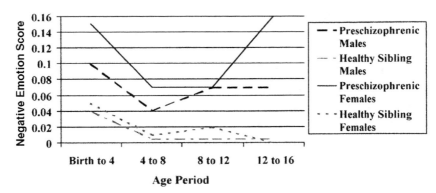

Fig. 1. Proportion of negative emotional expressions by age, sex, and diagnostic group. Modified from ref. *17*.

It appears that abnormalities in facial emotion are not secondary to the clinical syndrome of schizophrenia, rather they predate the onset of the illness. One prospective study revealed that preadolescent children at genetic risk for schizophrenia (offspring of schizophrenia parents) show less smiling and more blunted affect than offspring of healthy parents *(16)*. In a follow-back study of schizophrenia patients, Walker and colleagues found that facial expression deficits were detected as early as infancy *(17)*. By studying childhood home movies of adult-onset schizophrenia patients, these researchers found lower rates of positive affect displays and higher rates of negative affect. Both male and female preschizophrenic subjects showed more negative affect than their healthy siblings. This diagnostic group difference in negative emotion is illustrated in Fig. 1.

The study also showed sex differences in the positive facial expressions of preschizophrenic children: analyses revealed lower proportions of joy expressions among the preschizophrenic females when compared to same-sex healthy siblings. Among males, there were no significant diagnostic group differences in the expression of joy. Overall, when contrasted with healthy siblings, diagnostic group differences extended from infancy through childhood. Thus, emotional expression deficits may be linked with the congenital vulnerability to schizophrenia. Consistent with this assumption, when the relation between childhood facial displays and adult brain morphology was examined, the investigators found that higher rates of negative affect in early childhood were associated with greater ventricular enlargement in adulthood *(18)*.

Recognizing Emotion

The facial expression deficits associated with schizophrenia would certainly be expected to have implications for the ability of patients to accurately convey

their subjective emotional states and impede social interactions. Combined with this, numerous studies have demonstrated that schizophrenia patients are impaired in the identification, or *decoding*, of posed facial expressions of emotion, especially negative emotions (19,20). The deficit appears to be unrelated to medication (21), and is apparent in children with schizophrenia (20), as well as individuals with schizotypal personality disorder (21).

However, posed facial expressions may not have contextual validity; it is possible that they do not convey emotional information in the same way as genuine facial expressions. One recent investigation examined the ability of patients to identify both posed and genuine facial expressions and indicated that the deficit was restricted to the posed expressions (22). In fact, these investigators found that paranoid schizophrenia patients were better than normal controls in deciphering genuine facial expressions. We are not aware of any other study that has examined the ability of schizophrenia patients to identify genuine facial expressions of emotion, so this is an important issue to pursue in future research.

Another point of controversy in the literature on emotion recognition in schizophrenia concerns the extent to which the impairment is reflective of a generalized performance deficit, as opposed to a deficit that is specific to the recognition of nonverbal cues of emotion. Researchers have attempted to address this issue by administering "control" tasks that involve extracting nonemotional visual information from facial and nonfacial stimuli. The results have been mixed, with some concluding that the deficit is more pronounced for the decoding of emotional information (23,24), and others concluding that it is a nonspecific impairment (22,25). Nonetheless, it has been shown that patients' scores on certain measures of visual attention (e.g., the span of apprehension test) are correlated with performance on emotion perception tasks, indicating that emotion recognition deficits in schizophrenia are partially determined by attentional problems (26,27).

The debate about the specificity of emotion recognition deficits in schizophrenia is likely to persist until more effective psychometric approaches for establishing "task-specific" deficits are established. However, whether general or specific, the deficit would likely have ramifications for interpersonal functioning, independent of its origins. This assumption received support from studies that have found an association between recognition deficits and social functioning. Kohler and colleagues (28) showed that problems with facial emotion recognition, but not age recognition, were related to greater severity of negative and positive symptoms, as well as attention, verbal and spatial memory, and language deficits. In healthy controls, emotion recognition was not correlated with cognitive functions. Similarly, emotion recogntion deficits are associated with social incompetence and greater illness chronicity among schizophrenia patients (29).

It is of interest to note that studies examining both emotion recognition and expression in schizophrenia show little relation between the two (30,31). This

tentatively suggests that expression and recognition abilities are subserved by different mechanisms. Further research is needed to elucidate the relation between emotion encoding and decoding in both clinical populations and normals.

SOCIAL COGNITION

The ability to reason correctly about the meaning and consequences of social exchanges is another critical skill in social interaction. This is the essence of social cognition. Researchers who study social behavior in normal subjects have demonstrated that social cognitive ability is predictive of social adjustment. Given the clinical phenomenology of schizophrenia, it is not surprising that the illness is linked with sociocognitive impairments (32–34). Moreover, deficiencies in the ability to reason about social problems have implications for overt behavior (35). Using a battery of tasks measuring various facets of social cognition, Penn and colleagues found a significant association with the behavior of schizophrenia inpatients. Those with better sociocognitive skills were less behaviorally impaired. Moreover, this association held even when general cognitive ability was statistically controlled.

What is the origin of sociocognitive deficits? It appears that they may be partially determined by more general deficits in cognitive ability. Verbal expression ability, verbal memory, and vigilance are significant predictors of social problem solving in schizophrenia patients (36,37). Systematic interventions aimed at remediating these general cognitive deficits can improve sociocognitive abilities in schizophrenia patients. Corrigan, Hirshbeck and Wolfe (38) found that interventions aimed at improving memory and vigilance resulted in significant improvements in patients' ability to recognize nonverbal social cues. But it is important to note that sociocognitive deficits are not solely attributable to problems with basic cognitive processes, as the correlations are of moderate magnitude.

The phrase "theory of mind" has been used to refer to an individual's understanding of the independent and subjective mental activity of other persons, and ability to accurately infer others' intentions. Not typically measured in studies of social cognition, interest in theory of mind first arose in the field of autism research. More recently researchers have explored theory of mind in schizophrenia patients. The method of assessment involves the presentation of vignettes where a situation is described in which the knowledge or perspective one of the characters differs from the listener. The subject is asked to answer questions that require accurate inferences about the character's understanding of the situation. Schizophrenia patients have considerable difficulty with theory-of-mind tasks (39,40). Although the correlates of this deficit have not been identified, studies of the prodromal period, described later, indicate that it may be present prior to the onset of the clinical disorder.

THE DEVELOPMENTAL COURSE

Social Behavioral Precursors to Schizophrenia in Childhood and Adolescence

In order to study the behavioral precursors of schizophrenia, investigators have employed several methods, each of which has its own methodological limitations. *Retrospective studies* rely on the patient's and family's retrospective accounts of the behaviors preceding the onset of psychosis. Biased recall can be problematic with this method. *Follow-up studies* ascertain the outcome of individuals who either were the subject of previous research, or were treated in a clinical setting for adjustment problems. *Follow-back studies* look at the previous academic and/or medical records of adult subjects who have a diagnosis of schizophrenia. The usefulness of these studies is limited by the availability of archival sources of data (which are often incomplete or unavailable). On the other hand, the strength in this kind of study lies in the generalizability of the findings.

High-risk studies are prospective in nature, and follow individuals deemed to be at elevated risk of developing a psychotic disorder. High-risk criteria may include a family history of mental illness, and/or behavioral characteristics. A weakness of the former kind of study lies in its lack of generalizability; that is, most people with schizophrenia do not have a positive family history. In addition, many high-risk studies have not followed their cohorts through the entire risk period for schizophrenia. Losses to follow-up can be significant in this kind of research.

When examining the literature on behavioral precursors to schizophrenia during childhood and adolescence, it is important to recognize, first of all, that behavioral precursors are not universally present in people who will go on to develop the disorder. Thus the positive predictive value of social/behavioral abnormalities may be modest, depending on when the subjects are assessed *(41–43)*. Second, the behavioral precursors that have been documented in schizophrenia are not specific to the disorder. Rather, they are also present in some individuals who will go on to develop affective psychosis, other disorders, or no disorder. However, the severity of premorbid social problems tends to be greater for those who will later develop schizophrenia *(44)*. Also, predictive power increases with age, such that the divergence between preschizophrenic children and those with healthy adult outcomes is greatest in late adolescence.

Empirical data on the childhood and adolescent behavior of patients with adult-onset schizophrenia come from several sources, with parent and teacher reports being the two primary sources. Because parents are with their children in a variety of settings, they may have the opportunity to observe behavioral phenomena that would go undetected at school. But the parental reports used in research on premorbid behavior are more often retrospective in nature, and may, therefore, be

influenced by knowledge of the individual's psychiatric outcome. Behavioral observations of teachers are usually obtained from records that were established prior to the illness onset, and are thus not subject to retrospective bias.

In 1969, Offord and Cross published a comprehensive review of research on the childhood precursors of schizophrenia. The review left little doubt that many parents of patients with adult-onset schizophrenia recalled an elevated rate of childhood behavioral problems. More specifically, when they were asked to compare the child who eventually succumbed to a mental illness to his or her healthy siblings, parents tended to recall more adjustment problems in those who later developed a disorder. The rate of adjustment problems increased with age.

More recent studies of parents' perceptions of their preschizophrenic child have utilized standardized child behavior rating scales that cover a broad range of behaviors *(45–47)*. Consistent with earlier results, the findings indicate that a variety of behavioral problems precede the onset of schizophrenia, including anxiety, depression, thought abnormalities, attention problems, delinquent behavior, aggressive behavior, social withdrawal, and interpersonal problems. The developmental trajectories of these behavioral precursors vary; for example, attention problems are elevated from early childhood, whereas thought abnormalities do not distinguish the preschizophrenic children from controls until early adolescence. Also, according to parents, social problems are apparent throughout childhood, but become more severe in the teenage years. The developmental trajectory for social problems in preschizophrenic children is shown in Fig. 2.

The validity of these retrospective parental accounts is supported by evidence from studies that utilize parent ratings obtained *prior* to the onset of the child's illness. A prospective study conducted by Jones et al. *(48)* focused on preschizophrenic youth who had participated in a longitudinal investigation of a cohort of 13,687 individuals born in the United Kingdom in 1946. Parents reported that preschizophrenic subjects had a preference for solitary play at ages 4 and 6. These investigators also examined self-report measures, and found that at age 13 years the preschizophrenic youth reported feeling less socially confident than controls.

The trends revealed in parental reports converge with those based on teacher ratings. In a study based on the Danish high-risk project, Olin and Mednick *(49)* found that teachers more often judged students who later developed schizophrenia to be •emotionally labile and vulnerable to future psychotic breakdown'. Boys who went on to develop schizophrenia were more likely to be rated as •exhibiting disruptive classroom behavior'. They were also described as having disciplinary problems, anxiety, suffering from rejection by peers, and to have repeated a school year. The girls who subsequently developed schizophrenia were more likely to be nervous and withdrawn. For both sexes, the adjustment problems were greater in older children. Furthermore, among the group who went on to develop schizophrenia, teacher ratings predicted prognosis for both sexes *(50)*.

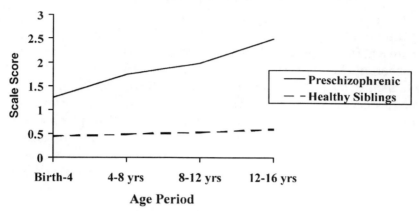

Fig. 2. Social Problem scale scores by age and diagnostic group. Data from studies by Baum et al. *(45)* and Walker et al. *(46)*.

In a later study from this high-risk project, Olin and colleagues *(50,51)* looked at childhood behavioral differences among preschizophrenics, those with healthy adult outcomes, and those later diagnosed with schizotypal personality disorder (SPD), or nonpsychotic mental illnesses. The investigators found that 75% of pre-schizotypal subjects exhibited classroom behaviors that distinguished them from other children. The children who subsequently developed SPD were more passive, socially unengaged, and hypersensitive to criticism. The premorbid behavioral factors that distinguished SPD from schizophrenia varied by gender. Males who went on to develop schizophrenia were more disruptive and excitable than males who were later diagnosed with SPD, but premorbid behavior did not differentiate girls who later developed schizophrenia vs SPD.

Other studies of the offspring of schizophrenic parents have yielded similar findings. The Israeli high-risk study showed that children at risk for schizophrenia manifest an elevated rate of interpersonal problems, particularly social withdrawal, during middle childhood and adolescence *(52)*. The risk for such problems was greater for male offspring, and was associated with motoric soft signs.

The findings from follow-back studies of schizophrenia patients mirror the results from the high-risk prospective studies. In the 1970s, Watt and colleagues *(53)* obtained the school records of adult schizophrenia patients and examined teachers' comments. The results indicated that preschizophrenic girls differed from same-sex controls beginning in the early elementary years, and were perceived as shy and withdrawn by their teachers. In contrast, preschizophrenic boys were described as disruptive and emotionally labile.

Jones et al. *(48)* examined teacher ratings of the preschizophrenic youth who had participated in a longitudinal study of 13,687 individuals born in the United Kingdom in 1946. They reported that at ages 13 and 15 years, these children

displayed more solitary and anxious behaviors (e.g., "timid in class," "avoids competition and rough games," "frequently day dreams in class"). Using a similar approach, Done et al. *(54)* obtained information on adult psychiatric outcome for a cohort of children who were born in March 1958 and then followed for a longitudinal study of development. They found that preschizophrenic children of both genders were rated by their teachers as having displayed socially maladaptive behavior. There were gender differences, however, with preschizophrenic boys manifesting more overreactive behavior than same-sex controls at ages 7 and 11 years. Among the girls, there were no diagnostic group differences at 7 years, but by the age of 11 preschizophrenic girls were rated by their teachers as underreactive, particularly as more withdrawn and depressed.

In summary, information drawn from a variety of sources provides converging support for significant deficits in the social behavior of children who later develop schizophrenia. These deficits vary in nature and severity by sex, and appear to become more pronounced as development proceeds, with adolescence being a particularly critical period for the emergence of problems. The fact that both parent and teacher ratings of childhood behavior are predictive of adult-onset schizophrenia suggests that they may have the potential to become a practical and inexpensive adjunctive tool for identifying individuals likely to develop psychotic disorders.

It is also noteworthy that there is reason to believe that the childhood behavioral precursors of schizophrenia are linked with congenital brain abnormalities. As mentioned, preschizophrenic infants who show more negative affect have greater ventricular enlargement in adulthood. Along these same lines, in the Danish study of high-risk children, reductions in behavioral responsivity in infancy were related to enlargement of the third ventricle in adulthood *(55)*. Thus the early premorbid social deficits observed in schizophrenia may be a consequence of brain dysfunction that is present at birth, although not detected until adulthood.

THE PSYCHOTIC PRODROME

There is certainly overwhelming evidence that many individuals who succumb to schizophrenia manifest various signs of impairment in social functioning during childhood. Subtle signs of emotional deficit may be apparent in infancy, and impaired social functioning becomes more pronounced as the individual passes through childhood and into adolescence. For many patients, the entry into adolescence is accompanied by a marked rise in adjustment problems, including difficulties with family and peers. These problems typically spiral into a subclinical syndrome as the first psychotic episode approaches.

The prodromal period is defined as the phase immediately preceding the onset of psychosis, where the first nonspecific indicators of the active illness become

evident. Of course *prodrome* is a retrospective concept. That is, one can only say with certainty that an individual's nonspecific neurotic and attenuated psychotic symptoms are the •prodrome' to a psychotic illness *after* the definitive characteristics of the disorder are present. As defined by the *DSM*, the prodrome includes deficits in social functioning and affective abnormalities, as well as unusual perceptual experiences and ideas. In many cases, the prodrome continues until the eruption of the psychotic syndrome. But at times the first prodromal phase may decrease in intensity, and thus not lead directly into clinical schizophrenia. In these cases, the prodromal syndrome is designated an "outpost" syndrome ("Vorpost Syndrome"). It appears that the outpost syndrome occurs in about half of schizophrenic patients, on average 10 years prior to the clinical onset of the illness *(56)*.

In a retrospective study of prodromal signs in first-episode psychosis patients, Yung and McGorry *(57)* found a broad range of indicators. The pattern and sequence of phenomena described varied, but most often consisted of initial nonspecific •neurotic' symptoms, with symptoms gradually becoming more deviant, and then evolving into psychosis. Many patients described reactive symptoms such as feeling depressed, anxious, or confused about internal and perceptual changes. Thus, prodromal features were reported in this study as consisting mainly of attenuated psychotic symptoms, nonspecific neurotic and mood-related symptoms, and behavioral changes, frequently in response to other experiential phenomena.

A more recent retrospective study of •the psychotic prodrome' in first-episode psychotic patients obtained information from multiple sources *(58)*. In this series of 19 patients, diagnosed with schizophrenia by *DSM–IV* criteria, prodromal phenomena were explored in depth using both patients and family members as informants. In addition, data were obtained from medical records. Repeated, open-ended interviews were conducted with subjects and family members, within 2 years of the initiation of the first treatment. Clinical diagnoses were made by structured clinical interview and consensus among clinicians. Diagnoses were reviewed and confirmed 1 . 2.5 years later by the current therapist and main researcher. The results indicated that *all* of the subjects (with a diagnosis of schizophrenia or schizoaffective disorder) had experienced a prodrome, ranging from 1 week to more than 11 years in duration (with a median duration of 50 weeks). Behavioral observations reported by family members included withdrawal from school or work, change of interests, and social passivity, withdrawal, or isolation. Distinct qualitative changes in subjective experience were reported long before behavioral consequences created serious family concern. Furthermore, most patients described serious difficulty with interpreting and communicating their early experiential changes. Among the changes reported by patients were a compromised capacity for self-observation and mental control, lack of adequate concepts and words to describe experiences, the perception of an unreal/strange self resulting in social/ emotional withdrawal, fear induced by confusing experiences, overvalued ideas

interfering with the •will' to communicate experiences, and preoccupation with overvalued ideas, which made social participation and communication unimportant. Given such experiences, it seems likely that these patients would have also manifested deficits in theory of mind during the prodromal period.

Of course, gender differences in the age of onset of schizophrenia have been consistently reported (59). Women tend to be diagnosed with the illness, on average, 3. 4 years later than men. In keeping with this, men also have a younger age of first hospitalization. These, and other findings, have led to the hypothesis that estrogen protects neural circuits in various ways and delays the onset of psychosis in predisposed individuals. In contrast, findings from a recent study suggest that there are no sex differences in the timing of the onset of the prodrome. Cohen, Gotowiec, and Seeman (60) examined the relative duration of the prepsychotic prodrome for male and female patients using an •Interview for the Retrospective Assessment of the Onset of Schizophrenia'. Time of first treatment was determined by hospital record. The first sign of behavioral disturbance occurred at approximately the same age in women and men (18.5..19.8 years). But the psychotic prodrome was almost twice as long for women as for men (7.1 vs 3.9 years). The duration of untreated psychosis did not differ between the sexes, and substance abuse did not influence the sex difference in the prepsychotic phase.

The Origins of Social Impairment in Schizophrenia

The evidence of social impairment in schizophrenia is extensive. Early in life it is manifested in subtle abnormalities in emotional expression. As development proceeds, it becomes increasingly apparent in interactions with family members and peers. We now turn to the question of its origins. We know that brain injury can result in profound changes in social and interpersonal behavior (61). Contemporary neuroimaging procedures are contributing to our understanding of the neural substrates of more subtle individual differences in socioemotional information processing.

Findings from functional neuroimaging show that the amygdala, and the circuits that link it with frontal and temporal regions, play an important role in facial emotion processing in normal subjects, both adults and children (62). In a functional magnetic resonance imaging (fMRI) study of facial emotion processing, researchers found that it was accompanied by increased activity in the temporal and hippocampal regions, amygdalohippocampal junction, and pulvinar nucleus (63). Requiring conscious (explicit) attention to the emotional features of the face evoked more activity in the temporal lobe, but when subjects were not instructed to attend to the emotion on the face, there was relatively greater activity in the amygdala region. The authors concluded that facial expressions are processed within the amygdalohippocampal complex, temporal lobe, visual cortex, and thalamus. Other studies have also yielded evidence that the amygdala and hippocampus are

implicated in the processing of emotional stimuli *(33,64,65)*. The medial frontal cortex appears to be involved when higher level processing of affective meaning is required *(61)*.

More recently, studies of the neural basis of emotion processing in clinical populations have been undertaken. This research has potential for elucidating the brain abnormalities that underlay the socioemotional deficits in psychiatric disorders. For example, autism appears to be linked with an abnormality in the neural basis of facial emotion processing. When compared to controls, subjects with autism show less activation of the cortical face processing areas while explicitly appraising expressions, and reduced activity in the left amygdala region when implicitly processing emotional facial expressions *(66)*.

To date, there have been only three published neuroimaging studies of socioemotional processes in schizophrenia, but the results are consistent in showing abnormalities in patterns of regional brain activity. In a study by Russell and colleagues *(65)*, mean brain activation in patients with schizophrenia was compared to that in normals during performance of a task involving attribution of mental state. The patients made more errors on the mental state attribution task, and showed less activity in the left frontal region while performing the task. Thus, deficits in higher level sociocognition in schizophrenia may result from frontal dysfunction.

Decreased activation of the amygdala may be implicated in the facial expression *encoding* deficits observed in schizophrenia. Using a mood induction task, Schneider and colleagues found that normals showed increased brain activity in the amygdala during negative affect induction, which is in line with previous neuroimaging findings *(67)*. In contrast, schizophrenia patients did not demonstrate amygdala activation, despite the fact that they indicated subjective feelings of negative mood similar to normal controls.

Schizophrenia patients also manifest abnormal patterns of brain activity when processing, or *decoding*, facial expressions of emotion. An fMRI study of brain activity in response to negative facial emotions revealed that patients showed less brain activation to these stimuli than normals *(68)*. Nonparanoid patients showed the greatest performance deficits and failed to activate neural regions that are normally linked with emotion recognition. Furthermore, they mislabeled disgust as either anger or fear more frequently than paranoids, and in response to disgust expressions showed greater activation in the amygdala, a region typically activated more by the perception of fearful faces.

It is obvious that the advent of functional neuroimaging has just recently set the stage for understanding of the origins of social deficits in schizophrenia. Nonetheless, extant data on brain dysfunction in schizophrenia provide a basis for generating hypotheses about the neural substrates that might play a role in the social impairment associated with the illness. Functional imaging studies of resting and task-related brain activity have generally revealed significant reductions in frontal

activity *(69–72)*, although some have reported abnormally heightened frontal activity under certain conditions *(69)*. Other findings suggest that hypofrontality may be task-specific. The processing of novel stimuli by schizophrenia patients results in less activity, compared to normals, in the thalamus and prefrontal cortex, whereas the recognition of previously presented visual stimuli results in increased prefrontal cortical activation in patients *(71,72)*.

Furthermore, the tendency toward frontal hypoactivity in schizophrenia may be especially pronounced in patients with the deficit syndrome *(72)*. Heckers and colleagues found that, during attempts to retrieve poorly encoded words, patients with the deficit syndrome recruited the frontal cortex significantly less than did patients without the deficit syndrome. When compared to normals, both schizophrenia subtypes showed an attenuation of activity in the hippocampus during memory retrieval.

In summary, studies of normal subjects have confirmed that the limbic regions, including the amygdala and hippocampus, as well as the prefrontal cortex, are activated in response to socioemotional stimuli. These brain regions, and the circuit that connect them, are known to undergo a protracted developmental course that extends into young adulthood *(73,74)*. Neuroimaging studies indicate that schizophrenia is associated with abnormalities in the activation of limbic and prefrontal cortical regions. Some of these areas, particularly the hippocampus, play a role in general cognitive processes, especially memory. Others are more specifically implicated in processing emotionally salient stimuli.

The fact that preschizophrenic infants differ from controls in facial expressions of emotion and general responsivity suggests that limbic system dysfunction is congenital in schizophrenia patients. Further evidence supporting this assumption is provided by studies that show a relation between these early behavioral signs and ventricular enlargement in brain scans conducted on the same patients in adulthood. Assuming that ventricular enlargement is a nonspecific indicator of abnormalities in periventricular brain regions, the findings are consistent with the notion that an abnormality in limbic-cortical circuitry is present at birth.

Abnormalities in limbic-cortical circuitry could arise from prenatal insult or from a genetic liability. Recent advances have been made in the identification of genotypes associated with disorders that affect socioemotional behavior. For example, the 22q deletion is a genetic mutation known to be linked with physical anomalies (the Velo-Cardio-Facial syndrome), brain abnormalities, and behavioral signs *(75,76)*. The behavioral deficits range from mild to severe, and include deficits in cognitive and social functions, and in some cases clinical schizophrenia. The characteristic social deficits are manifested in comprehending nonverbal social cues and awkwardness in initiating social interaction *(76)*. The rate of 22q deletion in schizophrenia patients is estimated to be about 2%. The fact that this genetic mutation produces brain abnormalities, as well as a characteristic

sociobehavioral syndrome, suggests the possibility that the social deficits observed in schizophrenia are a relatively direct manifestation of the specific neuropathology underlying the disorder.

Although brain abnormalities may be congenital, ensuing neuromaturational processes subsequently modulate the behavioral expression of the abnormality. The developmental literature on social aspects of premorbid behavior in schizophrenia suggests that deficits in interpersonal functions become more pronounced with age. The onset of adolescence is an especially critical period, with a marked increase in behavioral dysfunction. During the prodromal period, which typically has its onset in late adolescence/early adulthood, socioemotional deficits become more pronounced, signaling the impending onset of the clinical syndrome. It is plausible that this developmental trajectory is determined by neuromaturational processes that are taking place in the limbic-cortical circuitry that is pivotal in socioemotional maturation. Thus congenital abnormalities in limbic-cortical circuitry that gave rise to more subtle behavioral deficits in the early childhood of schizophrenia patients may have more devastating implications for behavior in young adulthood.

As mentioned, there is substantial evidence of sex differences in premorbid behavior, with females manifesting less pronounced deficits than males. It is possible that these differences are a consequence of the effects of gonadal hormones on the pace of limbic system maturation. For example, estrogen may serve to enhance the process of limbic maturation, and thereby mitigate dysfunction of limbic-cortical circuitry (73,74). Alternatively, testosterone might hasten the maturational process in these brain regions.

CONCLUSIONS

Socioemotional impairments in schizophrenia are not solely epiphenomenal consequence of the illness. Although suffering from such a devastating illness may lead to despair and social withdrawal, research has clearly demonstrated that the roots of social dysfunction are present early in life. Thus, socioemotional deficits are a key feature of the illness. They hold information about the neural substrate of schizophrenia, and may also have important implications for prevention and treatment.

The identification of the antecedents of psychotic disorders is of great importance. This is because schizophrenia and other psychotic disorders are associated with profound personal suffering, increased morbidity and mortality rates, significant functional impairment, and high direct and indirect costs to society. The suggested relationship between early treatment for psychosis and improved prognosis has made the notion of prevention before the onset of actual psychotic symptoms an area of considerable scientific interest (57). Investigations are under way in

North America, and abroad, with the aim of identifying trait and state risk factors that are associated with a heightened risk for the development of psychosis. It is likely that the identification of individuals at risk will ultimately be based on multiple indicators. The combination of behavioral signs with biological measures may prove to be optimal.

REFERENCES

1. Beels CC. Social support and schizophrenia. Schizophr Bull 1981; 7:58..72.
2. Erickson DH, Beiser M, Iacono WG. Social support predict 5-year outcome in 1st-episode schizophrenia. J Abnorm Psychol 1998; 107:681..685.
3. Seidman L, Sokolove RL, McElroy C, et al. Lateral ventricular size and social network differentiation in young, nonchronic schizophrenic patients. Am J Psychiatry 1987; 144:512..514.
4. Owens D. Lateral ventricular size in schizophrenia: relationship to the disease process and its clinical manifestations. Psychol Med 1985; 15:27..41.
5. Boecker F. Social integration and contact with people in the normal social environment during treatment in a psychiatric hospital: a follow-up of first-admission inpatients with schizophrenia and affective disorders. Eur Arch Psychiatry Neurol Sci 1984; 234:250..257.
6. Penn D, Kohlmaier JR., Corrigan PW. Interpersonal factors contributing to the stigma of schizophrenia: social skills, perceived attractiveness, and symptoms. Schizophr Res 2000; 45:37..45.
7. Brozgold A, Borod JC, Martin CC, Pick LH, Alpert M, Welkowitz J. Social functioning and facial emotional expression in neurological and psychiatric disorders. App Neuropsychol 1998; 5:15..23.
8. Martin C, Borod JC, Alpert M, et al. Spontaneous expression of facial emotion in schizophrenic and right-brain-damaged patients. J Comm Dis 1990; 23:287..301.
9. Berenbaum H, Oltmanns TF. Emotional experience and expression in schizophrenia and depression. In: Ekman ELR, ed. What the Face Reveals: Basic and Applied Studies of Spontaneous Expression Using the Facial Action Coding System (FACS). Series in affective science. New York: Oxford University Press, 1997:343..360.
10. Yecker S, Borod JC, Brozgold A, Martin C, Alpert M, Welkowitz, J. Lateralization of facial emotional expression in schizophrenic and depressed patients. J Neuropsychia Clin Neurosci 1999; 11:370..379.
11. Flack WJ, Laird JD, Cavallaro, LA. Emotional expression and feeling in schizophrenia: effects of specific expressive behaviors on emotional experiences. J Clin Psychol 1999; 55:1..20.
12. Kring A, Neale JM. Do schizophrenic patients show a disjunctive relationship among expressive, experiential, and psychophysiological components of emotion? J Abnorm Psychol 1996; 105:249..257.
13. Kring A, Kerr SL, Earnst KS. Schizophrenic patients show facial reactions to emotional facial expressions. Psychophysiology 1999; 36:186..192.
14. Ellgring, H. Nonverbal expression of psychological states in psychiatric patients. In Ekman ELR ed. What the Face Reveals: Basic and Applied Studies of Spontaneous Expression Using the Facial Action Coding System (FACS). Series in affective science. New York: Oxford University Press, 1997:386..397.
15. Ellgring H. Nonverbal expression of psychological studies in psychiatric patients. Eur Arch Psychiatry Neurol Sci 1986; 236:31..34.
16. Dworkin RH, Cornblatt BA, Friedmann R, et al. Childhood precursors of affective vs. social deficits in adolescents at risk for schizophrenia. Schizophr Bull 1993; 19:563..577.

17. Walker E, Grimes K, Davis D, Smith, D. Childhood precursors of schizophrenia: facial expressions of emotion. Am J Psychiatry 1993; 150:1654..1660.
18. Walker EF, Lewine RRJ, Neumann C. Childhood behavioral characteristics and adult brain morphology in schizophrenia. Schizophr Res 1996; 22:93..101.
19. Mandal M, Jain HNS, Weiss U, Schneider F. Generality and specificity of emotion-recognition deficit in schizophrenic patients with positive and negative symptoms. Psychiatry Res 1999; 87:39.46.
20. Walker E, Marwit S, Emory E. A cross-sectional study of emotion recognition in schizophrenics. J Abnorm Psychol 1980; 89:428.436.
21. Mueser K, Penn DL, Blanchard JJ, Bellack AS. Affect recognition in schizophrenia: a synthesis of findings across three studies. Psychiatry Interpers Biol Proc 1997; 60:301.308.
22. Davis PG, Gibson MG. Recognition of posed and genuine facial expressions of emotion in paranoid and nonparanoid schizophrenia. J Abnorm Psychol 2000; 109:445.450.
23. Feinberg TE, Rifkin A, Schaffer C, Walker E. Facial discrimination and emotional recognition in schizophrenia and affective disorders. Arch Gen Psychiatry 1986; 43:276.279.
24. Penn D, Combs DR, Ritchie M, et al. Emotion recognition in schizophrenia: further investigation of generalized versus specific deficit models. J Abnorm Psychol 2000; 109:512.516.
25. Kerr S, Neale JM. Emotion perception in schizophrenia: specific deficit or further evidence of generalized poor performance? J Ab Psychol 1993; 102:312.318.
26. Brysen G, Bell M, Lysaker P. Affect recognition in schizophrenia: a function of global impairment or a specific cognitive deficit. Psychiatry Res 1997; 71:105..13.
27. Kee KS, Kern RS, Green MF. Perception of emotion and neurocognitive functioning in schizophrenia: what's the link? Psychiatry Res 1998; 81:57..65.
28. Kohler CB, Hagendoorn M, Gur RE, Gur RC. Emotion recognition deficit in schizophrenia: association with symptomatology and cognition. Biol Psychiatry 2000; 48:127..136.
29. Haefner HRR., Hambrecht M, Maurer K, et al. IRAOS: an instrument for the assessment of onset and early course of schizophrenia. Schizophr Res 1992; 6:209.223.
30. Mueser K, Doonan R, Penn DL, et al. Emotion recognition and social competence in chronic schizophrenia. J Abnorm Psychol 1996; 105:271.275.
31. Shaw RJ, Dong M, Lim KO, Faustman WO, Pouget E R, Alpert M. The relationship between affect expression and affect recognition in schizophrenia. Schizophr Res 1999; 37:245..250.
32. Corrigan P, Nelson DR. Factors that affect social cue recognition in schizophrenia. Psychiatry Res 1998; 78:189..196.
33. Heckers S, Rauch SL, Goff D. Impaired recruitment of the hippocampus during conscious recollection in schizophrenia. Nat Neurosci 1998; 1:318..323.
34. Mueser KE, Tarrier N, eds. Handbook of Social Functioning in Schizophrenia. Boston: Allyn & Bacon, 1998.
35. Penn DL, Spaulding W, Reed D, Sullivan M. The relationship of social cognition to ward behavior in chronic schizophrenia. Schizophr Res 1996; 20:327.335.
36. Addington J, Addington D. Neurocognitive and social functioning in schizophrenia: a 25 year follow-up study. Schizophr Res 2000; 44:47..56.
37. Penn D, Spaulding W, Reed D, Sullivan M, Mueser KT, Hope DA. Cognition and social functioning in schizophrenia. Psychiatry Interpers Biol Proc 1997; 60:281.291.
38. Corrigan P, Hirschbeck J, Wolfe M. Memory and vigilance training to improve social perception in schizophrenia. Schizophr Res 1995; 17:257.265.
39. Doody G, Goetz M, Johnstone EC, Frith CD, Cunningham, M. Owens DG. Theory of mind and psychoses. Psychol Med 1998; 28:397.405.

40. Sarfati Y, Hardy-Bayle M, Brunet E, Widloecher D. Investigating theory of mind in schizophrenia: influence of verbalization in disorganized and non-disorganized patients. Schizophr Res 1999; 37:183..190.
41. Klosterkotter JSL, Gross G, Huber G, Steinmeyer EM. Early self-experienced neuropsychological deficits and subsequent schizophrenic diseases: an 8-year average follow-up prospective study. Acta Psychiatri Scand 1997; 95:396..404.
42. Malmberg A, Lewis G, David A, Allebeck, P. Premorbid adjustment and personality in people with schizophrenia. Br J Psychiatry 1998; 172:308..313.
43. Jones P, Croudace T. Predicting schizophrenia in adults from teacher's reports in adolescence: perspectives on population-based intervention and indicated prevention. Schizophr Res 2000; 41:177..178.
44. Jones P, Tarrant CJS. Specificity of developmental precursors to schizophrenia and affective disorders. Schizophr Res 1999; 39:121..125.
45. Baum K, Walker EF. Childhood behavioral precursors of adult symptom dimensions in schizophrenia. Schizophr Res 1995; 16:111..120.
46. Neumann C, Walker E. Developmental pathways to schizophrenia: behavioral subtypes. J Abnorm Psychol 1995; 104:1..9.
47. Lane R, Reiman EM, Bradley MM, et al. Neuroanatomical correlates of pleasant and unpleasant motion. Neuropsychologia 1997; 35:1437..1444.
48. Jones P, Rodgers B, Murray R, Marmot M. Child development risk factors for adult schizophrenia in the British 1946 birth cohort. Lancet 1994; 344:1398..1402.
49. Olin S, Mednick SA. Risk factors of psychosis: identifying vulnerable populations pre-morbidly. Schizophr Bull 1996; 22:223.240.
50. Olin S, Mednick S, Cannon T, et al. School teacher ratings predictive of psychiatric outcome 25 years later. Br J Psychiatry 1998; 172:7..13.
51. Olin SS, Raine A, Cannon TD, et al. Childhood behavior precursors of schizotypal personality disorder. Schizophr Bull 1997; 23:93..103.
52. Hans S, Marcus J, Henson L, et al. Interpersonal behavior of children at risk for schizophrenia. Psychiatry Interpers Biol Proc 1992; 55:314.335.
53. Watt N. Patterns of childhood social development in adult schizophrenics. Arch Gen Psychiatry 1978; 35:160..165.
54. Done DC, Johnstone EC, Sacker, A. Childhood antecedents of schizophrenia and affective illness: social adjustment at ages 7 and 11. Br Med J 1994; 309:699..703.
55. Dykes KL, Mednick SA, Machon RA, et al. Adult third ventricle width and infant behavioral arousal in groups at high and low risk for schizophrenia. Schizophr Res 1992; 7:13..18.
56. Parnas J. From predisposition to psychosis: progression of symptoms in schizophrenia. Acta Psychiatr Scand Supp 1999; 395:20.29.
57. Yung AM, McGerry P. The initial prodrome in psychosis: descriptive and qualitative aspects. Austr New Zeal J Psychiatry 1996; 30:587.599.
58. Moller P, Husby R. The initial prodrome in schizophrenia: searching for naturalistic core dimensions of experience and behavior. Schizophr Bull 2000; 26:217.232.
59. Yassa R, Uhr S, Jeste DV. The elderly with chronic mental illness. In: Light E, Barry D, eds. Gender Differences in Chronic Schizophrenia: Need for Further Research. New York: Springer, 1991:16.30.
60. Cohen RZG, Seeman, MV. Duration of pretreatment phases in schizophrenia: women and men. Can J Psychiatry 2000; 45:544.547.
61. Leduc M, Herron JE, Greenberg DR, Eslinger PJ, Grattan LM. Impaired awareness of social and emotional competencies following orbital frontal lobe damage. Brain Cog 1999; 40:174..177.

62. Davidson R, Slagter HA. Probing emotion in the developing brain: functional neuroimaging in the assessment of the neural substrates of emotion in normal and disordered children and adolescents. Men Retard Dev Disabilit Res Rev 2000; 6:166..170.

63. Critchley H, Daly E, Phillips M, et al. Explicit and implicit neural mechanisms for processing of social information from facial expressions: a functional magnetic resonance imaging study. Hum Brain Mapp 2000; 9:93..105.

64. Matsumoto A. Synaptogenic action of sex steroids in developing and adult neuroendocrine brain. Psychoneuroendocrinology 1991; 16:25..40.

65. Russell TR, Bullmore ET, Soni W, et al. Exploring the social brain in schizophrenia: left prefrontal underactivation during mental state attribution. Am J Psychiatry 2000; 157:2040..2042.

66. Critchley H, Daly EM, Bullmore E, et al. The functional neuroanatomy of social behaviour: changes in cerebral blood flow when people with autistic disorder process facial expressions. Brain 2000; 123:2203..2212.

67. Schneider FW, Kessler C, Salloum JB, Posse S, Grodd W, Muller-Gartner HW. Differential amygdala activation in schizophrenia during sadness. Schizophr Res 1998; 34:133..142.

68. Phillips M, Williams L, Senior C. A differential neural response to threatening and non-threatening negative facial expressions in paranoid and non-paranoid schizophrenics. Psychiatry Res 1999; 92:11..31.

69. Kindermann S, Karimi A, Symonds L, Brown GG, Jeste, DV. Review of functional magnetic resonance imaging in schizophrenia. Schizophr Res 1997; 27:143..156.

70. Volz H, Nenadic I, Gaser C, et al. Time estimation in schizophrenia: an fMRI study at adjusted levels of difficulty. Neuroreport 2001; 12:313..316.

71. Heckers SG, Schacter DL, Savage CR, Fischman AJ, Alpert NM, Rauch SL. Functional imaging of memory retrieval in deficit vs. nondeficit schizophrenia. Arch Gen Psychiatry 1999; 56:1117..1123.

72. Heckers S, Curran T, Goff D, et al. Abnormalities in the thalamus and prefrontal cortex during episodic object recognition in schizophrenia. Biol Psychiatry 2000; 48:651..657.

73. Benes F. Emerging principles of altered neural circuitry in schizophrenia. Brain Res Brain Res Rev 2000; 31:251..269.

74. Romeo R, Diedrich SL, Sisk CL. Effects of gonadal steroids during pubertal development on androgen and estrogenreceptor-alpha immunoreactivity in the hypothalamus and amygdala. J Neurobiol 2000; 44:361..368.

75. Eliez SA., Stylianos E, Morris MA, Dahoun SP, Reiss AL. Parental origin of the deletion 22q11.2 and brain development in velocardiofacial syndrome. Arch Gen Psychiatry 2001; 58: 64..68.

76. Eliez S, Palacio-Espasa F, Spira A, et al. Young children with velo-cardio-facial syndrome (CATCH-22). Psychological and language phenotypes. Eur Child Adol Psychiatry 2000; 9: 109..114.

9

Neuroimaging Studies of Nonpsychotic First-Degree Relatives of People With Schizophrenia

Toward a Neurobiology of Vulnerability to Schizophrenia

Larry J. Seidman, PhD,
Heidi E. Wencel, PhD,
Colm McDonald, MB, MRC Psych,
Robin M. Murray, MD, FRC Psych, DSc,
and Ming T. Tsuang, MD, PhD, DSc

SUMMARY

Studies of individuals with schizophrenia and their nonpsychotic ("unaffected") family members are valuable for several reasons. First, abnormalities found in close biological relatives of ill persons may provide clues to those underlying characteristics that are genetically transmitted. Second, unlike studies of patients with schizophrenia, studies of unaffected relatives are not confounded by antipsychotic drug treatment, chronic hospitalization, the potential neurotoxic effects of psychosis, and other health consequences of serious mental illness. Third, characteristic features found in relatives are likely to be more reliable than those found in patients because the patients are less stable over time. Fourth, identifying markers of the vulnerability to schizophrenia ("endophenotypes") may provide useful phenotypes for future molecular genetic studies. In this chapter, we summarize the evidence of brain abnormalities in first degree, nonpsychotic relatives of

From: *Early Clinical Intervention and Prevention in Schizophrenia*
Edited by: W. S. Stone, S. V. Faraone, and M. T. Tsuang © Humana Press Inc., Totowa, NJ

persons with schizophrenia, as reflected in neuroimaging studies. Most of the research has investigated brain structure, with a smaller number of functional and chemical (spectroscopic) imaging studies. This literature, consistent with that found using psychophysiological, and neurocognitive measures in unaffected relatives, indicates that subtle brain deviations are found in adult nonpsychotic relatives. A smaller literature demonstrates similar deviations in teenagers at high risk of developing the disorder. The strongest evidence so far, mainly from magnetic resonance imaging (MRI) studies of brain structure, implicates abnormal medial temporal lobe regions, as well as abnormal cortical-subcortical activation involved in neurocognitive functions. This supports an important hypothesis: *that many of the neurobiological abnormalities associated with schizophrenic psychosis will actually turn out to be manifestations of preillness neurobiological vulnerability ("schizotaxia") rather than part of the psychotic process* per se. An important question to be determined is whether biological differences observed between relatives and healthy controls are minor variants of abnormalities found largely in pathological populations or whether they are the tail end of a normal distribution?

AN OVERVIEW OF GENETIC LINKAGE STUDIES AND THE SEARCH FOR ROBUST ENDOPHENOTYPES

The precise etiology of schizophrenia remains elusive. However, technological and conceptual advances in genetics and neuroimaging have led to substantial gains in the characterization of the schizophrenia phenotype(s). Unlike Huntington's disease and other disorders that involve major gene effects, the pattern of inheritance in schizophrenia does not fit a classic Mendelian model of inheritance at a single gene locus. The patterns of inheritance, and indeed incidence, are better explained when an oligogenic ($\leq$10 gene) or multifactorial (~100 gene) model is assumed, in which multiple genes interact with environmental stressors to propel the individual over a threshold for the expression of the disorder *(1)*.

Early attempts to demonstrate linkage of schizophrenia to specific chromosomal loci were not consistently replicated. One reason postulated for this failure was the use of a broad phenotype (clinical diagnosis of schizophrenia) in molecular genetic studies. Studies using this approach were likely confounded by the low penetrance rate of the disorder as defined clinically as well as the presence of phenocopies *(2,3)*.

Nevertheless, more recent studies, using improved methods, and more refined phenotypic measures (e.g., electrophysiological markers) have been somewhat more successful in replicating genetic linkage. For example, genetic linkage studies of schizophrenia that have incorporated eye-tracking *(4)* and sensory gating

measures *(5)* have been reported to demonstrate positive linkage. Evidence of linkage to schizophrenia may be beginning to converge on loci on chromosome 1 (1q42.1, 1q14.3, 1q21-22, 1q32.2) *(6–10)*, chromosome 6 (6p24-22, 6q13-26) *(11–15)*, chromosome 8 (8p21-22) *(16)*, chromosome 11 (11q21-q23) *(16)*, chromosome 13 (13q14.1-q32) *(17–19)*, chromosome 15 (15q13-q15) in the region of the α-7 nicotinic acetylcholine receptor and its duplication (Dupalpha7) *(20–23)*, and chromosome 22q *(15,24,25)*. In exclusively white samples, linkage has also been reported on chromosome 10 (10p14-p12) *(26,27)*. Nevertheless, although these results are encouraging, it is too early to say how many of these findings will stand the test of time.

Future research will use new genomic and proteomic techniques and will focus on how critical genes interact with each other and with the environment to result in schizophrenia. It is likely that there are multiple developmental pathways, involving different combinations of genes and environment factors, that can result in schizophrenia. Indeed, it has been suggested that, because neurodevelopmental alterations are prominent in schizophrenia, the genetics of schizophrenia is the genetics of neurodevelopment *(28)*.

Since the the 1970s, the study of abnormal psychobiological traits in "unaffected" (nonpsychotic) first-degree relatives of persons with schizophrenia has developed. This approach enables a richer description of the potentially heritable characteristics found in families with schizophrenic members. It assumes that intermediate between the genes carrying risk of schizophrenia (the genotype) and the clinical symptoms that represent their behavioral product (the clinical phenotype), lie an interacting array of psychobiological outcomes ("endophenotypes") that are more proximal to their genetic (and in some cases their environmental) causes than are clinical symptoms or psychiatric diagnosis (see Fig. 1). The identification of robust endophenotypes is likely to result in better understanding of the neurobiological vulnerability (which we have previously termed "schizotaxia") to the illness. Moreover, the clarification of pathophysiological mechanisms should improve the prospects for advances in diagnosis and treatment *(29)*.

In this chapter, we summarize the neuroimaging studies of persons with schizophrenia and their unaffected biological relatives. We focus primarily on adult nonpsychotic relatives because when they have passed through the peak ages of risk (age 20. 35) for schizophrenia, they are likely to carry some of the traits associated with schizophrenia, independent of developing the full syndrome. The presence of abnormalities in the absence of psychosis identifies underlying trait markers of the disorder *(30)*. Studies of nonpsychotic adolescents who are at high risk for the illness (based on having a sibling or parent with schizophrenia) are very informative for prediction of illness and for distinguishing premorbid characteristics associated with vulnerability vs illness. However, that strategy mixes pro-

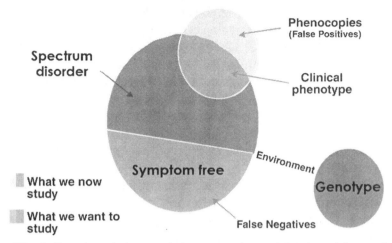

Fig. 1. Genetic and phenotypic heterogeneity model (adapted from ref. *122*).

spective cases and those who will remain unaffected through the period of risk thus clouding interpretation of findings. We review neuroimaging studies of children and adolescents at risk, but they are even fewer in number than studies of adult relatives.

We first review what is known about brain structural and functional abnormalities in schizophrenic patients to set a context for what might be expected to be found in unaffected relatives if such abnormalities are transmitted genetically or acquired through intrafamilial environmental exposures. We briefly summarize the literature on schizophrenia-related clinical conditions and psychobiological deficits in nonpsychotic family members. This is followed by a summary of neuroimaging abnormalities found in first-degree relatives. Finally, we briefly speculate about the possible mechanisms underlying some of these findings.

NEUROIMAGING OF BRAIN ABNORMALITIES IN SCHIZOPHRENIA: STRUCTURAL ABNORMALITIES

More than 200 in vivo, neuroimaging studies have documented the presence of structural brain abnormalities in schizophrenia patients *(31–34)*. Despite heterogeneous patient samples and methodologies, neuroimaging studies consistently implicate enlargement of the third and lateral ventricles, and very frequently, although not invariably, volume reduction of the temporal lobes (including the superior temporal gyrus gray matter) and medial limbic structures. Ventricular enlargement is prominent   a recent meta-analysis of 58 studies of subjects with schizophrenia reported a 26% enlargement in ventricular volume compared to

controls *(35)*. Although not all regional abnormalities are found consistently, subtly smaller volumes in medial limbic structures are generally found, especially of the hippocampus, parahippocampal gyrus, insula, amygdala, and cingulate gyrus *(33,35–39)*. Other less frequently replicated structural abnormalities include regions of the basal ganglia, thalamus, prefrontal cortex, and corpus callosum. We cannot currently say for certain which of these anatomical differences are minor variants of abnormalities found largely in pathological populations (e.g., ventricular enlargement) and which might represent the tail end of a normal distribution (e.g., hippocampal volume).

Rather than focusing on a small number of structures with a region of interest (ROI) approach to morphometry, some researchers have adopted alternative techniques involving whole-brain analysis in order to explore distributed morphological abnormalities. Goldstein et al. *(40)*, in a volumetric analysis of the entire cortex divided into 48 parcellation units per hemisphere, identified the greatest volume reductions in the paralimbic cortices including the anterior cingulate and paracingulate gyri and the insula. Studies using voxel-based morphometry have also identified volume reduction in the insula *(39,41–43)* as well as the left dorsolateral prefrontal cortex (DLPFC), fronto-medial cortex, superior temporal gyrus, and limbic/para-limbic regions. Voxel-based morphometry is a fully automated whole-brain analysis that involves segmentation and registration of magnetic resonance images in standard space, after which tissue densities throughout the brain can be compared across subject groups. Wright et al. *(41,44)* used such techniques to explore structural abnormalities of neural networks acting at a "supra-regional" level of organization. They identified abnormalities in two structural systems acting independently in schizophrenia: a global process involving reduced gray matter and increased ventricular size and a supra-regional process involving reduced gray matter in bilateral temporal. left frontal regions. They suggest that the latter may represent a network involved in auditory and linguistic processing.

Do these morphological abnormalities represent a process specific to schizophrenia or are they associated with other forms of psychosis? Although less extensively researched, there is some evidence from ROI studies that there are some similar structural brain abnormalities in patients with bipolar disorder especially with psychotic features *(45,46)*. When compared to healthy controls, subjects with bipolar psychotic disorder demonstrate ventricular enlargement and reduction of cortical grey matter, although these are not as prominent or found as consistently as those found in schizophrenia *(47,48)*. Ventricular enlargement and smaller intracranial volume and reduced thalamic volume similar to that found in schizophrenia has been reported in adolescent bipolar subjects *(49,50)*. There is some evidence for smaller hippocampal volumes in bipolar disorder at the onset of illness *(51,52)*, although hippocampal volume loss has also been reported to be

specific to schizophrenia when compared to bipolar disorder *(53)*. Differences seem to exist between the major functional psychoses. For example, abnormalities of regions involved in modulating mood, such as enlargement of the amygdala *(53,54)* and smaller volume of the subgenual prefrontal cortex *(55)* may be specific to bipolar disorder. On the other hand, loss of normal asymmetry and reduced volume of the posterior superior temporal gyrus *(56,57)*, involved in auditory processing and language, may be specific to schizophrenia. The exact nature of the similarities and differences in structural abnormalities has yet to be clearly elucidated.

Functional Neuroimaging Abnormalities

Studies of cerebral metabolism and blood flow have attempted to address fundamental questions regarding dysfunctional brain systems in schizophrenia. A wealth of literature will be briefly summarized here, including the results of positron emission tomography (PET), single positron emission computed tomography (SPECT), and functional MRI (fMRI) studies of both resting activity as well as function in response to neurocognitive probes. In general, functional imaging studies of schizophrenia are characterized by heterogeneity, and are confounded by several factors, including differences in the disease progression, symptomology, medication status, and cognitive performance of patients *(58,59)*. Here, we review the results of available meta-analyses and well-designed, recent studies. Three major brain dimensions have been examined: anterior/posterior; lateralization of brain activity, especially regarding the temporal lobe; and subcortical/cortical connections.

Most studies using neurocognitive probes have indicated reduced metabolism or blood flow in the inferior frontal, medial frontal, and DLFPC *(60–63)*. However, some findings of increased prefrontal activity have been reported *(64)*, consistent with the idea that prefrontal function is heterogeneous in schizophrenia *(65)*. In a recent study, Callicott et al. *(66)* attempted to address this issue, using a parametric version of the N-back working memory task. A subgroup of patients who performed the task relatively normally (with very mild, nonsignificant deficits) showed increased activation compared to normal controls, whereas those who performed poorly failed to activate the prefrontal cortex in response to the task *(66)*. Those patients showing increased task-elicited activation also had the lowest levels of *N*-acetyl-aspartate (NAA), a putative measure of prefrontal neuronal pathology, suggesting that the loss of normal working memory-induced prefrontal activation is related to the level of neuronal pathology in this region. However, in some studies, patients with good task performance still show reduced activation in the DLPFC *(67)*. Future studies of the effects of performance, length of illness, attention, motivation, and structural abnormalities are required to clarify why some patients appear to maintain their ability to activate the prefrontal cortex (albeit inefficiently) in some settings, whereas others do not.

Studies of the temporal lobe have also been distinguished by heterogeneity *(68)*. In PET and SPECT studies, many patients show normal temporal lobe function, whereas others show reduced functioning in this region. These deficits appear to be most robust in the bilateral superior temporal cortex *(68)*, are often more significant in the left hemisphere, and have been correlated with the presence of clinical thought disorder *(69–71)*. A recent fMRI study of the early stages of auditory processing in patients also revealed reduced activation in the superior temporal gyrus *(72)*. McGuire et al. suggested that reduced activation in the temporal lobe may be associated with failure to activate areas involved in the monitoring of inner speech, and that this may underlie verbal hallucinations *(73)*.

In a PET study of declarative memory, patients showed reduced task-elicited hippocampal activation compared to normal controls, but basal activity in this region was increased *(74)*. Similarly, decreased activity in the superior temporal gyrus was associated with increased metabolism in the parahippocampal/anterior fusiform gyrus of thought-disordered patients describing ambiguous scenes *(71)*. Finally, most fMRI studies of brain activity during auditory hallucinations show increased activity in the middle and superior temporal cortex, and Heschl's gyrus *(75–78)*. Together, these findings suggest that basal activity, cognitive task-elicited, and speech-elicited activity in the temporal lobe are poorly regulated. These findings are compatible with the hypothesis of fronto-temporal disconnection in schizophrenia.

Finally, functional abnormalities have been reported in subcortical structures, including regions of the striatum (i.e., basal ganglia) and thalamus. However, abnormalities in these regions appear to be dependent on the patient's medication status and the length of pharmacologic treatment. Reduction of blood flow to pallidum and caudate has also been reported in first-episode schizophrenia, as have increases in metabolism in the thalamic and striatal nuclei, hippocampus, paralimbic region, and cingulate cortex as the illness progresses *(79)*. The importance of abnormal connections among frontal, temporal, and subcortical structures in schizophrenia is illustrated by the finding that prefrontal dysfunction is associated with hippocampal volume reductions, especially in the left hippocampus *(80)*. Abnormal functional activity in prefrontal-hippocampal circuitry during performance of a declarative memory task is also relevant *(74)*.

In short, although abnormalities of brain function in schizophrenia have yet to be precisely characterized, it does appear that metabolism and blood flow are altered in schizophrenia, and therefore might be abnormal in unaffected relatives as well.

Chemical Neuroimaging Abnormalities

Proton (1H) and phosphorus (P31) magnetic resonance spectroscopy (MRS) and magnetic resonance spectroscopy imaging (MRSI) have been applied to study the in vivo biochemistry of brain regions that are implicated in schizophrenia.

The pathophysiologic significance of MRS measures is still under debate. NAA, phosphocreatine (CRE), and choline (CHO) ratios, measured by 1H-MRS, have been proposed and indeed used as putative measures of nondegenerative neuronal pathology (i.e., neuronal number and metabolism). Phosphomonoester (PME) and phosphodiester (PDE) resonance, measured by 31P-MRS, have been used to study membrane phospholipid metabolism and breakdown, as well as the turnover of high energy phosphates. Recent MRS techniques have enabled quantitation of neurotransmitters and macromolecules such as glutamate/glutamine (tGlx), γ-aminobutyric acid (GABA), membrane phospholipids and synaptic proteins *(81)*.

The majority of studies show reduced NAA/CRE and NAA/CHO ratios in the hippocampus *(82,83)*, hippocampal area/mesial temporal lobe region *(84–86)* and the DLPFC *(82,83,87–89)*. Although most studies only demonstrate significant differences in DLPFC and hippocampus, a handful of studies have also reported reduced NAA in thalamus *(90)*, anterior cingulate *(91)*, and pons *(92)*, with normal NAA in the basal ganglia *(93,94)*. Fukuzako et al. *(95)* claimed that patients with a family history of psychotic disorders show lower temporal lobe NAA/CRE than those without a family history, and reduced NAA/CRE has also been observed in the frontal lobes of children or adolescents with schizophrenia *(89,96)*. These latter findings suggest that NAA/CRE may be a marker of genetic vulnerability for schizophrenia that is not secondary to the long-term effects of psychosis *(97)*. Indeed, a recent study showed that treatment with antipsychotic drugs increased NAA in cortical neurons of the PFC *(98)*.

Phosphorous MRS studies of schizophrenics have revealed decreased PME resonance in both medicated, chronic and neuroleptic-naive, first-episode schizophrenia subjects, in both DLPFC *(99,100)* and temporal lobe *(101)*. Reduced PME resonance reflects reduced synthesis of membrane phospholipid precursors (e.g., phosphocholine, phosphothanolamine, and underlying, less mobile molecules, such as phosphorylated proteins, micelles, vesicles, and phospholipids, and is correlated with negative symptoms *(102)*, poor executive neurocognitive performance *(103)*, and reduced delta sleep *(104)*.

Increased PDE resonance, thought to reflect increased membrane breakdown products (e.g., glycerophosphocholine, glycerophosphoethanolamine), has also been observed in the DLPFC in unmedicated patients *(105)*. Studies of PDE resonance in medicated patients have been inconsistent *(102,106)*, but recent studies viewing the more broad components of PDE (using proton-decoupled 31P MRS) reveal increased PDE in chronic, medicated schizophrenics in both frontal *(107)* and parietal cortex *(108)*. Studies of ATP in the DLPFC have yielded inconsistent results *(99,102,105,106)*.

Consistent with postmortem immunohistochemical studies, MRS studies raise the possibility of glutamatergic dysfunction in schizophrenia *(109)*. Glutamate/glutamine (tGlx) concentration has been shown to be reduced in the DLPFC *(110–*

112) and anterior cingulate *(111)*; the reductions in DLPFC can be reversed by neuroleptic treatment *(110)*. Cecil et al. *(88)* showed increased amino acid concentration in the medial temporal lobe, potentially suggesting increased tGlx in this region as well. GABA+glutamate to creatine ratio was shown to be increased in the prefrontal cortex in two studies *(113)*, but the glutamine peak, thought to be a more sensitive marker of glutamatergic transmission *(110)*, was not included in this calculation. Advances in MRS quantification procedures may help to resolve individual spectral metabolites (glutamate, glutamine, GABA) and help to better characterize the in vivo interactions of these molecules.

Summary of Brain Abnormalities in Schizophrenia Measured by Neuroimaging

The accumulating findings from structural, metabolic, and fMRI studies indicate abnormal brain structure and function in schizophrenia, in prefrontal cortex (especially DLPFC), lateral (especially STG), and medial (especially hippocampus) temporal lobes, and also the insula and thalamus, and are reasonably consistent with morphological findings from postmortem studies. Furthermore, more precise cellular measurements of postmortem prefrontal cortex suggest that volume reductions may reflect a combination of decreased intraneuronal neuropil in the presence of increased neuronal intensity *(114)*. This indicates a reduction of dendritic and axonal processes in schizophrenia and, as a result, fewer neuronal connections *(115)*. These results are consistent with evidence from fMRI studies of loss of the normal frontal-temporal connectivity and with a significant contribution of neurodevelopmental alterations in brain development *(116)*; indeed, Bullmore et al. *(117)* suggested that the dysfunctional connectivity arises out of dysplastic development of neural networks. Although there is a growing but contradictory literature over whether there is some subtle loss of brain volume and increase in cerebral spinal fluid (CSF) during the first few years of the illness *(118–120)*, abnormalities present in the first episode indicate that at least some abnormalities may precede the illness. This combination of pre-existing abnormalities and deterioration after psychosis begins has led some investigators to propose that schizophrenia is a "progressive neurodevelopmental disorder" *(121)*. If there are indeed such progressive changes after onset of psychosis, this emphasizes the importance of studying nonpsychotic relatives who can provide a clearer (i.e., no medications, etc.) window into the neurobiological vulnerability to the illness, apart from effects of psychosis *per se*.

SCHIZOPHRENIA-RELATED CLINICAL CONDITIONS

Ever since Kraepelin first described schizophrenia ("dementia praecox"), an increased risk for schizophrenia and other psychotic disorders (notably schizoaffective disorders and psychosis not otherwise specified) in family members of

schizophrenic patients has been noted. In addition, clinicians have observed for many years that some nonpsychotic relatives had eccentric personalities. They also noticed poor social relations, anxiety in social situations, language and communication disturbances, and limited emotional responses among the family members of schizophrenics, similar to what are now called the "negative" symptoms of schizophrenia. Less frequently observed were mild forms of thought disorder, suspiciousness, magical thinking, illusions, and perceptual aberrations *(122)*.

These characteristics have been studied as dimensional traits (such as degree of schizotypy) using various psychometric measures *(123)* as well as diagnosable psychiatric disorders that appear to run more frequently in the families of schizophrenics than in control subjects. Schizophrenia-related psychiatric disorders are called "schizophrenia-spectrum disorders" to convey the idea of a continuum of disorders related to schizophrenia *(124)*.

Researchers have focused most on the familial prevalence of three diagnoses embodying most of the previously mentioned traits: schizotypal, schizoid, and paranoid personality disorders. Numerous studies have documented the increased prevalence of schizotypal personality disorder (SPD) in the biological relatives of chronic schizophrenic probands *(125)*. These results are consistent across family studies, adoption studies, and twin studies. Prevalence estimates of this disorder in first-degree relatives of persons with schizophrenia range between 4.2% and 14.6%. Strong evidence linking paranoid and schizoid personality disorders with schizophrenia has yet to be firmly established. Thus, among Axis II disorders, SPD is the strongest candidate for a relatively mild disorder that is genetically related to schizophrenia *(125)*. SPD has received an increasing amount of study in the past decade, including use of brain-imaging techniques to identify some brain abnormalities similar to those found in schizophrenia *(126)*.

NEUROBIOLOGIC ENDOPHENOTYPES RELATED TO SCHIZOPHRENIA

Despite advances in associating some Axis II disorders such as SPD with schizophrenia, a one-to-one correspondence between genetically influenced processes in the brain and the clinical phenomena that define diagnostic categories is unlikely. Because psychiatric signs and symptoms are relatively remote effects of the genotype, genetic studies might be more fruitful if they focused on measures tied more closely to brain function, regardless of diagnosis. Moreover, a putative indicator may reflect only one component of the schizophrenia genotype, if, as is likely, more than one gene contributes to the development of schizophrenia. The probability of this outcome increases if genes that are minor for schizophrenia are major for some aspect of central nervous system (CNS) dysfunction *(127)*.

We use the term "neurobiologic endophenotypes" to refer to measures of brain functioning that can be considered to reflect deviant or indeed abnormal brain

structure or function related to the schizophrenia genotype. The criterion for defining a neurobiologic phenotype is straightforward: the characteristic must occur in schizophrenia and be found more frequently among the biological relatives of schizophrenic patients than in healthy controls. This provides suggestive evidence that its expression is mediated by one or more of the genes that also lead to schizophrenia.

Adult nonpsychotic relatives of schizophrenic patients have been found to have an increased prevalence of clinical abnormalities and neurobiologic endophenotypes: schizotypal and paranoid personality traits *(128)*, flat affect *(122)*, thought disorder *(129)*, communication disturbance *(130)*, neurologic signs *(131)*, eye-tracking dysfunctions *(132)*, attentional impairment *(133)*, cognitive impairments in executive functions and memory *(3,134,135)*, backward-masking deficits *(136)*, abnormal auditory evoked potentials, such as P50 suppression *(137, 138)* and P300 latency *(139)*. These abnormalities also provide clues as to abnormal brain circuitry in unaffected and affected relatives.

NEUROIMAGING ABNORMALITIES
IN FIRST-DEGREE RELATIVES OF SCHIZOPHRENIC PATIENTS

Structural Brain Imaging

Compared to the large number of studies of other neurobiologic endophenotypes, imaging studies of unaffected relatives are relatively few in number. Most are studies of brain structure. The earliest studies, which used computed tomography (CT), demonstrated more abnormality (typically ventricular enlargement) in patients with schizophrenia ("probands") than in their unaffected relatives *(140–146)*. The initial studies used unaffected relatives as a comparison group for probands predominantly as a means of reducing the considerable genetic variation of ventricular size in the population, and several did not include an independent control group. Of those CT studies that did include an independent control group, some reported ventricular enlargement in unaffected siblings *(140)*, whereas others did not *(142,146)*. In one cohort study of 97 adult offspring of mothers with schizophrenia (who had largely lived through the risk period for schizophrenia, with a mean age of 42) and 60 controls *(147)*, the offspring had enlargement of ventricular and sulcal CSF spaces in accordance with their genetic risk rising from none to one to both parents affected with schizophrenia-spectrum disorders. The results were unchanged when the analysis was conducted after excluding those 15 individuals who later developed schizophrenia.

The CT studies were limited to relatively gross linear and area measurements, and could not detect subtle differences and alterations in important, but small, brain regions of interest. MRI studies have the advantage of greater spatial resolution, particularly for identification and measurement of deep gray structures.

The relatively recent application of MRI to the investigation of brain structure in relatives has confirmed and extended findings obtained by CT. That is, the general tendency is to find greater volume loss in the brains of schizophrenic patients than in their nonpsychotic relatives *(148,149)*, although the unaffected relatives may also be impaired, particularly those with SPD or an especially strong genetic loading for schizophrenia *(148)*.

In the Maudsley Family Study, one of the largest neuroimaging family studies of schizophrenia *(148)*, volumetric MRI measurements were investigated in 31 subjects with schizophrenia from multiply affected ("multiplex") families (defined as two or more first- or second-degree relatives with schizophrenia), 57 of their nonpsychotic first-degree relatives, and 39 normal controls. The group of relatives included nine parents who were considered "presumed obligate carriers," because they appeared to transmit the liability for schizophrenia to their affected children because (a) they also had a sibling and/or parent affected and (b) transmission of liability was unilineal within each of these families; i.e., family history of psychosis was absent from the presumed obligate carrier's spouse. The probands had significantly enlarged lateral ventricles as did the presumed obligate carrier group. Furthermore, the probands demonstrated loss of the normal pattern of cerebral asymmetry when compared to the controls, who displayed normal cerebral asymmetry (where the right frontal region is larger than the left and the left occipital region is larger then the right). The presumed obligate carrier group displayed loss of cerebral asymmetry to a lesser degree, whereas the other relatives had loss of cerebral asymmetry in just one of the four regions measured; i.e., loss of cerebral asymmetry appeared to correlate with the putative likelihood of carrying genes for schizophrenia in the subjects. These studies suggested that ventricular enlargement and loss of the normal pattern of cerebral asymmetry are markers for genetic liability to schizophrenia. No such evidence was found when loss of planum temporale asymmetry *(150)* or reduced size of the corpus callosum *(151)* were similarly investigated in these subjects. The asymmetry findings, although intriguing, require replication.

Cannon et al. *(152)*, using MRI, demonstrated reduced cortical gray matter and enlarged sulcal CSF spaces in patients with schizophrenia or schizoaffective disorder, which was shared by their unaffected siblings. This gray-matter reduction was particularly pronounced in frontal and temporal regions. However, only the patients, and not their siblings, demonstrated significant ventricular enlargement and reduced white-matter volume, suggesting that cortical gray-matter loss might represent an endophenotypic marker for schizophrenia.

The subjects in the initial Harvard-MMHC study *(153,154)* were never psychotic, and nonschizotypal, first-degree adult relatives of schizophrenics and normal controls. Cortical and subcortical gray and white matter, and CSF were segmented using a semiautomated intensity contour mapping algorithm *(155)*. Analyses of

covariance of the volumes of brain regions, controlling for expected intellectual (i.e., reading) ability, sex, and diagnosis were used to compare the groups. The most robust findings were that, compared to controls, relatives had significant volume reductions bilaterally in the amygdala-hippocampal region and thalamus. Unlike patients with schizophrenia or the obligate carriers *(148)*, there was no significant enlargement of the lateral ventricles. The third ventricle was slightly enlarged but this effect was attenuated when controlling for comorbid psychiatric diagnoses. Unlike the Maudsley study, the Harvard-MMHC study evaluated first-degree relatives from families where only one person was diagnosed with schizophrenia ("simplex" families).

Subsequently, Seidman et al. *(156)* expanded this study to include an additional sample of 17 first-degree relatives, almost all of whom were siblings, from families with at least two first-degree relatives with schizophrenia (the Harvard-MMHC definition of "multiplex"). Four hypotheses were tested:

1. Hippocampal volume is smaller in nonpsychotic relatives than in controls, particularly in the left hemisphere.
2. Hippocampi will be smaller in multiplex, as compared to simplex relatives, and both will be smaller than in controls.
3. Hippocampal volumes and verbal declarative memory function will be positively correlated.
4. Hippocampi will be smaller in schizophrenic patients than in their nonpsychotic relatives, or than controls.

Subjects were 45 nonpsychotic adult first-degree relatives, from families with either two ("multiplex," $n = 17$) or one ("simplex," $n = 28$) person diagnosed with schizophrenia, 18 schizophrenic relatives, and 48 normal controls. Compared to controls, relatives, particularly from multiplex families, had significantly smaller left hippocampi. Verbal memory and left hippocampal volumes were significantly and positively correlated. Within families, hippocampal volumes did not differ between schizophrenics and their nonpsychotic relatives. Results support the hypothesis that the vulnerability to schizophrenia includes smaller left hippocampi and verbal memory deficits, and these reflect the degree of genetic liability to schizophrenia. O'Driscoll et al. *(157)* found similar anatomical. functional relationships in a smaller sample of nonpsychotic relatives of schizophrenics and controls. They reported a smaller amygdala-anterior hippocampal region and worse verbal declarative memory in relatives than controls, and again these measures were significantly associated.

Staal et al. reported that both schizophrenic patients and their unaffected siblings displayed third ventricular enlargement and reduced volume in the thalamus *(158,159)*. Patients with schizophrenia had significantly reduced cerebral volumes compared to controls whereas their siblings had cerebral volumes that

were intermediate between patients and controls, not significantly differing from either. They suggested that thalamic volume reduction, with associated third ventricular enlargement, and possibly reduced cerebral volume were markers of genetic liability for schizophrenia.

There are only three MRI studies in the literature on adolescents and young adults at high risk for schizophrenia *(160–163)*. In a pilot study of offspring at risk for schizophrenia *(160)*, adolescent offspring of persons with schizophrenia were found to have reduced left amygdala volume, enlarged third ventricle volume, and smaller overall brain volume. This is essentially consistent with that reported in a substantially larger study (*n* = 146) *(162,163)*, which showed that high-risk subjects (age 15. 25) had significantly reduced mean volumes of the left and right amygdalo-hippocampus (especially left) and thalamus, as compared to healthy control subjects. The investigators noted smaller total brain volumes in a subgroup of the high-risk subjects who reported some psychotic symptoms. However, their report does not make it clear whether the smaller brain volumes were present before the onset of psychotic symptoms. In a small study of 15 adolescent offspring of schizophrenic parents and matched teenage controls *(161)*, offspring had significant reduction of the right hippocampus-amygdala complex compared to controls.

Thus, although there is disagreement in the literature, there is evidence from the studies on unaffected relatives of schizophrenic patients for a familial, and likely genetic, contribution to several of the structural brain abnormalities associated with schizophrenia (*see* Table 1). A variety of ROIs have been studied with either negative or inconclusive results, but the total number of subjects is too small, and the clinical and MRI methodological differences too great between studies, to base firm conclusions on the existing literature. The strongest trend thus far implicates the hippocampus-amygdala region and to a lesser extent the thalamus. The absence of significant volume differences (aside from statistical power considerations) does not rule out cellular abnormalities, nor does it eliminate the possibility of neuronal dysfunctions in those ROIs. Some of the disagreement in the literature may be related to reliability problems associated with measuring certain subcortical structures, such as the thalamus, where segmenting gray from white matter is particularly difficult. Such difficulties will be compounded in studies that may lack statistical power: because structural changes are likely to be more subtle in relatives than probands, larger numbers of subjects are required to demonstrate a statistically significant result in studies of relatives than studies comparing only probands with controls.

Functional Brain Abnormalities

To our knowledge, there are only a few PET and fMRI studies of relatives of persons with schizophrenia *(135,164–166)*. Berman et al. *(164)* used PET to com-

Table 1

Structural MRI Findings in Nonpsychotic First-Degree Relatives of Persons With Schizophrenia Compared With Normal Controls

Region of Interest (Volume)	Positive Findings: Adult Relatives	Negative Findings: Adult Relatives	Positive Findings: Offspring/Siblings Up to Age 25	Negative Findings: Offspring/Siblings Up to Age 25
Hippocampus-amygdala	Seidman et al. (1999) (154); O'Driscoll et al. (2001) (157); Seidman et al. (2002) (156) (left)	Staal et al. (2000) (159)	Lawrie et al. (2001) (163); Keshavan et al. (1997) (160) (left); Schreiber et al. 1999 (161) (right)	
Parahippocampal gyrus				
Thalamus	Seidman et al. (1999) (154); Staal et al. (1998) (158)	Staal et al. (2000) (159)		
Prefrontal lobe	Cannon et al. (1998) (152) (cortex)	Staal et al. (2000) (159)	Lawrie et al. (2001) (163)	Lawrie et al. (2001) (163); Schreiber et al. (1999) (161)
Temporal lobe	Cannon et al. (1998) (152) (cortex)	Sharma et al. (1998) (148)		Lawrie et al. (2001) (163); Schreiber et al. (1999) (161)
Cerebellum		Staal et al. (2000) (159); Sharma et al. (1998) (148)		
Caudate nucleus		Seidman et al. (1999) (154); Staal et al. (2000) (159)		Lawrie et al. (2001) (163)
Lenticular nucleus	Seidman et al. (1999) (154) (pallidum)	Seidman et al. (1999) (154) (putamen)		Lawrie et al. (2001) (163)
Corpus callosum area		Chua et al. (2000) (151)		
Lateral ventricle	Orlova et al. (1999) (186); Sharma et al. (1998) (148)	Cannon et al. (1998) (152); Staal et al. (2000) (159)		Schreiber et al. (1999) (161); Lawrie et al. (2001) (163); Schreiber et al. (1999) (161)
Third ventricle			Keshavan et al. (1997) (160)	
Fourth ventricle		Seidman et al. (1999) (154); Sharma et al. (1998) (148); Seidman et al. (1999) (154)		
Total cerebral volume	Staal et al. (2000) (159)	Seidman et al. (1999) (154); Sharma et al. (1998) (148); Seidman et al. (1999) (154)	Keshavan et al. (1997) (160)	Lawrie et al. (2001) (163)
Total cortical gray matter	Cannon et al. (1998) (152)			Lawrie et al. (2001) (163)
Sulcal CSF		Staal et al. (2000) (159)		
Total cerebral white matter	Cannon et al. (1998) (152)	Cannon et al. (1998) (152); Seidman et al. (1999) (154)		
Loss of planum temporale asymmetry		Frangou et al. (1997) (139)		
Loss of normal cerebral asymmetry	Sharma et al. (1999) (187)			

Note: Only results from quantitative MRI studies are presented.
Only statistically significant results are presented as positive. Where trends were present, studies were taken as being neither positive nor negative (e.g., ref. 154; third ventricle volume).

pare regional cerebral blood flow in monozygotic (MZ) twins discordant for schizophrenia while they completed the Wisconsin Card Sorting Test (WCST). All of the twins with schizophrenia had relatively reduced prefrontal blood flow compared with their unaffected co-twins, and hypofrontality was correlated with reduced anterior hippocampal volumes *(80)*. Although they did not statistically analyze the data, when unaffected co-twins of patients with schizophrenia were compared with twins who were both normal, no obvious differences were observed. Nevertheless, this study was quite small and reported only a qualitative sense of the data, leaving it ambiguous as to whether the unaffected twins are different than controls (*see* Table 2).

In a subsequent PET study of verbal fluency in nonpsychotic, presumed obligate carrier parents, relatives showed increased right DLPFC activation, and a reduced relationship of left DLPFC activation to activation in the left superior temporal gyrus and precuneus *(165)*. This study suggests impaired prefrontal modulation of temporal and parietal activation, as indicated by the lack of the normal relationship between activation in these structures which had been observed in controls. Additionally, increased activation in the right prefrontal cortex in the relatives may suggest either (a) functional compensation via recruitment of "more" top-down inputs from the right hemisphere, and/or (b) abnormal structural development and lateralization of cortico-cortical and/or thalamocortical projections to and from the prefrontal cortex associated with altered lateralization of function.

The results from the London group *(165)* are similar to pilot work from the Harvard-MMHC group, which has used fMRI to study auditory sustained attention and working memory in adult siblings of schizophrenic patients *(135,166)*. A series of tasks were designed to activate the distributed networks underlying attention and working memory *(167)*. Brain activation was compared in 10 relatives of schizophrenic patients and 10 normal controls, and analyzed using two statistical methods *(135,166)*. On cognitive performance prior to and during scanning, relatives were not significantly different on simple vigilance and working memory without interference ("MEM"), but were significantly impaired on a working memory task that required interference suppression ("INT"). In preliminary analyses, which focused on the whole cortex, relatives and controls showed predicted activation in prefrontal and parietal cortices in response to the working memory tasks. However, patterns of whole-brain activation differentiated relatives and controls on both the "MEM" and the "INT" task, even in the absence of performance deficits by relatives on the "MEM" task. Specifically, relatives showed less activation in the inferior and lateral prefrontal cortex than controls, had greater magnitude and spatially larger areas of activation in the fronto-orbital cortex, the superior parietal lobules, the anterior cingulate, and the thalamus *(135)*. Moreover, there was a different association in relatives than in controls between

Table 2
Functional MRI Findings in First-Degree Relatives
of Persons With Schizophrenia Compared With Normal Controls

Functional Region of Interest	Positive Findings: Adult Relatives	Negative Findings: Adult Relatives
Hippocampus	Wencel et al. (2001) *(166)* (working memory-CPT, fMRI)	Weinberger et al. (1992) *(80)* (WCST, PET)
Thalamus	Wencel et al. (2001) *(166)* (working memory-CPT, fMRI) Seidman et al. (1997) *(135)* (working memory-CPT, fMRI)	
Prefrontal Cortex	Spence et al. (2000) *(165)* (verbal fluency, PET) Seidman et al. (1997) *(135)* (working memory-CPT, fMRI)	
Anterior Cingulate	Seidman et al. (1997) *(135)* (working memory-CPT, fMRI)	
Parietal Cortex	Seidman et al. (1997) *(135)* (working memory-CPT, fMRI)	
Fronto-orbital Cortex	Seidman et al. (1997) *(135)* (working memory-CPT, fMRI)	

Note: There are not studies of adolescent offspring or siblings using fMRI.

volumes of the hippocampus, thalamus, and anterior cingulate, and brain activity in response to cognitive challenges *(166)*.

Thus, similar to Spence et al. *(165)*, this work suggests the following: (a) abnormal task-elicited prefrontal activation, (b) increased activation in other regions of cortex and limbic system (i.e., parietal cortex, anterior cingulate cortex, and hippocampus, specific to performance of working memory and interference suppression tasks), (c) increased activation in the sensory thalamus (pulvinar nucleus) and sensory-motor thalamus (posterior lateral nucleus) *(166)*, and (d) potentially abnormal cortico-cortical and/or corticothalamic-thalamocortical connectivity. Results suggest impaired prefrontal modulation of cortical and limbic system activation. The specific site of cortical overactivation appears to be a function of both the sensory and motivational demands of the task. Abnormal cortical responses to sensory stimuli may be related, in part (or in some persons), to a failure of prefrontal modulation of early sensory gating in the thalamus. Thus, it is possible that abnormal cortico-cortical, cortico-limbic, and cortico-thalamic structure and/or function may reflect a trait marker that is common to persons with schizophrenia

Table 3
Magnetic Resonance Spectroscopic Findings in First-Degree Relatives
of Persons With Schizophrenia Compared With Normal Controls (NC)

Region of Interest (Volume)	Positive Findings Adult Relatives	Negative Findings: Adult Relatives	Positive Findings: Offspring/Siblings Up to Age 25	Negative Findings: Offspring/Siblings Up to Age 25
Hippocampus	Calicott et al. (1998) *(97)* (NAA/CRE[a])			
Anterior Cingulate			Keshavan et al. (1997) *(160)* (NAA/CHO[b])	
Frontal Lobe			Klemm et al. (2001) *(168)* (PME/PDE[c], PDE)	

[a]NAA/CRE = *N*-acetyl-aspartate to creatine ratio. [b]NAA/CHO = *N*-acetyl-aspartate to choline ratio. [c]PME/PDE = Phosphomonoester to phosphodiester ratio.

and their first-degree relatives. This pilot research requires substantially larger samples of unaffected biological relatives and replication of findings.

Chemical Brain Imaging Abnormalities

In studies of offspring at risk for schizophrenia, utilizing proton and P31 MRS (*see* Table 3), nonpsychotic adolescent offspring of persons with schizophrenia had a trend toward decreased NAA/CHO ratios in the anterior cingulate *(160)*, and lower mean ratios of phosphomonoesters to phosphodiesters and higher mean phosphodiester values in the frontal lobes *(168)*. Callicot et al. *(97)* demonstrated significant reductions in levels of the neuronal marker NAA in the hippocampus of unaffected adult siblings of patients with schizophrenia. This preliminary evidence suggests that deviations in both NAA, a measure sensitive to neuronal integrity, and meaures of phospholipid breakdown are observed in prefrontal, hippocampal, and possible anterior cingulate regions of unaffected relatives of patients with schizophrenia. In a case report, it was noted that alterations of phospholipid metabolites measured by MRS were observed in a presumed healthy control subject who was studied 2 years before her first psychotic episode *(169)*, again suggesting that such abnormalities may be markers of vulnerability to the disorder. This literature is obviously very small and much work is needed to determine the robustness of the preliminary findings.

ETIOLOGY AND TIMING OF THE BRAIN
ABNORMALITIES IN UNAFFECTED RELATIVES

A number of questions arise from the evidence of brain abnormalities in relatives:

1. Are these abnormalities an expression of the genetic liability to schizophrenia?
2. When do the abnormalities occur?
3. Are the brain abnormalities stable traits or do they fluctuate like psychotic symptoms?
4. Are the abnormalities specific to schizophrenia or characteristic of other psychotic disorders such as bipolar disorder?

The excess presence of a characteristic in the nonpsychotic members of families with a schizophrenic member suggests but cannot prove genetic etiology, because family studies cannot distinguish genetic from environmental factors. Twin studies, or linkage studies using brain abnormalities as markers, are needed to determine whether the impairments are a result of sharing the same family environment or of inheritance of the same genes. Evidence from a number of designs that manipulated genetic loading (147,148) suggests that genetic factors are indeed involved. As specific brain abnormalities become clearly identified as risk factors for schizophrenia, the search for candidate molecules and genes influencing altered brain development will likely quicken (28,170). However, we must also consider the possibility that the abnormalities in unaffected relatives originate from environmental etiological factors in schizophrenia, such as pre- and peri- natal complications (PPCs) (171,172). MRI studies of MZ twins discordant for schizophrenia have shown that the ill twin had significantly more brain abnormalities (especially hippocampal volume reduction and ventricular enlargement) contrasted with the nonschizophrenic twin (141,149,173,174). Differences between MZ twins are most likely due to nongenetic factors such as PPCs. Despite sharing the same intrauterine environment, twins can experience different prenatal conditions such as inequalities in blood flow with resultant lack of oxygen or other nutrients or indeed more exposure to blood borne noxious agents such as infections. Such differences in the prenatal environment may also render one twin more vulnerable to the effects of perinatal hypoxia, although experienced by both (173). Perinatal hypoxia-ischemia could lead to periventricular haemorrhage, ventricular enlargement, and hippocampal volume reduction, possibly mediated by glutamatergic excitotoxic damage (175). Could this process also occur in nonpsychotic relatives?

Much of the data pertaining to the issue of the prevalence of PPCs in nonpsychotic relatives of schizophrenic patients comes from studies of offspring of schizophrenic parents (especially mothers) and it is still unclear whether the offspring are more likely to experience PPCs. The prevailing view had been that there is no excess of PPCs among high-risk offspring (176). This has been questioned

in a recent meta-analysis of 14 case-control studies with information on offspring of parents with schizophrenia (177), and which concluded that such individuals incur a small but significantly increased risk of PPCs, low birthweight, and poor neonatal condition. Rosso et al. (178) also observed slightly elevated rates of PPCs in adult nonpsychotic first-degree relatives of schizophrenic patients. Moreover, there is also evidence suggesting that when PPCs do occur, offspring of schizophrenics are more susceptible to the negative effects from them in proportion with their likely genetic risk. Hence in the study reported by Cannon et al. (147), ventricular enlargement in association with birth complications became more prominent as genetic liability increased, as indicated by having none, one, or both parents affected with schizophrenia-spectrum disorders. Thus it is possible that unaffected adult offspring of schizophrenics suffer subtle brain abnormalities from PPCs. Given that most of the relatives in the studies reviewed were siblings and not offspring of schizophrenic patients, this model cannot be applied with certainty. Identification of PPCs in the histories of unaffected relatives who have passed through the peak age of risk for schizophrenia, and who have brain abnormalities measured in vivo, is needed to answer this question.

Other possible etiologies for brain abnormalities in relatives, other than genetic causes or PPCs, includes later acquired brain injury or possible effects of stress, which may be most relevant to the prominence of abnormalities in the hippocampus (179). Currently, there are no empirical studies demonstrating either association in nonpsychotic relatives of schizophrenia patients.

Another unresolved issue is when do the abnormalities occur? A number of studies have demonstrated abnormalities occurring in an adolescent and young at-risk group, ages 10.25 (160–163). This suggests that damage or dysfunction is likely to be present in some persons by early teenage years at the latest. One possibility, based on the abnormalities seen in patients with schizophrenia, is that early brain development is altered on the basis of genes controlling neurodevelopment or early environmental insult (PPCs) as previously described. Of course, we cannot rule out the possibility of later occurring alterations in developmental processes such as synaptic pruning or abnormal myelination that could account for the observations such as smaller hippocampi. However, consistent with occurrence of earlier abnormal brain development, abnormalities in children at risk for schizophrenia, including signs of childhood neurological, cognitive, and social-affective maladjustment, are observed as early as the preschool years (180). Thus, our working model is that the abnormalities are present from before or shortly after birth.

Another issue pertains to whether the brain abnormalities found in unaffected relatives are stable or whether they fluctuate or "turn on" during certain developmental periods (endogenously or in response to stress) as proposed for schizophrenia by Weinberger (116). Our working assumption is that the structural brain abnormalities are stable "traits," whereas the functional and chemical abnormal-

ities could reflect either stable traits or fluctuating characteristics. Pertaining to the latter point, data from studies of children at risk for schizophrenia demonstrate that there are fluctuations in the presence or absence of neurologic signs in childhood and adolescence *(181)*. As there are currently few studies of brain abnormalities in unaffected relatives of persons with schizophrenia, and all are single-assessment, cross-sectional studies, we cannot yet provide any empirical data on this question from the literature.

Are the abnormalities in unaffected relatives specific to schizophrenia or characteristic of other psychotic disorders such as bipolar disorder? There are no data currently published on this question but our research groups are carrying out such studies. Although the literature on specificity of neuropsychological abnormalities is also relatively sparse, there are some data indicating more severe deficits in relatives of schizophrenics compared to relatives of patients with bipolar psychoses *(182,183)*. This might suggest that nonpsychotic relatives of bipolar psychotic patients are less afflicted by brain abnormalities than nonpsychotic relatives of schizophrenic patients.

Summary and Future Directions

Much prior work indicates that the nonpsychotic relatives of schizophrenic patients are vulnerable to subtle expressions of the schizophrenia syndrome including neuropsychological and psychophysiological deficits, and negative symptoms. New research, including that by our own groups (the Maudsley and Harvard-MMHC family brain studies), suggests that structural, functional, and chemical brain abnormalities are also found in some first-degree relatives of schizophrenic patients. These studies are currently few in number and require replication, but are promising because the findings are fairly consistent. The strongest evidence so far, mainly from structural MRI studies, indicates altered medial temporal lobe (especially hippocampal) and thalamic volumes, and abnormal functional brain activity in cortical-subcortical circuitry regulating executive neurocognitive functions. This appears to be a subtler version of the findings syndrome observed in patients with schizophrenia. Of note is the relative lack of significant enlargement of the lateral ventricles in relatives in most of the studies except those with heavily genetically loaded "obligate carriers" *(148)*, and also observed in well MZ co-twins who are, of course, genetically even closer. These results, also observed in teenagers at risk for schizophrenia, suggest an increasingly clear conclusion; *that many of the brain abnormalities considered to be associated with schizophrenic psychosis are actually associated with the vulnerability to the illness.*

To date, the results of psychophysiological and neuroimaging studies suggest that there are a few, fairly robust neurophysiological similarities in persons with schizophrenia and their first-degree relatives, and that some of those endopheno-

typic traits vary with genetic load for the disorder. These include the following: (a) hippocampal abnormalities and related cognitive problems, including reduced hippocampal volume, deviant NAA ratios and impairments on encoding and retrieval components of verbal memory tests; (b) reduced thalamic volume and associated psychophysiological responses, including abnormal P50; and (c) abnormal prefrontally mediated cognitive functions, such as abnormal saccadic eye movements and impaired performance on high-load working memory, encoding, and retrieval tasks. Although many adult relatives have some of these endophenotypic traits, most never develop psychotic symptoms. Thus, a key question in understanding the onset of schizophrenia, and ultimately its prevention, is identifying what causes a vulnerable person to shift from such subtle and presumably fairly stable deviations into frank psychosis.

Substantially more research, with larger samples, studying teenagers or children through the peak ages of risk for schizophrenia, is necessary to determine the robustness, stability, and predictive power of the deficits. Because there are no postmortem studies of nonpsychotic relatives, there is no precise correlation of cellular abnormalities with those observed in vivo. Moreover, the current data cannot determine why some relatives with brain pathology similar to that seen in persons with schizophrenia do not develop the illness. Further work is needed to determine whether relatives have less severe pathology or if they have not been exposed to environmental triggers of the illness. We believe such research would be invaluable in distinguishing the deficits associated with schizotaxic vulnerability vs schizophrenic illness.

The abnormalities described in this chapter may also contribute to our understanding of the clinical difficulties faced by some of the family members related to a schizophrenic person. Although psychiatric genetic research has yet to produce new therapies for schizophrenic patients, it is likely that in the long run, the discovery of susceptibility genes will facilitate the development of more effective treatments *(184)*. Improved diagnostic techniques also raise the possibility of designing primary prevention and other early-intervention strategies for preschizophrenic individuals, and for helping nonpsychotic family members *(29,30)*. Although the major clinical contributions of genetic neurobiologic research in schizophrenia may be decades away, this line of research will lead to advances in diagnosis, treatment, and genetic counseling that should eventually be useful to the practicing clinician as well as to schizophrenic patients and their family members *(29,185)*. In addition, the brain abnormalities described here may be useful for genetic studies that may ultimately lead to interventions designed to prevent schizophrenia.

ACKNOWLEDGMENTS

Preparation of this chapter was supported in part by: Stanley Foundation and the National Association for Research in Schizophrenia and Depression (NARSAD)

grants to Dr. Larry J. Seidman and Dr. Robin Murray; NIMH Institutional National Research Service Award "Clinical Research Training Program in Biological and Social Psychiatry" to Dr. Heidi E. Wencel, MH16259 (PI: Stuart T. Hauser, MD, PhD), a Research Training Fellowship in Mental Health from The Wellcome Trust to Dr. Colm McDonald, by NARSAD and National Institute of Mental Health grants MH 43518, 46318 and 50647 to Dr. Ming T. Tsuang, and by a Stanley Foundation Centre Grant to Dr. Robin Murray.

REFERENCES

1. Tsuang MT, Stone WS, Faraone SV. Schizophrenia: a review of genetic studies. Harv Rev Psychiatry 1999; 7:185..207.
2. Karayiorgou M, Gogos JA. A turning point in schizophrenia genetics. Neuron 1997; 19:967..979.
3. Tsuang MT, Seidman LJ, Faraone SV. New approaches to the genetics of schizophrenia: neuropsychological and neuroimaging studies of nonpsychotic first degree relatives of people with schizophrenia. In: Gattaz WF, Hafner H, eds. The Fourth Symposium on the Search for the Causes of Schizophrenia. Vol. IV. Berlin: Springer, 1999:191..207.
4. Arolt V, Lencer R, Nolte A, et al. Eye tracking dysfunction is a putative phenotypic susceptibility marker of schizophrenia and maps to a locus on chromosome 6p in families with multiple occurrence of the disease. Am J Med Genet Neuropsychiat Genet 1996; 67:560..563.
5. Coon H, Plaetke R, Holik J, et al. Use of a neurophysiological trait in linkage analysis of schizophrenia. Biol Psychiatry 1993; 34:277..289.
6. St. Clair D, Blackwood D, Muir W, et al. Association within a family of a balanced translocation with major mental illness. Lancet 1990; 336:13..16.
7. Kosower N, Gerad L, Goldstein M, et al. Constitutive heterochromatin of chromosome 1 and Duffy blood group alleles in schizophrenia. Am J Med Genet 1995; 60:133..138.
8. Millar JK, Christie S, Semple CA, Porteous DJ. Chromosomal location and genomic structure of the human translin-associated factor X gene (TRAX; TSNAX) revealed by intergenic splicing to DISC1, a gene disrupted by a translocation segregating with schizophrenia. Genomics 2000; 67:69..77.
9. Hovatta I, Varilo T, Suvisaari J, et al. A genomewide screen for schizophrenia genes in an isolated Finnish subpopulation, suggesting multiple susceptibility loci. Am J Med Genet 1999; 65:1114..1124.
10. Brzustowicz LM, Hodgkinson KA, Chow EW, Honer WG, Bassett AS. Location of major susceptibility locus for familial schizophrenia on chromosome 1q21-q22. Science 2000; 288:678..682.
11. Antonarakis SE, Blouin JL, Pulver AE, et al. Schizophrenia susceptibility and chromosome 6p24-22. Nat Genet 1995; 11:235..236.
12. Schwab SG, Albus M, Hallmayer J, et al. Evaluation of susceptibility gene for schizophrenia on chromosome 6p by multipoint affected sib-pair linkage analysis. Nat Genet 1995; 11: 325..327.
13. Maziade M, Bissonnette L, Rouillard E, et al. 6p24-22 region and major psychoses in the Eastern Quebec population. Am J Med Genet 1997; 74:311..318.
14. Levinson DF, Holmans P, Straub RE, et al. Multicenter linkage study of schizophrenia candidate regions on chromosomes 5q, 6q, 10p, and 13q: schizophrenia linkage collaborative group III. Am J Med Genet 2000; 67:652..663.
15. Pulver AE, Karayiorgou M, Wpolyneic P, et al. Sequential strategy to identify a susceptibility gene for schizophrenia: report of potential linkage on chromosome 22q12-q13:1: part 1. Am J Med Genet 1994; 54:36..43.

16. Gurling HM, Kalsi G, Brynjolfson J, et al. Genomwide genetic linkage analysis confirms the presence of susceptibility loci for schizophrenia, on chromosomes 1q32.2, 5q33.2, and 8p21-22 and provides support for linkage to schizophrenia, on chromosomes 11q23.3-24 and 20q12.1-11.23. Am J Med Genet 2001; 68:661..673.

17. Lin MW, Curtis D, Williams N, et al. Suggestive evidence for linkage of schizophrenia to markers on chromosome 13q14.1-q32. Psychiatr Genet 1995; 5:117..126.

18. Kalsi G, Sherrington R, Mankoo BS, et al. Linkage study of the D5 dopamine receptor (DRD5) in multiplex Icelandic and English schizophrenia pedigrees. Am J Psychiatry 1996; 153: 107..109.

19. Blouin JL, Dombrowski BA, Nath SK, et al. Schizophrenia susceptibility loci on chromosomes 13q32 and 8p21. Nat Genet 1998; 20:70..73.

20. Freedman R, Adams CE, Leonard S. The alpha-7 nicotinic acetylcholine receptor and the pathology of hippocampal neurons in schizophrenia. J Chem Neuroanat 2000; 20:299..306.

21. Freedman R, Leonard S, Gault JM, et al. Linkage disequilibrium for schizophrenia at the chromosome 15q13-14 locus of the alpha7-nicotinic acetylcholine receptor subunit gene (CHRNA7). Am J Med Genet 2001; 105:20..22.

22. Craddock N, Lendon C. Chromosome Workshop: chromosomes 11, 14 and 15. Am J Med Genet 1999; 88:244..254.

23. Leonard S, Kuldau JM, Breier JI, et al. Cumulative effect of anatomical risk factors for schizophrenia: an MRI study. Biol Psychiatry 1999; 46:374..382.

24. Moises HW, Yang L, Kristbjarnarson H, et al. Potential linkage disequilibrium between schizophrenia and locus D22S278 on the long arm of chromosome 22. Am J Med Genet 1995; 60:465..467.

25. Lasseter VK, Pulver AE, Wolyniec PS, et al. Follow-up report of potential linkage for schizophrenia on chromosome 22q: Part 3. Am J Med Genet 1995; 60:172..173.

26. Faraone SV, Matise C, Svrakic D, et al. Genome scan of European-American schizophrenia pedigree; results of the NIMH Genetics Initiative and Millenium Consortium. Am J Med Genet 1998; 81:290..295.

27. Straub RE, MacLean CJ, Martin RB, et al. A schizophrenia locus may be located in region 10p15-p11. Am J Med Genet 1998; 81:296..301.

28. Jones P, Murray RM. The genetics of schizophrenia is the genetics of neurodevelopment. Br J Psychiatry 1991; 158:615..623.

29. Tsuang MT, Stone WS, Seidman LJ, et al. Treatment of schizotaxia with Risperidone: four case studies. Biol Psychiatry 1999; 45:1412..1418.

30. Faraone SV, Green AI, Seidman LJ, Tsuang MT. Clinical implications for schizotaxia: a new direction for research. Schizophr Bull 2001; 27:1..18.

31. Bogerts B. Recent advances in the neuropathology of schizophrenia. Schizophr Bull 1993; 19:431..445.

32. Shenton ME, Wible CG, McCarley RW. A review of magnetic resonance imaging studies of brain abnormalities in schizophrenia. In: Krishnan KRR, Doraiswamy PM, eds. Brain Imaging in Clinical Psychiatry. New York: Marcel Dekker, 1997:297..380.

33. McCarley RW, Wible CG, Frumin M, et al. MRI anatomy of schizophrenia. Biol Psychiatry 1999; 45:1099..1119.

34. Harrison PJ. The neuropathology of schizophrenia: a critical review of the data and their interpretation. Brain 1999; 122:593..624.

35. Wright IC, Rabe-Hesketh S, Woodruff PWR, David AS, Murray RM, Bullmore ET. Meta-analysis of regional brain volumes in schizophrenia. Am J Psychiatry 2000; 157:16..25.

36. Nelson MD, Saykin AJ, Flashman LA, Riordan HJ. Hippocampal volume reduction in schizophrenia as assessed by magnetic resonance imaging a meta-analytic study. Arch Gen Psychiatry 1998; 55:433..440.
37. Noga JT, Aylward E, Barta PE, Pearlson G. Cingulate gyrus in schizophrenic patients and normal volunteers. Psychiatry Res 1995; 61:201..208.
38. Lawrie SM, Abukmeil SS. Brain abnormality in schizophrenia: a systematic and quantitative review of volumetric magnetic resonance imaging studies. Br J Psychiatry 1998; 172: 110..120.
39. Crespo-Facorro B, Kim J, Andreasen NC, O'Leary DS, Bockholt HJ, Magnotta V. Insular cortex abnormalities in schizophrenia: a structural magnetic resonance imaging study of first-episode patients. Schizophr Res 2000; 46:35..43.
40. Goldstein JM, Goodman JM, Seidman LJ, et al. Cortical abnormalities in schizophrenia identified by structural magnetic resonance imaging. Arch Gen Psychiatry 1999; 56:537..547.
41. Wright IC, Ellison ZR, Sharma T, Friston KJ, Murray RM, McGuire PK. Mapping of grey matter changes in schizophrenia. Schizophr Res 1999; 35:1..14.
42. Wilke M, Kaufmann C, Grabner C, Putz B, Wetter TC, Auer DP. Gray matter changes and correlates of disease severity in schizophrenia: a statistical parameter mapping study. Neuroimage 2001; 13:814..824.
43. Sigmundsson T, Suckling J, Maier M, et al. Structural abnormalities in frontal, temporal, and limbic regions and interconnecting white matter tracts in schizophrenic patients with prominent negative symptoms. Am J Psychiatry 2001; 158:234..243.
44. Wright I, Sharma T, Ellison ZR, et al. Supra-regional brain systems and the neuropathology of schizophrenia. Cereb Cortex 1999; 9:366..378.
45. Norris SD, Krishnan KR, Ahearn E. Structural changes in the brain of patients with bipolar affective disorder by MRI: a review of the literature. Prog Neuropsychopharmacol Biol Psychiatry 1997; 21:1323..1337.
46. Soares JC, Mann JJ. The anatomy of mood disorder review of structural neuroimaging studies. Biol Psychiatry 1997; 41:86..106.
47. Elkis H, Friedman L, Wise A, Meltzer HY. Meta-analyses of studies of ventricular enlargement and cortical sulcal prominence in mood disorders. Comparisons with controls or patients with schizophrenia. Arch Gen Psychiatry 1995; 52:735..746.
48. Lim KO, Rosenbloom MJ, Faustman WO, Sullivan EV, Pfefferbaum A. Cortical gray matter deficit in patients with bipolar disorder. Schizophr Res 1999; 40:219..227.
49. Friedman L, Findling RL, Kenny JT, et al. An MRI study of adolescent patients with either schizophrenia or bipolar disorder as compared to healthy control subjects. Biol Psychiatry 1999; 46:78..88.
50. Dasari M, Friedman L, Jesberger J, et al. A magnetic resonance imaging study of thalamic area in adolescent patients with either schizophrenia or bipolar disorder as compared to healthy controls. Psychiatry Res 1999; 91:155..162.
51. Velakoulis D, Pantelis C, McGorry PD, et al. Hippocampal volume in first-episode psychoses and chronic schizophrenia a high-resolution magnetic resonance imaging study. Arch Gen Psychiatry 1999; 56:133..141.
52. Hirayasu Y, Shenton ME, Salisbury DF, et al. Lower left temporal lobe MRI volumes in patients with first-episode schizophrenia compared with psychotic patients with first-episode affective disorder and normal subjects. Am J Psychiatry 1998; 155:1384..1391.
53. Altshuler LL, Bartzokis G, Grieder T, et al. An MRI study of temporal lobe structures in men with bipolar disorder or schizophrenia. Biol Psychiatry 2000; 48:147..162.

54. Strakowski SM, DelBello MP, Sax KW, et al. Brain magnetic resonance imaging of structural abnormalities in bipolar disorder. Arch Gen Psychiatry 1999; 56:254..260.
55. Drevets WC, Price JL, Simpson JR, et al. Subgenual prefrontal cortex abnormalities in mood disorders. Nature 1997; 386:824..827.
56. Pearlson GD, Barta PE, Powers RE, et al. Ziskind-Somerfeld Research Award 1996. Medial and superior temporal gyral volumes and cerebral asymmetry in schizophrenia versus bipolar disorder. Biol Psychiatry 1997; 41:1..14.
57. Hirayasu Y, McCarley RW, Salisbury DF, et al. Planum temporale and Heschl gyrus volume reduction in schizophrenia: a magnetic resonance imaging study of first-episode patients. Arch Gen Psychiatry 2000; 57:692..699.
58. Bullmore E, Brammer MJ, Williams CR, et al. Functional MR imaging of confouded hypofrontality. Hum Brain Mapp 1999; 8:86..91.
59. Curtis VA, Bullmore ET, Morris RG, et al. Attenuated frontal activation in schizophrenia may be task dependent. Schizophr Res 1999; 37:35..44.
60. Weinberger DR, Berman KF, Zec RF. Physiologic dysfunction of dorsolateral prefrontal cortex in schizophrenia I. Regional cerebral blood flow evidence. Arch Gen Psychiatry 1986; 43: 114..124.
61. Stevens AA, Goldman-Rakic PS, Gore JC, Fulbright RK, Wexler BE. Cortical dysfunction in schizophrenia during auditory word and tone working memory demonstrated by functional magnetic resonance imaging. Arch Gen Psychiatry 1998; 55:1097..1103.
62. Carter CS, Perlstein W, Ganguli R, Brar J, Mintun M, Cohen JD. Functional hypofrontality and working memory dysfunction in schizophrenia. Am J Psychiatry 1998; 155:1285..1287.
63. Curtis VA, Bullmore ET, Brammer MJ, et al. Attenuated frontal activation during a verbal fluency task in patients with schizophrenia. Am J Psychiatry 1998; 155:1056..1063.
64. Manoach DS, Gollub RL, Benson ES, et al. Schizophrenic subjects show aberrant fMRI activation of dorsolateral prefrontal cortex and basal ganglia during working memory performance. Biol Psychiatry 2000; 48:99..109.
65. Zakzanis KK, Heinrichs RW. Schizophrenia and the frontal brain: a quantitative review. J Int Neuropsychol Soc 1999; 5:556..566.
66. Callicott JH, Bertolino A, Mattay VS, et al. Physiological dysfunction of the dorsolateral prefrontal cortex in schizophrenia revisited. Cereb Cortex 2000; 10:1078..1092.
67. Weinberger DR, Mattay V, Callicott J, et al. fMRI applications in schizophrenia research. Neuroimage 1996; 4:S118..S126.
68. Zakzanis KK, Poulin P, Hansen KT, Jolic D. Searching the schizophrenic brain for temporal lobe deficits: a systematic review and meta-analysis. Psychol Med 2000; 30:491..504.
69. Woodruff PWR, Wright IC, Bullmore C, et al. Auditory hallucinations and the temporal cortical response to speech in schizophrenia: a functional magnetic resonance imaging study. Am J Psychiatry 1997; 154:1676..1682.
70. Kircher TT, Liddle PF, Brammer MJ, Williams SC, Murray R, McGuire M. Neural correlates of formal thought disorder in schizohprenia: preliminary findings from a functional magnetic resonance imaging study. Arch Gen Psychiatry 2001; 58:769..774.
71. McGuire PK, Quested DJ, Spence SA, Murray RM, Frith CD, Liddle PF. Pathophysiology of positive thought disorder in schizophrenia. Br J Psychiatry 1998; 173:231..235.
72. Wible CG, Kubicki M, Yoo SS, et al. A functional magnetic resonance imaging study of auditory mismatch in schizophrenia. Am J Psychiatry 2001; 158:938..943.
73. McGuire PK, Silbersweig DA, Wright IC, et al. Abnormal monitoring of inner speech: a physiological basis for auditory hallucinations. Lancet 1995; 346:596..600.

74. Heckers S, Rauch SL, Goff D, et al. Impaired recruitment of the hippocampus during conscious recollection in schizophrenia. Nat Neurosci 1998; 1:318..323.
75. Dierks T, Linden DE, Jandl M, et al. Activation of Heschl's gyrus during auditory hallucinations. Neuron 1999; 22:615..621.
76. Lennox BR, Park SB, Medley I, Morris PG, Jones PB. The functional anatomy of auditory hallucinations in schizophrenia. Psychiatry Res 2001; 100:13..20.
77. Shergill SS, Cameron LA, Brammer MJ, Wililams SC, Murray RM, McGuire PK. Modality specific neural correlates of auditory and somatic hallucinations, areas involved in the processing of external speech. J Neurol Neurosurg Psychiatry 2001; 71:688..690.
78. Shergill SS, Brammer MJ, Williams CR, Murray RM, McGuire PK. Mapping auditory hallucinations in schizophrenia using functional magnetic resonance imaging. Arch Gen Psychiatry 2000; 57:1033..1038.
79. Early TS, Posner MI, Reiman EM, Raichle ME. Hyperactivity of the left striatopallidal projection II. Phenomenology and thought disorder. Psychiatric Dev 1989; 2:109..121.
80. Weinberger DR, Berman KF, Suddath R, Torrey EF. Evidence of dysfunction of a prefrontal-limbic network in schizophenia: a magnetic resonance imaging and region cerebral blood flow study of discordant monozygotic twins. Am J Psychiatry 1992; 149:890..897.
81. Keshavan MS, Stanley JA, Pettegrew JW. Magnetic resonance spectroscopy in schizophrenia: methological issues and findings part II. Biol Psychiatry 2000; 48:369..380.
82. Bertolino A, Nawroz S, Mattay VS, et al. Regionally specific pattern of neurochemical pathology in schizophrenia as assessed by multislice proton magnetic resonance spectroscopic imaging. Am J Psychiatry 1996; 153:1554..1563.
83. Deicken RF, Zhou L, Schuff N, Fein G, Weiner MW. Hippocampal neuronal dysfunction in schizophrenia as measured by proton magnetic resonance spectroscopy. Biol Psychiatry 1998; 43:483..488.
84. Renshaw PF, Yugelun-Todd DA, Tohen MS. Temporal lobe proton magnetic resonance of patients with first-episode psychosis. Am J Psychiatry 1995; 152:444..446.
85. Yurgelun-Todd DA, Renshaw PF, Gruber SA, Ed M, Waternaux C, Cohen BM. Proton magnetic resonance of the temporal lobes in schizophrenics and normal controls. Schizophr Res 1996; 19:55..59.
86. Fukuzako H, Takeuchi K, Hokazono Y, et al. Proton magnetic resonance spectroscopy of the left medial temporal and frontal lobes in chronic schizophrenia: preliminary report. Psychiatry Res Neuroimaging 1995; 61:163..200.
87. Buckley PF, Moore C, Long H, et al. 1H-Magnetic resonance spectroscopy of the left temporal and frontal lobes in schizophrenia: clinical neurodevelopmental and cognitive correlates. Biol Psychiatry 1994; 36:792..800.
88. Cecil KM, Lenkinski RE, Gur RE, Gur RC. Proton magnetic resonance spectroscopy in the frontal and temporal lobes of neuroleptic naive patients with schizophrenia. Neuropsychopharmacology 1998; 20:131..140.
89. Brooks WM, Hodde-Vargas J, Hodde-Vargas LA, Yeo RA, Ford CC, Hendren RL. Frontal lobe of children with schizophrenia spectrum disorders: a proton magnetic resonance spectroscopic study. Biol Psychiatry 1998; 43:263..269.
90. Heimberg C, Komoroski R, Lawson WB, Cardwell D, Karson CN. Regional proton magnetic resonance spectroscopy in schizophrenia and exploration of drug effect. Psychiatr Res 1998; 83:105..115.
91. Deicken RF, Zhou L, Schuff N, et al. Proton magnetic resonance spectroscopy of the anterior cingulate region in schizophrenia. Schizophr Res 1997; 27:65..71.

92. Eluri R, Paul C, Roemer R, Boyko O. Single-voxel proton magnetic resonance spectroscopy of the pons and cerebellum in patients with schizophrenia: a preliminary study. Neuroimage 1998; 84:17.26.

93. Sharma R, Venkatasubramanian PN, Barany M, Davis JM. Proton magnetic resonance spectroscopy of the brain in schizophrenic and affective patients. Schizophr Res 1992; 81:43.49.

94. Shioiri T, Hamakawa H, Kato T, et al. Proton magnetic resonance spectroscopy of basal ganglia in chronic schizophrenia. Biol Psychiatry 1996; 40:14..18.

95. Fukuzako H. Heritability heightens brain metabolite differences in schizophrenia. J Neuropsychiatry Clin Neurosci 2000; 12:95..97.

96. Bertolino A, Callicott JH, Elman I, et al. Regionally specific neuronal pathology in untreated patients with schizophrenia: a proton magnetic resonance spectroscopic imaging study. Biol Psychiatry 1998; 43:641..648.

97. Callicott JH, Egan MF, Bertolino A, et al. Hippocampal N-acetyl aspartate in unaffected siblings of patients with schizophrenia: a possible intermediate neurobiological phenotype. Biol Psychiatry 1998; 44:941..950.

98. Bertolino A, Callicott JH, Mattay VS, et al. The effect of treatment with antipsychotic drugs on brain N-acetylaspartate measures in patients with schizophrenia. Biol Psychiatry 2001; 49:39..46.

99. Stanley JA, Williamson PC, Drost DJ, et al. An in vivo study of the prefrontal cortex of schizophrenia patients at different stages of illness via phosphorous magnetic resonance spectroscopy. Arch Gen Psychiatry 1995; 52:399..406.

100. Kato T, Shioiri T, Murashita J, Hamakawa H, Inubushi T, Takahashi S. Lateralized abnormality of high-energy phosphate and bilateral reduction of phosphomonoester measured by phosphorous-31 magnetic resonance spectroscopy of the frontal lobes in schizophrenia. Psychiatry Res 1995; 61:151..160.

101. Fukuzako HH, Kodama S, Fukuzako T, et al. Subtype-associated metabolite differences in temporal lobe in schizophrenia detected by proton magnetic resonance spectroscopy. Psychiatric Res 1999; 92:45..56.

102. Shioiri T, Kato T, Inubushi T, Murashita J, Takahashi S. Correlations of phosphomonoesters measured by phosphorous-31 magnetic resonance spectroscopy in the frontal lobes and negative symptoms of schizophrenia. Psychiatry Res 1994; 55:223..235.

103. Deicken RF, Merrin EL, Floyd TC, Weiner MW. Correlation between left frontal phospholipids and Wisconsin Card Sort Test performance in schizophrenia. Schizophr Res 1995; 14:177..181.

104. Keshavan MS, Pettegrew JW, Reynolds CF, et al. Biological correlates of slow wave sleep deficits in functional psychoses: 31P-magnetic resonance spectroscopy. Psychiatry Res 1995; 57:91..100.

105. Pettegrew JW, Keshavan MS, Panchalingam K, et al. Alterations in brain high-energy phosphate and membrane phospholipid metabolism in first-episode, drug-naive schizophrenics. A pilot study of the dorsolateral prefrontal cortex by in vivo phosphorous 31 nuclear magnetic resonance spectroscopy. Arch Gen Psychiatry 1991; 48:563..568.

106. Volz HP, Rzanny R, May S, et al. 31P magnetic resonance spectroscopy in the dorsolateral prefrontal coretx of schizophrenics with a volume selective technique preliminary findings. Biol Psychiatry 1997; 42:644..648.

107. Potwarka JJ, Drost DJ, Williamson PC, et al. A 1H-decoupled 31P chemical shift imaging study of medicated schizophrenic patients and healthy controls. Biol Psychiatry 1999; 45:687..693.

108. Bluml S, Tan J, Harris K, et al. Quantitative proton-decoupled 31P MRS of the schizophrenic brain in vivo. J Comput Assist Tomogr 1999; 23:272..275.

109. Tamminga C. Glutamatergic aspects of schizophrenia. Br J Psychiatry 1999; 37(Suppl):12..15.
110. Stanley JA, Williamson PC, Drost DJ, et al. An in vivo proton magnetic resonance spectroscopy study of schizophrenia patients. Schizophr Bull 1996; 22:597..609.
111. Bartha R, Williamson TC, Drost DJ, et al. Measurement of glutamate and glutamine in the medial prefrontal cortex of never-treated schizophrenic patients and healthy controls by proton magnetic resonance spectroscopy. Arch Gen Psychiatry 1997; 54:959..965.
112. Bartha R, al-Sernaan YM, Williamson PC, et al. A short echo proton magnetic resonance spectroscopy study of the left mesial temporal lobe in first-onset schizophrenia patients. Biol Psychiatry 1999; 45:1403..1411.
113. Choe BY, Suh TS, Shinn KS, Lee CW, Lee C, Paik IH. Observation of metabolic changes in chronic schizophrenia after neuroleptic treatment by in vivo hydrogen magnetic resonance spectroscopy. Invest Radio 1996; 31:345..352.
114. Selemon LD, Rajkowska G, Goldman-Rakic PS. Abnormally high neuronal density in the schizophrenic cortex. A morphometric analysis of prefrontal area 9 and area 17. Arch Gen Psychiatry 1995; 52:805..818.
115. Selemon LD, Goldman-Rakic PS. The reduced neuropil hypothesis: a circuit based model of schizophrenia. Biol Psychiatry 1999; 45:17..25.
116. Weinberger DR. Implications of normal brain development for the pathogenesis of schizophrenia. Arch Gen Psychiatry 1987; 44:660..669.
117. Bullmore ET, Frangou S, Murray RM. The dysplastic net hypothesis: an integration of developmental and dysconnectivity theories of schizophrenia. Schizophr Res 1997; 28:143..156.
118. Delisi LE, Sakuma M, Tew W, Kushner M, Hoff AL, Grimson R. Schizophrenia as a chronic active brain process: a study of progressive brain structural change subsequent to the onset of schizophrenia. Psychiatry Res 1997; 74:129..140.
119. Gur RE, Cowell P, Turetsky BI, et al. A follow-up magnetic resonance imaging study of schizophrenia. Relationship of neuroanatomical changes to clinical and neurobehavioral measures. Arch Gen Psychiatry 1998; 55:145..152.
120. Lieberman J, Chakos M, Wu H, et al. Longitudinal study of brain morphology in first episode schizophrenia. Biol Psychiatry 2001; 49:487..499.
121. Woods BT. Is schizophrenia a progressive neurodevelopmental disorder? Towards a unitary pathogenetic mechanism. Am J Psychiatry 1998; 155:1661..1670.
122. Tsuang MT, Gilbertson MW, Faraone SV. Genetic transmission of negative and positive symptoms in the biological relatives of schizophrenics. In: Marneros A, Andreasen NC, Tsuang MT, eds. Negative Versus Positive Schizophrenia. Berlin: Springer-Verlag, 1991: 265..291.
123. Chapman LJ, Chapman JP. Strategies for resolving the heterogeneity of schizophrenics and their relatives using cognitive measures. J Abnorm Psychol 1989; 98:357..336.
124. Kety SS, Rosenthal D, Wender PH, Schulsinger F, Jacobson B. Mental illness in the biological and adoptive families of adopted individuals who have become schizophrenic: a preliminary report based on psychiatric interviews. In: Rieve RR, Rosenthal D, Brill H, eds. Genetic Research in Psychiatry. Baltimore, MD: Johns Hopkins University Press, 1975:147..165.
125. Kendler KS, McGuire M, Gruenberg AM, A OH, Spellman M, Walsh D. The Roscommon family study. III. Schizophrenia-related personality disorders in relatives. Arch Gen Psychiatry 1993; 50:781..788.
126. Dickey CC, McCarley RW, Voglmaier MM, et al. Schizotypal personality disorder and MRI abnormalities of temporal lobe gray matter. Biol Psychiatry 1999; 45:1393..1402.
127. Matthysse S. Genetic linkage and complex diseases: a comment. Genet Epidemiol 1990; 7: 29..31.

128. Lenzenweger MF. Psychometric high-risk paradigm, perceptual aberrations, and schizotypy: an update. Schizophr Bull 1994; 20:121..136.
129. Shenton ME, Solovay MR, Holzman PS, Coleman M, Gale HJ. Thought disorder in the relatives of psychotic patients. Arch Gen Psychiatry 1989; 46:897..901.
130. Docherty NM. Linguistic reference performance in parents of schizophrenic patients. Psychiatry 1995; 58:20..27.
131. Erlenmeyer-Kimling L, Cornblatt B, Friedman D, et al. Neurological, electrophysiological, and attentional deviations in children at risk for schizophrenia. In: Henn FA, Nasrallah HA, eds. Schizophrenia as a Brain Disease. New York: Oxford University Press, 1982:61..98.
132. Levy DL, Holzman PS, Matthysse S, Mendell NR. Eye tracking and schizophrenia: a selective review. Schizophr Bull 1994; 20:47..62.
133. Cornblatt BA, Kelip JG. Impaired attention, genetics and the pathophysiology of schizophrenia. Schizophr Bull 1994; 20:31..46.
134. Kremen WS, Seidman LJ, Pepple JR, Lyons MJ, Tsuang MT, Faraone SV. Neuropsychological risk indicators for schizophrenia: a review of family studies. Schizophr Bull 1994; 20:96..108.
135. Seidman LJ, Goldstein JM, Breiter H, et al. Functional MRI of attention in relatives of schizophrenic patients. Schizophr Res 1997; 49(Suppl):172.
136. Green MF, Nuechterlein KH, Breitmeyer B. Backward masking performance in unaffected siblings of schizophrenic patients. Arch Gen Psychiatry 1997; 54:465..472.
137. Friedman D, Squires-Wheeler E. Event-related potentials (ERPs) as indicators of risk for schizophrenia. Schizophr Bull 1994; 20:63..74.
138. Leonard S, Adams C, Breese C, et al. Nicotinic receptor function in schizophrenia. Schizophr Bull 1996; 22:431..445.
139. Frangou S, Sharma T, Alarcon G, et al. The Maudsley Family Study, II: Endogenous event-related potentials in familial schizophrenia. Schizophr Res 1997; 23:45..53.
140. Weinberger DR, DeLisi LE, Neophytides AN, Wyatt RJ. Familial aspects of CT scan abnormalities in chronic schizophrenic patients. Psychiatry Res 1981; 4:65..71.
141. Reveley AM, Reveley MA, Clifford CA, Murray RM. Cerebral ventricular size in twins discordant for schizophrenia. Lancet 1982; 1:540..541.
142. Delisi LE, Goldfin LR, Hamovit JR, Maxwell ME, D, Gershon ES. A family study of the association of increased ventricular size with schizophrenia. Arch Gen Psychiatry 1986; 43:148..153.
143. Cannon TD, Marco E. Structural brain abnormalities as indicators of vulnerability to schizophrenia. Schizophr Bull 1994; 20:89..102.
144. Honer WG, Bassett AS, Smith GN, Lapointe JS, Falkai P. Temporal lobe abnormalities in multigenerational families with schizophrenia. Biol Psychiatry 1994; 36:737..743.
145. Zorilla LTE, Cannon TD, Kronenberg S, et al. Structural abnormalities in schizophrenia: a family study. Biol Psychiatry 1997; 42:1080..1086.
146. Silverman JM, Smith CJ, Guo SL, Mohs RC, Siever LJ, Davis KL. Lateral ventricular enlargement in schizophrenic probands and their siblings with schizophrenia-related disorders. Biol Psychiatry 1998; 43:97..106.
147. Cannon TD, Mednick SA, Parnas J, Schulsinger F, Praestholm J, Vestergaard A. Developmental brain abnormalities in the offspring of schizophrenic mothers: contributions of genetic and perinatal factors. Arch Gen Psychiatry 1993; 50:551..564.
148. Sharma T, Lancaster E, Lee D, et al. Brain changes in schizophrenia: volumetric MRI study of families multiply affected with schizophrenia-the Maudsley family study 5. Br J Psychiatry 1998; 173:132..138.

149. Suddath RL, Christison GW, Torrey EF, Casanova MF, Weinberger DR. Anatomical abnormalities in the brains of monozygotic twins discordant for schizophrenia. N Engl J Med 1990; 332:789..800.
150. Frangou S, Sharma T, Sigmudsson T, Barta P, Pearlson G, Murray RM. The Maudsley Family Study IV. Normal planum temporale asymmetry in familial schizophrenia a volumetric MRI study. Br J Psychiatry 1997; 170:328..333.
151. Chua SE, Sharma T, Takei N, Murray RM, Woodruff PWR. A magnetic resonance imaging study of corpus callosum size in familial schizophrenic subjects, their relatives, and normal controls. Schizophr Res 2000; 41:397..403.
152. Cannon TD, Van Erp TGM, Huttunen M, Lonnqvist J, Salonen O, Valanne L. Regional gray matter, white matter, and cerebrospinal fluid distributions in schizophrenic patients, their siblings and controls. Arch Gen Psych 1998; 55:1084..1091.
153. Seidman LJ, Faraone SV, Goldstein JM, et al. Reduced subcortical brain volumes in nonpsychotic siblings of schizophrenic patients: a pilot MRI study. Am J Med Genet: Neuropsychiatric Genet 1997; 74:507..514.
154. Seidman LJ, Faraone SV, Goldstein JM, et al. Thalamic and amygdala-hippocampal volume reductions in first degree relatives of schizophrenic patients: an MRI-based morphometric analysis. Biol Psychiatry 1999; 46:941..954.
155. Filipek P, Richelme C, Kennedy DN, Caviness VS. The young adult human brain: an MRI-based morphometric analysis. Cereb Cort 1994; 4:344..360.
156. Seidman LJ, Faraone SV, Goldstein JM, et al. Left hippocampal volume as a vulnerability indicator for schizophrenia: a MRI morphometric study of non-psychotic first degree relatives. Arch Gen Psychiatry 2002; 59:839..849.
157. O'Driscoll GA, Florencio PS, Gagnon D, et al. Amygdala-hippocampal volume and verbal memory in first-degree relatives of schizophrenic patients. Psychiatry Res 2001; 107:75..85.
158. Staal WG, Hulshoff HE, Schnack H, Van der Schot AC, Kahn RS. Partial volume decrease of the thalamus in relatives of patients with schizophrenia. Am J Psychiatry 1998; 155:1784..1786.
159. Staal WG, Hulshoff Pol HE, Schnack HG, Hoogendoorn ML, Jellema K, Kahn RS. Structural brain abnormalities in patients with schizophrenia and their healthy siblings. Am J Psychiatry 2000; 157:416..421.
160. Keshavan MS, Montrose DM, Pierri J, et al. Magnetic resonance imaging and spectroscopy in offspring at risk for schizophrenia: preliminary studies. Biol Psychiatry 1997; 21:1285..1295.
161. Screiber H, Baur-Seack K, Kornhuber HH, et al. Brain morphology in adolescents at genetic risk for schizophrenia assessed by qualitative and quantitative magnetic resonance imaging. Schizophr Res 1999; 40:81..84.
162. Lawrie SM, Whalley H, Kestelman JN, et al. Magnetic resonance imaging of brain in people at high risk of developing schizophrenia. Lancet 1999; 353:30..33.
163. Lawrie SM, Whalley HC, Abukmeil SS, et al. Structure, genetic liability, and psychotic symptoms in subjects at high risk of developing schizophrenia. Biol Psychiatry 2001; 49:811..823.
164. Berman KF, Torrey EF, Daniel DG, Weinberger DR. Regional cerebral blood flow in monozygotic twins discordant and concordant for schizophrenia. Arch Gen Psychiatry 1992; 49: 927..934.
165. Spence SA, Liddle PF, Stefan MD, et al. Functional anatomy of verbal fluency in people with schizophrenia and those at genetic risk: focal dysfunction and distributed disconnectivy reappraised. Br J Psychiatry 2000; 176:52..60.
166. Wencel HE, Seidman LJ, Kennedy D, Makris N, Tsuang MT. Relationship of hippocampal and thalamic volume to dorsolateral prefrontal cortex activation in first-degree relatives of persons with schizophrenia. Schizophr Res 2001; 49(Suppl):189.

167. Seidman LJ, Breiter H, Goodman JM, et al. A functional magnetic resonance imaging study of auditory vigilance with low and high information processing demands. Neuropsychology 1998; 12:505..518.

168. Klemm S, Rzanny R, Riehmann S, et al. Cerebral phosphate metabolism in first-degree relatives of patients with schizophrenia. Am J Psychiatry 2001; 158:958..960.

169. Keshavan MS, Pettegrew JW, Panchalingam K, Kaplan D, Bozik E. Phosphorous 31 magnetic resonance spectroscopy detects altered brain metabolism before onset of schizophrenia. Arch Gen Psychiatry 1991; 48:1112..1113.

170. Weickert CS, Weinberger DR. A candidate molecule approach to defining developmental pathology in schizophrenia. Schizophr Bull 1998; 24:303..316.

171. Lewis SW, Murray RM. Obstetric complications, neurodevelopmental deviance, and risk for schizophrenia. J Psychiatric Res 1987; 21.

172. Tsuang MT, Faraone SV. The case for heterogeneity in the etiology of schizophrenia. Schizophr Res 1995; 17:161..175.

173. McNeil TF, Cantor-Graae E, Weinberger DR. Relationship of obstetric complications and differences in size of brain structures in monozygotic twin pairs discordant for schizophrenia. Am J Psychiatry 2000; 157:203..212.

174. Baare WF, van Oel CJ, Hulshoff Pol HE, et al. Volumes of brain structures in twins discordant for schizophrenia. Arch Gen Psychiatry 2001; 58:33..40.

175. Fearon P, Cotter D, Murray RM. Is the association between obstetric complications and schizophrenia mediated by glutamatergic excitotoxic damage to the fetal/neonatal brain? In: Reveley M, Deakin B, eds. Psychopharmacology of Schizophrenia. London: Chapman & Hall, 2000, pp. 21..24.

176. McNeil TF. Obstetric complications in schizophrenic parents. Schizophr Res 1991; 5:89..101.

177. Sacker A, Done DJ, Crow TJ. Obstetric complications in children born to parents with schizophrenia: a meta-analysis of case-control studies. Psychol Med 1996; 26:279..287.

178. Rosso IM, Cannon TD, Huttunen T, Huttunen MO, Lonnqvist J, Gasperoni TL. Obstetric risk factors for early-onset schizophrenia in a Finnish birth cohort. Am J Psychiatry 2000; 157:801..807.

179. McEwen BS, Magarinos AM. Stress effects on morphology and function of the hippocampus. Ann NY Acad Sci 1997; 821:271..284.

180. Olin SS, Mednick SA. Risk factors of psychosis: identifying vulnerable populations premorbidly. Schizophr Bull 1996; 22:223..240.

181. Marcus J, Hans SL, Lewow E, Wilkinson L, Burack CM. Neurological findings in high-risk children: childhood assessment and 5-year follow-up. Schizophr Bull 1985; 11:85..100.

182. Kremen WS, Faraone SV, Seidman LJ, Pepple JR, Tsuang MT. Neuropsychological risk indicators for schizophrenia: a preliminary study of female relatives of schizophrenic and bipolar probands. Psychiatry Res 1998; 79:227..240.

183. Gilvarry CM, Takei N, Russell A, Rushe T, Hemsley D, Murray RM. Premorbid IQ in patients with functional psychosis and their first degree relatives. Schizophr Res 2000; 41:417..429.

184. Moldin SO, Gottesman II. Genes, experience, and chance in schizophrenia-positioning for the 21st century. Schizophr Bull 1997; 23:547..561.

185. Tsuang MT, Faraone SV. Schizophrenia. In: Jameson L, ed. Textbook of Molecular Medicine. Totowa, NJ: Humana, 1998:989..994.

186. Orlova VA, Trubnikov VI, Odintsova SA, et al. Genetic analysis of anatomical and morphological traits of the brain, determined by magnetic resonance imaging in families of schizophrenic patients. Genetika 1999; 35:998..104.

187. Sharma T, Lancaster E, Sigmundsson T, et al. Lack of normal pattern of cerebral asymmetry in familial schizophrenic patients and their relatives The Maudsley Family Study. Schizophr Res 1999; 40:111..120.

10 Neurophysiological Endophenotypes in Early Detection of Schizophrenia

Marina Myles-Worsley, PhD

Previous chapters have discussed the concept of vulnerability indicators or "endophenotypes" for schizophrenia, biobehavioral traits that reflect an underlying genetic liability for schizophrenia (1,2). In terms of early detection, intervention, and prevention, these vulnerability indicators have the potential to identify individuals at increased risk for developing schizophrenia and predict course and outcome in recent-onset patients.

To function as an endophenotype for schizophrenia, a trait marker should fulfill a number of criteria. One of the most crucial criteria is a higher than normal prevalence of the dysfunction not only in schizophrenia patients but also in their unaffected biological relatives. In recent years, considerable research effort has been directed toward investigating the ability of various biobehavioral traits to fulfill this criterion. This research has predominantly studied siblings of probands but some studies have extended their investigations to include a broader range of relatives, particularly when the study is using genetic linkage analysis to examine genetic etiology in large multiplex schizophrenia families. These studies have revealed several excellent neurophysiological candidates that may serve as vulnerability markers for schizophrenia by showing that a significant proportion of first-degree relatives who remain clinically unaffected throughout their lives exhibit impairments in neurophysiological functioning similar to those found in schizophrenia patients.

The two domains of neurophysiological functioning that have been most widely investigated in the search for endophenotypes for schizophrenia are ocular motor functioning (OMD) and event-related potentials (ERPs). Neurophysiological measures within these two domains are reviewed first. A briefer review of other neurophysiological abnormalities associated with schizophrenia that are not included in these two categories follows.

From: *Early Clinical Intervention and Prevention in Schizophrenia*
Edited by: W. S. Stone, S. V. Faraone, and M. T. Tsuang © Humana Press Inc., Totowa, NJ

OCULAR MOTOR DYSFUNCTION

Ocular motor functioning includes several different types of eye movements. The OMDs most frequently associated with schizophrenia are eye-tracking dysfunction (ETD), also known as smooth-pursuit abnormalities, and impairments in the saccadic eye-movement system.

Eye-Tracking Dysfunction

Pursuit eye movements are elicited by tasks that require the subject to visually follow a target that moves either sinusoidally or at a constant velocity. During an eye-tracking task, the pursuit system stabilizes the image of the moving target on the fovea by matching eye velocity to target velocity. During a pursuit task, saccadic eye movements may occur. Compensatory saccades serve to reposition the target on the fovea when the eyes move either slower or faster than the target, whereas intrusive saccades such as anticipatory saccades disrupt correct eye position. More than 25 years of research on ETD in schizophrenia has convincingly shown a significantly higher prevalence of ETD in schizophrenia patients and their biological relatives than in normal and psychiatric controls *(3,4)*. Furthermore, twin studies strongly support genetic control of eye-tracking performance *(5–9)*. Thus, ETD fulfills the main criteria for a candidate endophenotype for schizophrenia.

Several studies of first-episode patients have confirmed the presence of ETD at rates comparable to those found in samples of acutely ill, chronic, and remitted schizophrenic patients. Sweeney et al. *(10)* found that pursuit eye-movement impairments are present in both first- and multiple-episode patients but are less severe in first-episode patients. Lieberman et al. *(11)* reported that 51% of patients in their first episode of schizophrenia showed abnormal pursuit eye movement, suggesting that ETD occurs independently of the effects of chronic illness and neuroleptic exposure. Hutton et al. *(12)* examined ETD as well as saccadic abnormalities in first-episode schizophrenic patients and found that both types of OMD occurred only in the subset of untreated patients who had received no medication.

ETD is one of the few psychophysiological measures that have been studied in young high-risk subjects. However, sample sizes have been relatively small, and the ETD measures that discriminate normal from abnormal performance in high-risk subjects are not the same as the more global pursuit measures that consistently distinguish schizophrenic patients from normal controls. Mather *(13)* found significant levels of ETD as measured by intrusive saccades in the teenage children of schizophrenic patients. Ross et al. *(14)* found ETD in a sample of 13 young offspring of schizophrenic parents who were 6..15 years of age at the time of testing. However, the particular pursuit abnormality that most clearly distinguished high-risk children from normal children was different from the pursuit

abnormalities that distinguish schizophrenic patients from controls. These results raise questions about the suitability of pursuit tasks for children who have not yet reached the age at which the ocular motor system has matured. The New York High Risk Project (NYHRP) conducted a study of the offspring of parents with either schizophrenia (HRScz) or an affective disorder (HRAff), but eye-tracking performance was not assessed until these subjects had reached adulthood. Global measures of eye-tracking performance, which distinguish schizophrenia patients from normals, were found to be the same in both offspring groups. The only measure that distinguished the HRScz from the HRAff group was number of intrusive anticipatory saccades *(15)*.

Several of the recently initiated high-risk studies include eye-tracking measures in their assessment protocol *(16)*. One of these high-risk studies, the Hillside Study of Risk and Early Detection in Schizophrenia, is beginning to generate ETD data. Preliminary results were reported at the 1999 International Congress of Schizophrenia Research based on 20 adolescent schizophrenia patients and 20 of their adolescent siblings compared to 20 adult schizophrenia patients *(17)*. These preliminary findings indicate that ETD can be measured reliably in adolescent patients and their young siblings, ETD is comparable across age of onset and duration of illness, and ETD is independent of clinical status at the time of testing. Large-scale prospective studies like the Hillside Study are clearly needed to determine which measures of ETD are most reliable in predicting risk for developing schizophrenia.

Saccadic Eye Movements

A particular saccadic measure that has consistently revealed abnormalities in schizophrenic patients is performance on the antisaccade (AS) task. AS tasks measure ocular motor response inhibition and require voluntary control over prepotent reflexive saccades. In reflexive visually guided saccade tasks, subjects are instructed to move their eyes in response to a target that jumps from one location to another, typically from a central fixation point to either the right or the left in an unpredictable series. In antisaccade tasks, subjects are required to inhibit a reflexive glance toward the target and instead voluntarily direct their eyes in an equal and opposite direction.

A number of studies have shown that schizophrenic patients have difficulty inhibiting reflexive glances during an AS task *(18–27)*. Furthermore, many studies have shown that AS impairments occur at a significantly elevated rate in the first-degree relatives of schizophrenic patients compared to normal control subjects *(22,25,28–30)*. Several of these studies have shown that AS performance is worse in relatives of poorly performing patients suggesting that the abnormality runs in families and is under genetic control *(28,30)*. Despite the consistency of these reports, a recent study by Levy et al. *(31)* failed to replicate the finding that the AS performance of biological relatives of schizophrenics differs from controls.

Similarly, Ettinger et al. *(32)* studied recent-onset schizophrenia patients, their healthy siblings, and normal controls and reported that recent-onset patients had a significantly higher error rate than their siblings and normal controls but siblings did not differ from controls. These failures to replicate the presence of AS performance deficits in first-degree relatives may reflect subtle differences in the AS task parameters pertaining to the timing of onset and offset of the central fixation point and the peripheral cues that significantly affect performance *(27,29)*.

Although further investigation of the reasons for the discrepancies in findings is clearly needed, research is proceeding to evaluate AS performance as a vulnerability marker for schizophrenia. Although studies confirming the presence of AS performance deficits in first-episode patients are beginning to appear *(32,33)*, the AS task is not known to be part of the ocular motor measurement protocol in any ongoing high-risk studies. An important issue to be considered in a high-risk study is age-related changes in task performance. Recent studies of normal subjects have reported significant improvement of AS task performance with age *(34,35)*. Therefore, the effects of age on AS performance would have to be partialed out in studies of child or adolescent high-risk subjects, which could seriously reduce effect sizes and thus power.

EVENT-RELATED POTENTIALS

ERPs are a reflection of the brain's electrical response to sensory stimulation. ERP studies in schizophrenia are designed to elucidate the underlying neurophysiological correlates of the characteristic cognitive impairments associated with the illness such as attention and working memory deficits. Because ERPs provide a means of studying brain function in human subjects that is noninvasive, ERP techniques can be used in a variety of subjects ranging from patients at various stages of illness to unaffected individuals at risk, including children.

ERP components are generally categorized by latency. The early and middle latency components of the ERP that occur during the first 200 ms after the stimulus are termed exogenous because they are primarily affected by the physical characteristics of that stimulus and the individual's response is involuntary. The later components such as P300 are considered to be endogenous because their amplitude and latency are primarily determined by the individual's voluntary attention to the stimulus rather than by its sensory characteristics.

Two distinct ERP paradigms, P50 sensory gating based on an exogenous component and P300 deficits based on an endogenous component, have dominated schizophrenia research. However, other ERP components such as mismatch negativity have begun to generate interesting results that could have an important bearing on early detection and intervention in schizophrenia.

P50 Sensory Gating

One of the more widely recognized psychophysiological abnormalities associated with schizophrenia is deficient gating of the P50 component of the auditory ERP. Regulation of sensitivity to sensory stimuli, commonly termed sensory gating, is a critical neurophysiological mechanism in brain function underlying the individual's ability to process information selectively and filter out extraneous stimuli from meaningful sensory inputs. A deficit in sensory gating refers to a dysfunction in the mechanisms responsible for modulating the brain's sensitivity to sensory stimuli, possibly because of dysfunction in inhibitory neurocircuitry *(36–39)*.

The P50 experimental paradigm is designed to measure auditory sensory gating. Using electroencephalographic (EEG) techniques, the P50 component of the ERP wave is recorded in a conditioning-testing paradigm. EEG responses are recorded to pairs of auditory clicks that are presented about 500 ms apart. A grand average of all resulting data is digitally filtered and a computer algorithm *(40)* is used to identify the EEG waves occurring approx 50 ms after each stimulus in the pair. The amplitudes of these P50 waves are measured, and the ratio of the second "test" wave to the first "conditioning" wave amplitude is computed. This P50 ratio measures gating of the P50 auditory evoked response, with lower values indicative of increased sensory gating.

A number of independent studies have shown that schizophrenia patients and their first-degree relatives show less suppression or gating of the second P50 wave *(38,41–42)*. Approximately 75% of schizophrenic patients show deficient auditory sensory gating as measured by the P50 ratio. Furthermore, about 50% of the first-degree relatives of schizophrenia patients show the P50 sensory gating abnormality compared to about 10% of normal controls *(43,44)*. Therefore, the P50 sensory gating deficit appears to meet one of the most important criteria for an endophenotypic marker for schizophrenia, namely, its elevated prevalence in an unaffected relatives of schizophrenia patients. The ability of the P50 sensory gating deficit to function as an endophenotype in family-genetic studies of schizophrenia was further strengthened when Freedman et al. *(45)* reported significant linkage of the P50 deficit to a chromosome 15q locus.

To date, there have been remarkably few published studies of P50 sensory gating in the populations of interest for early detection and intervention. Yee et al. *(46)* compared the P50 sensory gating performance of 22 recent-onset schizophrenia patients to 11 normal controls and revealed that P50 gating is indeed impaired in outpatients with a recent onset of the illness, just as it is in chronic schizophrenia patients. In terms of genetically at-risk subjects, the only published studies are of the first-degree relatives of schizophrenia probands, which include their unaffected adult siblings *(43,44)*. These studies have consistently shown the presence of the P50 sensory gating impairment in approximately half of the relatives.

The suitability of the P50 paradigm for young high-risk subjects was established in a study of developmental and genetic influences on P50 sensory gating *(47)*. Based on a sample of 127 subjects ranging from 10 to 39 years of age, this study found that the distribution of P50 ratios was similar across age groups suggesting that P50 sensory gating deficits can be reliably assessed in subjects as young as 10 years of age.

A recently initiated prospective study of the adolescent members of large multiplex families in Palau, Micronesia, who are at increased genetic risk for developing schizophrenia includes an assessment of P50 sensory gating performance *(48)*. This study will build upon the results of a recent assessment of P50 sensory gating in the multiplex schizophrenia families that have been identified in Palau *(49)*. A total of 85 schizophrenia patients (56 medicated with typical antipsychotics and 29 unmedicated), 83 of their first-degree relatives, and 29 normal comparison subjects were evaluated. Auditory sensory gating as measured by the P50 ratio was similarly impaired in medicated and unmedicated schizophrenia patients compared to the normal subjects, and medication dose had no significant effect on any P50 variable. This impairment extended to first-degree relatives, who also showed significantly higher P50 ratios than the normal subjects. Abnormal P50 ratios were found in 64.7% of the schizophrenia patients and 51.8% of their first-degree relatives but only 10.3% of the normal subjects. Thus, P50 sensory gating deficits were confirmed in these Palauan schizophrenia families, and rates of abnormal P50 sensory gating in first-degree relatives vs normal subjects resulted in a risk ratio of 5.0. Impairment was independent of medication effects, indicating that the P50 paradigm measures a stable neurobiological trait unaffected by treatment with typical antipsychotics. The P50 sensory gating deficits found in these multiply affected Palauan families are expected to be transmitted to the high-risk adolescent offspring and may represent an important predictor of transition to schizophrenia.

P300 Abnormalities

Reduction of the amplitude of the P300 component of the ERP has been one of the most widely replicated findings in neurophysiological research on brain dysfunction in schizophrenia *(50–52)*. The P300 wave is an endogenous, long-latency ERP component that is elicited by unexpected, novel, or cognitively significant events. P300 can be elicited by auditory, visual, and somatosensory stimulation, but most studies in schizophrenia have examined the auditory P300. P300 is traditionally elicited in an "oddball" paradigm in which subjects are required to detect infrequent, task-relevant target stimuli embedded in a series of frequently occurring, nontarget stimuli.

Studies of schizophrenic patients at various stages of illness indicate that whereas P300 amplitude does fluctuate significantly with clinical state, the auditory P300

amplitude reduction persists as a trait marker of schizophrenia *(52,53)*. Because P300 amplitude does covary with clinical state, this state marker may be able to provide valuable information about course, prognosis, and treatment effects in recent-onset patients.

A well-designed P300 study by Salisbury et al. *(54)* compared first-episode patients with a diagnosis of either schizophrenia or affective psychosis to normal control subjects. The results confirmed the presence of reduced P300 amplitude at midline in both groups of first-episode patients relative to controls. However, the schizophrenia group differed significantly from the affective psychosis group in P300 amplitude over the left temporal lobe suggesting that a left-sided P300 abnormality is specific to schizophrenia and present at illness onset.

P300 amplitude reduction is also seen in the unaffected biological relatives of schizophrenic patients *(55–58)* suggesting that this ERP measure may function as a vulnerability marker for schizophrenia. However, the study of P300 amplitude reduction in the offspring of schizophrenic patients has failed to generate the expected results. Schreiber et al. *(59,60)* reported that P300 latencies were longer in children at risk for schizophrenia compared to age-matched normal controls but P300 amplitude did not differ between groups. After Friedman et al. *(61)* reported failure to find any significant group differences in P300 generation in subjects participating in the NYHRP, Squires-Wheeler et al. *(62)* examined the relationship between P300 amplitude and subsequent clinical assessments made when the subjects reached adulthood. No link was found between reduced P300 amplitude and subsequent clinical status even when a broad spectrum of schizophrenia-related diagnoses were included. Consequently, the use of the auditory P300 ERP measure in high-risk studies has not fulfilled expectations and has not been included in recently initiated prospective high-risk studies *(16)*.

Mismatch Negativity Impairment

The P300 component of the ERP is preceded by several components that reflect earlier stages of information processing *(63)*. Mismatch negativity (MMN) is a short-latency cognitive ERP component that represents the earliest cortical response to stimulus novelty. Like the P300, MMN is usually elicited in an auditory oddball paradigm. MMN to target stimuli defined by pitch or intensity occurs with a peak latency of about 150 ms *(63)*.

A series of studies by Javitt and colleagues have shown that schizophrenic patients have marked impairments in the generation of MMN as well as P300 *(64,65)*. A comparison of chronic and recent-onset schizophrenic patients with normal controls showed that recent-onset patients have the same decreased MMN amplitude that chronic patients exhibit but their MMN latency is in the normal range *(66)*. Furthermore, Schreiber et al. *(67)* in a study of children at risk for schizophrenia vs normal controls used a selective-attention paradigm to examine the MMN

response in an ERP paradigm and found that MMN was reduced in the high-risk children compared to normal controls. However, a recent study that replicated the MMN impairment in patients found that the impairment did not extend to their unaffected first-degree relatives *(68)*. Additional research with the biological relatives of schizophrenics is clearly needed to determine whether the MMN impairment alone can fulfill this important criterion for an endophenotype for schizophrenia.

An advantage of the MMN measure is its strong association with working memory functioning, which has consistently been shown to be disrupted in schizophrenia patients as well as their biological relatives *(69)* including their high-risk offspring *(70)*. A recent study by Hirsch et al. *(71)* reported that MMN abnormalities were most frequent in schizophrenic patients with working memory deficits. Consequently, a combination of an MMN assessment and a comprehensive working memory assessment in high-risk and recent-onset studies could potentially provide important information about the neurobiological underpinnings of working memory deficits in schizophrenia.

OTHER NEUROPHYSIOLOGICAL ABNORMALITIES ASSOCIATED WITH SCHIZOPHRENIA

Two additional neurophysiological measures to be considered are prepulse inhibition (PPI) of the startle reflex and autonomic responsivity.

Braff, Geyer, and colleagues *(72–75)* have used neurophysiological measurement techniques to record PPI and habituation of the blink reflex component of startle as a means to assess sensorimotor gating in schizophrenia. Their studies have consistently shown that PPI and habituation of the blink reflex are impaired in schizophrenic patients. A recent study by Taiminen et al. *(76)* has replicated this result in a sample of first-episode patients, indicating that the impairment is present at the time of illness onset and is not a function of chronicity and neuroleptic exposure. However, the PPI impairment extended to patients with psychotic depression, indicating a more general association with psychotic illness rather than the kind of specific association with schizophrenia that is required for an endophenotype for schizophrenia. The PPI paradigm has not been used in any high-risk studies to date possibly because there are significant gender and age effects on PPI and habituation of the blink reflex.

Studies of electrodermal responsiveness in schizophrenia raised the possibility that abnormalities in autonomic nervous system activity might be a vulnerability marker for schizophrenia *(77,78)*. However, subsequent studies revealed that these abnormalities fluctuated with active symptomatology and thus represented more of a state marker than a trait or vulnerability marker for schizophrenia. Cannon et al. *(79,80)* extensively reanalyzed the autonomic nervous system

data that had been collected in the Copenhagen High Risk Project when subjects had reached a mean age of 15 years. He found that electrodermal nonresponsiveness interacted with genetic risk and birth complications to predict negative symptoms in adult schizophrenics. In contrast, heightened electrodermal responsiveness interacted with genetic risk and an unstable rearing environment to predict predominantly positive symptoms in adult schizophrenics. Although these findings renewed interest in autonomic nervous system functioning as a marker for schizophrenia, measures in this domain have generally been considered lacking in the levels of sensitivity and specificity required for inclusion in large-scale longitudinal studies of high-risk and first-episode patients.

SUMMARY

In terms of early detection, intervention, and prevention, neurophysiological abnormalities such as OMD and ERP impairments may have the potential to identify individuals at increased risk for developing schizophrenia and predict course and outcome in recent onset patients. In order to do so, the positive predictive value of these psychophysiological abnormalities for identifying high-risk individuals who transition to schizophrenia will need to be established by prospectively studying young people at high risk for developing schizophrenia and first-episode schizophrenia patients. Although this has not yet been done, recently initiated high-risk studies such as the Hillside Study, which will collect ETD data, and the Palau Family Genetic Study, which will collect P50 sensory gating data, can begin to generate this information over the next decade.

No single neurophysiological measure stands out as a superior for understanding the brain dysfunctions associated with liability for schizophrenia. Each of the neurophysiological measures covered by this review has both strengths and weaknesses. Consequently, large-scale longitudinal studies of high-risk children and adolescents and recent-onset schizophrenia patients likely need multiple neurophysiological measures to be used in combination with the most promising neuropsychological and cognitive measures. Combining measures across several domains of functioning should increase the positive predictive value of these measures so that meaningful composite indices for predicting onset and course of illness can be developed.

In the NYHRP, the systematic longitudinal investigation of attentional deficits in children at risk for schizophrenia, which used multiple measures of attentional/working memory functioning, led to the development of a global attentional deviance score with a positive predictive value of 80% in identifying subjects who eventually developed schizophrenia (81–83). This research effort, which extended over two decades, has set a high standard for researchers investigating vulnerability markers for schizophrenia. Neurophysiological measures such as OMD and

ERP impairments should be able to make an important contribution to the further development of vulnerability markers for schizophrenia, which can meet and possibly exceed this standard.

REFERENCES

1. Gottesman II, Shields J. Schizophrenia and Genetics: A Twin Study Vantage Point. Orlando, FL: Academic, 1972.
2. Gottesman II, Shields J. Schizophrenia: The Epigenetic Puzzle. New York: Cambridge University Press, 1982.
3. Levy DL, Holzman PS, Matthysse S, Mendell NR. Eye tracking dysfunction and schizophrenia: a critical perspective. Schizophr Bull 1993; 19:461.536.
4. Levy DL, Holzman PS, Matthysse S, Mendell NR. Eye tracking and schizophrenia   a selective review. Schizophr Bull 1994; 20:47..62.
5. Holzman PS, Kringlen E, Levy DL, Haberman S, Proctor LR, Yasillo NJ. Abnormal pursuit eye movements in schizophrenia: evidence for a genetic indicator. Arch Gen Psychiatry 1977; 34:802..805.
6. Holzman PS, Kringlen W, Levy DL, Haberman SM. Deviant eye tacking in twins discordant for psychosis: a replication. Arch Gen Psychiatry 1980; 37:627..631.
7. Iacono WG, Lyken DT. Electro-oculographic recording and scoring of smooth-pursuit and saccadic eye tracking: a parametric study using monozygotic twins. Psychophysiology 1979; 16:94..107.
8. Iacono WG, Lykken DT. Eye tracking and psychopathology: new procedures applied to a sample of normal monozygotic twins. Arch Gen Psychiatry 1979; 36:1361..1369.
9. Kendler KS, Ochs AL, Gorman AM, Hewitt JK, Rose DE, Mirsky AF. The structure of schizotypy: a pilot multitrait twin study. Psychiatry Res 1991; 36:19..36.
10. Sweeney JS, Haas GL, Li S. Neuropsychological and eye movement abnormalities in first episode and chronic schizophrenia. Schizophr Bull 1992; 18:283..293.
11. Lieberman JA, Jody D, Alvir JMJ, et al. Brain morphology, dopamine, and eye-tracking abnormalities in first-episode schizophrenia. Arch Gen Psychiatry 1993; 50:357.368.
12. Hutton S, Crawford TJ, Puri BK, et al. Smooth pursuit and saccadic abnormalities in first-episode schizophrenia. Psychol Med 1998; 28:685..692.
13. Mather JA. Eye-movements of teenage children of schizophrenics   a possible inherited marker of susceptibility to the disease. J Psychiatr Res 1985; 19:523.532.
14. Ross RG, Hommer D, Radant A, Roath M, Freedman R. Early expression of smooth-pursuit eye movement abnormalities in children of schizophrenic parents. J Am Acad Child Adolesc Psychiatry 1996; 35:941..949.
15. Rosenberg DR, Sweeney JA, Squires-Wheeler E, Keshavan MS, Cornblatt BA, Erlenmeyer-Kimling L. Eye-tracking dysfunction in offspring from the New York High-Risk Project: diagnostic specificity and the role of attention. Psychiatry Res 1997; 66:121..130.
16. Cornblatt B, Obuchowski M. Update of high-risk research: 1987..1997. Int Rev Psychiatry 1997; 9:437.447.
17. Obuchowski M, Goldman R, Smith C, et al. Neurocognitive deficits in adolescents prodromal for schizophrenia. Schizophr Res 1999; 36:146.
18. Fukushima J, Fukushima K, Chiba T, Tanaka S, Yamashita I, Kato M. Disturbances of voluntary control of saccadic eye movements in schizophrenic patients. Biol Psychiatry 1988; 23: 670..677.

19. Fukushima J, Morita N, Fukushima K, Chiba T, Tanaka S, Yamashita I. Voluntary control of saccadic eye movements in patients with schizophrenic and affective disorders. J Psychiatr Res 1990; 24:9..24.

20. Fukushima J, Fukushima K, Miyasaka K, Yamashita I. Voluntary control of saccadic eye movement in patients with frontal cortical lesions and Parkinsonian patients in comparison with that in schizophrenics. Biol Psychiatry 1994; 36:21..30.

21. Thaker GK, Nguyen JA, Tamminga CA. Increased saccadic distractibility in tardive dyskinesia: functional evidence for subcortical GABA function. Biol Psychiatry 1989; 25:49..59.

22. Clementz BA, McDowell JE, Zisook S. Saccadic system functioning among schizophrenia patients and their first-degree relatives. J Abnorm Psychol 1994; 103:277..287.

23. Crawford TJ, Haeger B, Kennard C, Reveley MA, Henderson L. Saccadic abnormalities in psychotic patients. I. Neuroleptic-free psychotic patients. Psychol Med 1995; 25:461..471.

24. Sereno A, Holzman PS. Antisaccades and smooth pursuit eye movements in schizophrenia. Biol Psychiatry 1995; 37:394..401.

25. McDowell JE, Clementz BA. The effect of fixation condition manipulation on antisaccade performance in schizophrenia: studies of diagnostic specificity. J Exp Brain Res 1997; 115: 333..344.

26. Katsanis J, Kortenkamp S, Iacono WG, Grove WM. Antisaccade performance in patients with schizophrenia and affective disorder. J Abnorm Psychol 1997; 106:468..472.

27. Levy DL, Mendell NR, LaVancher CA, et al. Disinhibition in antisaccade performance in schizophrenia. In: Lenzenweger MF, Dworkin RH, eds. Origins and Development of Schizophrenia. Washington, DC: American Psychological Association, 1998.

28. Crawford TJ, Sharma T, Puri BK, Murray RM, Berridge DM, Lewis SW. Saccadic eye movements in families multiply affected with schizophrenia: the Maudsley family study. Am J Psychiatry 1998; 155:1703..1710.

29. McDowell JE, Myles-Worsley M, Coon H, Byerley W, Clementz BA. Measuring liability for schizophrenia using optimized antisaccade stimulus parameters. Psychophysiology 1999; 36: 138..141.

30. Curtis CE, Calkins ME, Grove WM, Feil KJ, Iacono WG. Saccadic disinhibition in patients with acute and remitted schizophrenia and their first-degree biological relatives. Am J Psychiatry 2001; 158:100..106.

31. Levy DL, Brownstein J, Krastoshevsky O, Matthysse S, Holzman PS, Mendell NR. Is antisaccade performance a co-familial trait? Schizophr Res 2001; 49:216.

32. Ettinger U, Kumari V, Corr PJ, Das M, Zachariah E, Crawford TJ, Sharma T. Smooth pursuit and saccadic eye movements in patients with schizophrenia and their unaffected siblings. Schizophr Res 2001; 49:214.

33. Hutton SB, Dibnah C, Kennard C, Barnes TR, Joyce EM. The temporal stability of smooth pursuit and saccadic eye movement dysfunction: the West London first-episode schizophrenia study. Schizophr Res 2001; 49:215.

34. Fischer B, Biscaldi M, Gezeck S. On the development of voluntary and reflexive components in human saccade generation. Brain Res 1997; 754:285..297.

35. Klein D, Foerster F. Development of prosaccade and antisaccade task performance in participants aged 6 to 26 years. Psychophysiology 2001; 38:179..189.

36. Eccles JC. The Inhibitory Pathways of the Central Nervous System. Liverpool, England: University, 1969.

37. Freedman R, Adler LE, Waldo M, Pachtman E, Franks RD. Neurophysiological evidence for a defect in inhibitory pathways in schizophrenia: comparison of medicated and drug-free patients. Biol Psychiatry 1983; 18:537..551.

38. Freedman R, Adler LE, Gerhardt GA, Waldo M, Baker N, Rose GM, Drebing C, Nagamoto H, Bickford-Wimer P, Franks R. Neurobiological studies of sensory gating in schizophrenia. Schizophr Bull 1987; 13:669..678.
39. Braff DL, Geyer MA. Sensorimotor gating and schizophrenia: human and animal model studies. Arch Gen Psychiatry 1990; 47:181..188.
40. Nagamoto HT, Adler LE, Waldo MC, Freedman R. Sensory gating in schizophrenic and normal controls: effects of changing stimulation interval. Biol Psychiatry 1989; 25:549..561.
41. Judd LL, McAdams L, Budnick B, Braff DL. Sensory gating deficits in schizophrenia: new results. Am J Psychiatry 1992; 149:488..493.
42. Clementz BA, Geyer MA, Braff DL. Poor P50 suppression among schizophrenia patients and their first-degree biological relatives. Am J Psychiatry 1998; 155:1691..1694.
43. Siegel C, Waldo M, Mizner G, Adler LE, Freedman R. Deficits in sensory gating in schizophrenic patients and their relatives: evidence obtained with auditory evoked responses. Arch Gen Psychiatry 1984;41:607..612.
44. Clementz BA, Geyer MA, Braff DL. Multiple site evaluation of P50 suppression among schizophrenia and normal comparison subjects. Schizophr Res 1998; 30:71..80.
45. Freedman R, Coon H, Myles-Worsley M, et al. Linkage of a neurophysiological deficit in schizophrenia to a chromosome 15 locus. Proc Natl Acad Sci USA 1997; 94:587..592.
46. Yee CM, Nuechterlein KH, Morris SE, White PM. P50 suppression in recent-onset schizophrenia: clinical correlates and risperidone effects. J Abnorm Psychol 1998; 107:691..698.
47. Myles-Worsley M, Coon H, Byerley W, Waldo M, Young D, Freedman R. Developmental and genetic influences on the P50 sensory gating phenotype. Biol Psychiatry 1996; 39:289..295.
48. Myles-Worsley M, Blailes F, Tiobech J, Ord L, Lainhart J. The Palau family genetic project: early detection of prodromal adolescents in multiply affected schizophrenia families. Schizophr Res 2001; 49:77.
49. Myles-Worsley M. P50 sensory gating in multiplex schizophrenia families from a Pacific Island isolate. Am J Psychiatry 2002; 159:2007..2012.
50. McCarley RW, Faux SF, Shenton ME, Nestor PG, Adams J. Event-related potentials in schizophrenia: their biological and clinical correlates and a new model of schizophrenic pathophysiology. Schizophr Res 1991; 4:209..231.
51. Ford JM, Roth WT, Pfefferbaum A. P3 and schizophrenia. Ann NY Acad Sci 1992; 658: 146..162.
52. Ford JM. Schizophrenia: the broken P300 and beyond. Psychophysiology 1999; 36:667..682.
53. Mathalon DH, Ford JM, Pfefferbaum A. Trait and state aspects of P300 amplitude reduction in schizophrenia: a retrospective longitudinal study. Biol Psychiatry 2000; 47:434..449.
54. Salisbury DF, Shenton ME, Sherwood AR, et al. First-episode schizophrenic psychosis differs from first-episode affective psychosis and controls in P300 amplitude over left temporal lobe. Arch Gen Psychiatry 1998; 55:173..180.
55. Saitoh O, Niwa SI, Hiramasatsu KI, Kameyama T, Rymar K, Itoh K. Abnormalities in late positive components of event-related potentials may reflect a genetic predisposition to schizophrenia. Biol Psychiatry 1984; 19:293..303.
56. Blackwood DH, St-Clair DM, Muir WJ, Duffy JC. Auditory P300 and eye tracking dysfunction in schizophrenic pedigrees. Arch Gen Psychiatry 1991; 48:899..909.
57. Weisbrod M, Hill H, Niethammer R, Sauer H. Genetic influence on auditory information processing in schizophrenia: P300 in monozygotic twins. Biol Psychiatry 1999; 46:721..725.
58. Turetsky BI, Cannon TD, Gur RE. P300 subcomponent abnormalities in schizophrenia: III. Deficits in unaffected siblings of schizophrenic probands. Biol Psychiatry 2000; 47: 380..390.

59. Schreiber H, Stolz G, Rothmeier J, Kornhuber HH, Born J. Prolonged latencies of the N2 and P3 of the auditory event-related potential in children at risk for schizophrenia. A preliminary report. Eur Arch Psychiatry Neurol Sci 1989; 238:185..188.

60. Schreiber H, Stolz-Born G, Rothmeier J, Kornhuber A, Kornhuber HH, Born J. Endogenous event-related brain potentials and psychometric performance in children at risk for schizophrenia. Biol Psychiatry 1991; 30:177..189.

61. Friedman D, Cornblatt B, Vaughan HG, Erlenmeyer-Kimling L. Event-related potentials in children at risk for schizophrenia during two continuous performance tests. Psychiatry Res 1986; 18:161..177.

62. Squires-Wheeler E, Friedman D, Skodol AE, Erlenmeyer-Kimling L. A longitudinal study relating P3 amplitude to schizophrenia spectrum disorders and to global personality functioning. Biol Psychiatry 1993; 33:774..785.

63. Naatanen R. The role of attention in auditory information processing as revealed by event-related potentials and other measures of cognitive function. Behav Brain Sci 1990; 13:201..288.

64. Javitt DC, Doneshka P, Zylberman I, Ritter W, Vaughan HG Jr. Impairment of early cortical processing in schizophrenia: an event-related potential replication study. Biol Psychiatry 1993; 33:513..519.

65. Javitt DC, Doneshka P, Grochowski S, Ritter W. Impaired mismatch negativity generation reflects widespread dysfunction of working memory in schizophrenia. Arch Gen Psychiatry 1995; 52:550..558.

66. Javitt DC, Shelley A-M, Silipo G, Lieberman JA. Deficits in auditory and visual context-dependent processing in schizophrenia. Arch Gen Psychiatry 2000; 57:1131..1137.

67. Schreiber H, Stolz-Born G, Heinrich H, Kornhuber HH, Born J. Attention, cognition, and motor perseveration in adolescents at genetic risk for schizophrenia and control subjects. Psychiatry Res 1992; 44:125..140.

68. Virdi GK, Bramon E, Croft RJ, McDonald C, Pang D, Gruzelier JG, Murray RM. Mismatch negativity in schizophrenia: a family study. Schizophr Res 2001; 49:211.

69. Park S, Holzman PS. Schizophrenics show working memory deficits. Arch Gen Psychiatry 1992; 49:975..982.

70. Erlenmeyer-Kimling L, Adamo UH, Rock D, et al. The New York High-Risk Project: prevalence and comorbidity of axis I disorders in offspring of schizophrenic parents at 25-year follow-up. Arch Gen Psychiatry 1997; 54:1096..1102.

71. Hirsch SR, Baldeweg T, Krljes S, Faruqui RA. Mismatch negativity as an indicator of an abnormality of the brain plasticity in schizophrenia. International Congress on Schizophrenia Research, Whistler, British Columbia, Canada, 2001.

72. Braff DL, Stone C, Callaway E, Geyer MA, Glick I, Bali L. Prestimulus effects on human startle reflex in normals and schizophrenics. Psychophysiology 1978; 5:339..343.

73. Geyer MA, Braff DL. Habituation of the blink reflex in normals and schizophrenic patients. Psychophysiology 1982; 19:1..6.

74. Braff DL, Geyer MA. Sensorimotor gating and schizophrenia human and animal model studies. Arch Gen Psychiatry 1990; 47:181..188.

75. Braff DL, Grillon C, Geyer MA. Gating and habituation of the startle reflex in schizophrenic patients. Arch Gen Psychiatry 1992; 49:206..215.

76. Taiminen T, Jaaskelainen S, Ilonen T, et al. Habituation of the blink reflex in first-episode schizophrenia, psychotic depression and non-psychotic depression. Schizophr Res 2000; 44: 69..79.

77. Nuechterlein KH, Dawson ME. Information processing and attentional functioning in the developmental course of schizophrenic disorders. Schizophr Bull 1984; 10:160..203.

78. Dawson ME, Nuechterlein KH, Schell AM, Gitlin M, Ventura J. Autonomic abnormalities in schizophrenia state of trait indicators? Arch Gen Psychiatry 1994; 51:813..824.
79. Cannon TD, Mednick SA, Parnas J, Schulsinger F, Praestholm J, Vestergaard A. Developmental brain abnormalities in the offspring of schizophrenic mothers. I. Contributions of genetic and perinatal factors. Arch Gen Psychiatry 1993; 50:551..564.
80. Cannon TD, Mednick SA, Parnas J, Schulsinger F, Praestholm J, Vestergaard A. Developmental brain abnormalities in the offspring of schizophrenic mothers. II. Structural brain characteristics of schizophrenia and schizotypal personality disorder. Arch Gen Psychiatry 1994; 51:955..962.
81. Cornblatt BA, Erlenmeyer-Kimling L. Global attentional deviance as a marker for schizophrenia: specificity and predictive validity. J Abnorm Psychol 1985; 94:470..486.
82. Erlenmeyer-Kimling L, Cornblatt B. The New York High-Risk Project: a followup report. Schizophr Bull 1987; 13:451..461.
83. Erlenmeyer-Kimling L, Cornblatt BA, Rock D, Roberts S, Bell M, West A. The New York High-Risk Project: anhedonia, attentional deviance, and psychopathology. Schizophr Bull 1993; 19:141..153.

11 Is the Development of Schizophrenia Predictable?

Paola Dazzan, MD, MSc, MRCPsych,
Eugenia Kravariti, MA, MSc, PhD,
Paul Fearon, MB, MSc, MRCPI, MRCPsych,
and Robin M. Murray, MD, FRCPsych, DSc

The evidence that people who develop schizophrenia have features that precede the onset of psychosis dates back at least to the early years of the 20th century. Bleuler *(1)*, who coined the term, wrote that patients with schizophrenia "already stood out as children because they were unable to play with others and followed their own ways instead." In recent years, a number of studies have attempted to establish which attributes "characterize" these preschizophrenic children, and which, therefore, might predict the development of the condition. According to McNeil *(2)* an *ideal* predictive factor should be relatively easily identifiable, should be amenable to intervention, and should not carry a social stigma.

Satisfying McNeil's first criterion in schizophrenia is far from easy. None of the risk factors associated with this illness has, in isolation, been identified as a reliable *predictor* of future schizophrenia. The risk factors identified so far each carry only a small effect, and are largely nonspecific. Thus, they are found not only in those destined to develop schizophrenia but also, to a lesser extent, in those who will develop other psychiatric disorders, and also, although more rarely, who will remain entirely well. Because of this, many studies have examined high-risk populations, either those at increased genetic risk of schizophrenia, or those already presenting with some prodromal symptoms of the disorder. Nevertheless, even in these high-risk populations, the best prediction of future psychosis usually comes from considering the co-occurrence of several risk factors, rather than from the presence of any single one.

From: *Early Clinical Intervention and Prevention in Schizophrenia*
Edited by: W. S. Stone, S. V. Faraone, and M. T. Tsuang © Humana Press Inc., Totowa, NJ

We are even further from satisfying McNeil's second criterion. In the main, intervention means offering individuals who have not yet experienced psychotic symptoms, an antipsychotic drug similar to those used in the full-blown illness, rather than a treatment that acts on the risk factor. Given that such antipsychotic drugs have considerable side effects, and are difficult to justify even in high-risk samples, it is hardly surprising that primary prevention in the general population is not yet feasible.

This brings us to McNeil's last criterion, namely that the identification of a predictor in an individual should not carry social stigma. Given current social attitudes to schizophrenia, this is difficult to achieve. To minimize any stigma, the predictor should identify only individuals who *really* are at risk. Thus the number of false positives should be low; in other words, there should be a high specificity (specificity equals the false-positives rate). Indeed, the ideal predictor should show good specificity, sensitivity, and positive predictive value.

Before proceeding further, we need to define these terms. In this context, *specificity* is the probability of testing negative for the predictor if the illness will never develop, whereas *sensitivity* is the probability of testing positive for the predictor if the disease will truly develop. The *positive predictive value* is the probability of a person actually developing the disorder if they test positive for the predictor, whereas the *negative predictive value* is the probability of a person not developing the disease if they test negative for the predictor.

Unfortunately, in real life, a screening test (or *predictor* in our case) is rarely characterized by both high sensitivity and high specificity, and it is often necessary to compromise in favor of one of the two, depending on the characteristics of the disorder. For example, for lethal diseases it is sensible to compromise on the specificity of the screening factor in favor of a better sensitivity, so that as many as possible of those people who are at risk of dying are identified. However, for an illness with low mortality and a high risk of stigmatization such as schizophrenia, the ideal predictor should have a high specificity. This would mean that the number of people exposed to the worry and stigma of living with the potential of developing such an incapacitating illness would be reduced to a minimum. Unfortunately, on the basis of the evidence concerning those risk factors that are known to date, a sizeable proportion of people identified as "positive" would never develop the illness. This disadvantage would, therefore, need to be counterbalanced by a powerful benefit of an early intervention.

THE SEARCH FOR SCHIZOPHRENIA PREDICTORS

In this chapter we examine the potential of various risk factors for schizophrenia in predicting the disorder. Special emphasis is placed on (a) biological predictors of schizophrenia that operate during development, such as familial/genetic

factors and early environmental insults to the brain; (b) neuropsychological and educational risk factors, e.g., intellectual dysfunction and poor educational achievement; and (c) psychosocial predictors, such as social adversity. Finally, we consider how accurate these factors are in identifying subjects who develop schizophrenia.

Where possible, we report a measure of the effect size (the strength of the association between the predictor and the development of schizophrenia) for each risk factor considered. We report two main measures of effect size. The relative risk (RR; in cohort studies) indicates the likelihood of developing the disease in exposed (positive for the predictor in this context) relative to nonexposed (negative for the predictor) individuals. The odds ratio (OR; in case-control studies) is the ratio of the odds of exposure: this quantifies the increased likelihood (how many times more likely) of developing the illness in subjects positive for the predictor. We also consider results from meta-analytic studies, as these often offer the best cumulative evidence of the effect size of a single measure (e.g., Cohen's d) (see Table 1, footnote d). Wherever possible, we also include measures of sensitivity, specificity, and positive/negative predictive values of the factor considered.

THE EARLY DEVELOPMENTAL RISK FACTORS OF SCHIZOPHRENIA

Familial Risk

The most powerful risk factor predisposing an individual to later schizophrenia is being related to an individual already suffering from the disorder. The risk for broadly defined schizophrenia rises from approx 0.8% in the general population to about 10% in first-degree relatives of an affected person (Table 1), and to nearly 50% in the monozygotic co-twin of an individual with schizophrenia *(3)*. When operational definitions of schizophrenia are used, the risks are lower in all groups, but the general principle remains that the risk rises as an individual's genetic relationship to schizophrenia becomes closer *(4,5)*.

Unfortunately, no genes have yet been identified that reliably specify this risk. Nevertheless, being related to a person with schizophrenia is an important marker of risk and, as such, it has been frequently used in studies that attempt to identify individuals in the so-called prodrome of the condition *(see* below). It is particularly useful when combined with other markers, for example, in children of a schizophrenic parent who also show certain neuropsychological abnormalities.

Pre- and Perinatal Complications

Pregnancy and delivery complications (also grouped under the term obstetric complications [OCs]) have been repeatedly shown to collectively comprise a risk factor for developing schizophrenia *(6,7)*, with an odds ratio of about 2 for OCs in general *(8)* (Table 1). A stronger association between OCs and schizophrenia

Table 1
Predicting Schizophrenia: Familial and Pre/Perinatal Factors

Risk Factor	Effect Size
Familial Risk *(3)*[a]:	
Parent	OR 6
Sibling	OR 10
Child	OR 13
First-degree relative	OR 9.6
Total OCs:	
Present vs absent OCs exposure *(8)*[b]	OR 2.0
Pregnancy and birth complications *(22)*[c]	$d\ 0.32^{d}$
Individual OCs *(107)*[e]:	
Premature rupture of membranes	OR 3.1
Deviant gestational age	OR 2.4
Resuscitation/incubation	OR 2.2
Low birthweight	OR 1.5
Forceps delivery	OR 1.5
Excess winter births *(22)*[f]	$d\ 0.05^{d}$
Maternal exposure to influenza *(22)*[g]	$d\ 0.02^{d}$

OR = odds ratio; *d* = Cohen's *d*, OCs = obstetric complications.
[a]Relationship to person with schizophrenia. Risk is expressed as morbid risk when population risk is 1%.
[b]Meta-analysis including 700 patients.
[c]Meta-analysis including 15 studies.
[d]The effect size is expressed with Cohen's *d*. This is the result of the subtraction of the average of one sample from the average of the other sample, divided by the pooled standard deviation; it directly reflects the magnitude of the difference between the groups in exam.
[e]Meta-analysis including 12 case-control studies. Individual information was obtained on 700 schizophrenia subjects and on 835 controls. OCs were measured with the Lewis-Murray Scale.
[f]Meta-analysis including 17 studies. Winter birth rates were compared in subjects with schizophrenia and in healthy controls.
[g]Meta-analysis including four studies. Schizophrenia rates were compared between offspring of mothers exposed to the virus, and offspring of mothers without the exposure.

has been observed in patients with an early onset *(9–11)*, and possibly in male patients *(12–14)*. Attention has particularly focused on those complications associated with a risk of hypoxic-ischemic brain damage *(9)*, which could be one of the possible causes for the ventricular enlargement *(15,16)* and the reduced

hippocampal size *(17,18)* observed in schizophrenia. Some authors have suggested that the excito-toxic effects of hypoxia on the fetal brain might be particularly powerful in those subjects with a genetic liability for schizophrenia *(10)*.

Maternal fever in the latter part of pregnancy has also been identified as a risk factor *(19)*. Together with the finding of a relatively increased number of schizophrenic patients born in the months after influenza epidemics *(20,21)*, this would suggest that a range of illnesses in the mother may slightly impair the cortical development of her baby, and in turn increase the risk of later schizophrenia.

Unfortunately, although OCs increase the risk for schizophrenia, they are of little practical help in identifying individuals who will develop the illness. After an extensive research of the literature, Heinrichs *(22)* performed a meta-analysis of a range of pre- and perinatal variables associated with schizophrenia. He concluded that such complications are only modestly associated with schizophrenia (Cohen's $d = 0.32$), whereas maternal exposure to influenza (Cohen's $d = 0.02$) and the excess of winter births (Cohen's $d = 0.05$) represent some of the weakest findings in schizophrenia research (Table 1). Because each of these factors confers at best only a minor increase in risk, their individual value as predictive factors is negligible.

Developmental Deviations of the Body and Brain

MINOR PHYSICAL ANOMALIES AND DERMATOGLYPHICS

Minor physical *(23,24)* and dermatoglyphic *(25,26)* anomalies are found in excess in patients with schizophrenia. Minor physical anomalies (minor abnormalities of the head, hands, and feet) originate from alterations of ectodermal development during the first and second trimesters of intrauterine life; those of the craniofacial region are known to be related to brain development *(27)*. Although minor physical anomalies are not uncommon in the general population, an elevated number of these (≥ 6) discriminates between patients with schizophrenia and healthy controls (OR = 26.6), with a specificity reported as high as 95% *(28)* (Table 2). Physical anomalies that appear to be more common in schizophrenia include curved fifth finger, epicanthus, high/steepled palate, hyperconvex fingernails, and thin upper lip.

Abnormal dermatoglyphics, such as a reduction of the a-b ridge count *(25)*, have also been reported in subjects with schizophrenia (OR = $[1.3]^3 = 2.2$) (Table 2). Dermatoglyphics are epidermal ridges that develop between the 12th and 24th weeks of intrauterine life, and, therefore, they represent a stable abnormality that is identifiable well before the onset of schizophrenia. Unfortunately, the small effect size implies that they can be useful in prediction only if combined with other risk factors.

Table 2
Predicting Schizophrenia: Early Developmental Factors

Risk Factor	Effect Size	Sensitivity	Specificity	Positive Predictive Value	Negative Predictive Value
Minor physical anomalies (MPA):					
≥6 minor physical anomalies (28)[a]	OR 26.6	60%	95%		
Dermatoglyphics:					
Total a-b ridge count (25)[b]	OR 2.2				
Brain structural abnormalities:					
Cavum Septum Pellucidum (30)[c]	OR 3.8	2%	99%	23%	92%
Adult brain: (32)[d]					
Mean cerebral volume	d −0.19[d]				
Total ventricular volume	d 0.49[d]				
Left amygdala	d −0.72[d]				
Right amygdala	d −0.79[d]				
Left hippocampus/amygdala	d −0.24[d]				
Right hippocampus/amygdala	d −0.28[d]				
Left parahippocampus	d −0.69[d]				
Right parahippocampus	d −0.40[d]				
Neuromotor Development:					
Delayed milestones at 2 years (43)[e]	OR 4.8	7%	98%	3%	99%
Better performance in sports and handicrafts (7.9 years) (44)[f]	OR 0.8[f]				
Gross motor skills (41)[g]	OR 20[g]	75%	73%	33%	94%
Adult neurological soft signs (47)[h]	OR 2.4	20%	91%	80%	37%

OR = odds ratio; d = Cohen's d.

[a]Ismail et al. (28) studied 60 schizophrenia patients and 75 normal comparison subjects. MPAs (Waldrop scale plus 23 other MPAs) in hand, eye, and mouth discriminated best between patients and controls.

[b]Fearon et al. (25) compared 150 schizophrenia patients with 92 healthy controls. There was a significant linear trend for lower total a-b ridge count and increasing incidence of schizophrenia. This implied a continuous increase in the risk of schizophrenia with reduction in total a-b ridge count.

[c]Lewis et al. (30) evaluated 4454 consecutive psychiatric, neurological, and neurosurgical patients. The rate of functional psychosis in patients with a cavum (6 out of 26) was significantly higher than in subjects without a cavum ($p < 0.01$).

[d]Meta-analysis including 58 structural MRI studies and 1588 schizophrenia patients, reporting on volume measurements of a number of brain regions. Effect size was expressed with Cohen's d (see Table 1, footnote[d]).

[e]Jones et al. (43) analyzed prospective data on a stratified random sample (n = 4746 alive at 16 years) of 13,687 births in Britain during the week March 3..9, 1946. The psychiatric outcome was established between 16 and 43 years, and the comparison group included the entire risk set after excluding those identified as cases of schizophrenia (n = 4716).

[f]In this case-control study, nested in a population-based birth cohort study (of all individuals born in Helsinki, Finland, between 1951 and 1960), the authors obtained elementary school (age: 7..11 years) records for 400 subjects diagnosed with schizophrenia, and for 408 controls. Subjects who developed schizophrenia performed worse on factors that indicated a motor-coordination deficit. The risk is expressed as mean odds ratio.

[g]Erlenmeyer-Kimling et al. (41) evaluated neurobehavioral deficits at 7..12 years of age in the offspring of schizophrenic and healthy parents. By conducting different path analyses, using logistic regression equations, they attempted to clarify the relationship of childhood deficits to adulthood schizophrenia-related psychoses. The odds ratio expressed here results from the combination of both genetic risk and gross motor skill abnormalities. Specificity, sensitivity, and positive/negative predictive values refer specifically to gross motor skill dysfunction.

[h]Boks et al. (47) reviewed 17 studies and reported on the weighted mean prevalence of neurological soft sings in adult schizophrenia patients (n = 386) and in healthy controls (n = 202).

231

Structural Brain Abnormalities

An excess of congenital brain lesions is reported in schizophrenia, including agenesis of the corpus callosum *(29)*, cavum septum pellucidum *(30)*, and aqueduct stenosis *(31)*. Although these do convey significantly increased risk, they are extremely rare: reports to date mainly consist of small case series, which make any risk estimate difficult to evaluate. An attempt was made in the study of Lewis et al. *(30)* on cavum septum pellucidum. Among their 4454 consecutive psychiatric, neurological, and neurosurgical patients, those who were diagnosed as having psychosis were more likely than the rest of the group to have a cavum septum pellucidum (OR = 3.8) (Table 2). However, its positive predictive value was quite low (23%), and this makes it unlikely to be a good predictor of schizophrenia.

Neuroimaging has mainly been used to investigate brain structure in schizophrenic subjects after the illness has become apparent   enlarged ventricular size, decrease in the volumes of cortex, temporal lobe, and hippocampus, and abnormal hemispheric asymmetry have been reported *(32)* (Table 2). Imaging has been applied to nonpsychotic high-risk subjects in an attempt to clarify whether these brain abnormalities precede the onset of schizophrenia. Studies reported to date have confirmed an increase in ventricular volume and a reduction in medial temporal lobe structures in asymptomatic subjects at increased genetic risk for schizophrenia *(33,34)*. However, neuroimaging is expensive, and increased cerebral ventricular size and sulcal enlargement are not specific to schizophrenia: they have also been reported in affective psychosis *(35,36)*, although this association seems to be less marked than for schizophrenia *(37)*.

At present, a number of factors limit the possibility of using brain structural abnormalities as predictors of schizophrenia. First, the brain abnormalities identified so far are subtle, nonspecific to schizophrenia, and may just represent deviations within the normal range. Second, it is possible that some structural abnormalities appear only with the transition to psychosis, and are, therefore, not visible until the full-blown illness appears. Finally, it remains unclear how many high-risk nonpsychotic individuals who present subtle brain abnormalities will ever develop the disorder.

NEUROMOTOR DEVELOPMENT

Studies on children at genetic risk for schizophrenia *(38–41)* and general-population birth cohort studies *(42,43)* have reported impairments of motor development and fine motor coordination. In the 1946 British Birth Cohort Study *(43)*, 4746 children were followed up for 43 years. Those who developed schizophrenia were 4.8 times more likely to have delayed milestones at age 2 (particularly walking, which was delayed by 1.2 months) (Table 2). However, the authors indicated that in their cohort "no child destined to develop schizophrenia could be

singled out as a late walker." In fact, as shown in Table 2, the probability that a late walker would develop schizophrenia (positive predictive value) was only 3%. More recently, Cannon and colleagues *(44)* reviewed the school records of 400 Finnish individuals with schizophrenia and showed that these subjects performed significantly worse than a group of 408 controls in activities requiring motor coordination (odds ratio of 0.8 indicates that children who did not develop schizophrenia had a better performance in sports and handicrafts) (Table 2).

Walker and Lewine *(45)* retrospectively observed home videos recorded during the first 2 years of life of children who later developed schizophrenia. They reported that the presence of postural and upper-limb neuromotor abnormalities, particularly localized on the left side of the body, tended to disappear after that age. Similar findings came from studies of children at high risk for schizophrenia. Erlenmeyer-Kimling et al. *(41)* evaluated neuromotor performance in the offspring of schizophrenic parents and compared it with that of healthy controls. Impairment in gross motor skills showed a reasonably high sensitivity and specificity. However, patients with abnormal gross motor skills had only 33% probability of developing schizophrenia (Table 2).

Patients with schizophrenia have a higher prevalence of neurological soft signs (NSS) in comparison with normal controls or subjects with other psychiatric disorders *(46,47)* (Table 2). However, no specific category of neurological sign has been identified as characteristic of schizophrenia. Furthermore, some of these signs are found also in a significant proportion of the nonpatient population, and in patients with affective disorder and nonschizophrenic psychosis *(48,49)*. Therefore, when they are considered alone, their accuracy in identifying subjects with schizophrenia, let alone those destined to develop it, remains poor.

NEUROPSYCHOLOGICAL DEVELOPMENTAL RISK FACTORS
Population-Based Studies

Prospective investigations of population-based samples have provided relatively unbiased estimates of associations between putative neuropsychological risk indicators of schizophrenia and the subsequent development of the disorder *(43,50–55)*. These studies have reported persistent intellectual deficits, language pathology, and educational failures in preschizophrenic children and adolescents, with the respective functional abnormalities showing relative stability across developmental periods *(50,52)*. The above longitudinally ascertained findings have been supplemented by cognitive data collected routinely in late adolescence from national male samples tested for eligibility for military service *(56,57)*.

Intellectual abnormalities in individuals destined to develop schizophrenia in the Philadelphia 1959..1966 birth cohort have been documented as early as 4 and

7 years of age; IQ category at either age emerged as a significant predictor of adult schizophrenia in this population *(52)*. These findings have been supplemented by the 1946 and 1958 British birth cohort studies *(50)*, which reported deficits in intellectual capacity, verbal and nonverbal reasoning, reading comprehension, and mathematics at various age points between 7 and 16 years of age in preschizophrenic individuals. Repeating a school grade or receiving special education at age 14 (mainly because of low IQ) also predicted future schizophrenia in the Northern Finland 1966 birth cohort study *(54)*. Similarly, poor intellectual functioning in a national sample of 18-year-old male conscripts to the Swedish army emerged as a strong predictor of future schizophrenia *(56)* (Table 3), a finding replicated in the national Israeli cohort of 16- to 17-year-old males discussed above *(57)*. In the latter, combining intellectual ratings with measures of social functioning and organizational ability gave rise to an impressive predictive model of 75% sensitivity, 100% specificity, and 72% positive predictive value. Individuals scoring 0.5 SD below the norm on intellectual functioning, 1 SD below the norm on social functioning, and below the norm to any extent on at least one additional personality or behavioral measure were reported to have at least 80% chance of developing schizophrenia. Using this rule of thumb yielded a model of 30% sensitivity and 100% validated specificity.

A common finding in nearly all of the above studies is a linear association between intellectual functioning and the risk for schizophrenia: the latter appears to be a function of performance over the entire range of population scores, increasing progressively as ability declines *(43,50–52,56,57)*. The Philadelphia birth cohort study, for example, reported a 30. 60% increase in schizophrenia risk per unit decrease in ability category (divided into five performance levels), such that individuals scoring in the deficient range were five to six times more likely to become schizophrenic than those scoring in the high-average to superior range *(51)*. Similarly, David et al. *(56)* reported a ninefold increase in schizophrenia risk among conscripts scoring in the lowest IQ band compared to those falling within the highest one.

Despite the significant increase in schizophrenia risk in the lower end of the IQ distribution, in no study did the disorder arise solely from a population subgroup with low IQ, nor was there evidence of a subgroup of cases with very low scores *(43,50–52,56,57)*. Rather, the IQ distribution of the schizophrenia population as a whole is shifted downward in a systematic fashion, most likely reflecting an effect on each individual. This effect is rather subtle: IQ data at age 11 examined together for the 1946 and 1958 birth cohorts revealed a shift of the schizophrenia population mean by less than half a standard deviation *(50)*. No single child destined to develop schizophrenia in the former cohort could be singled out as having learning difficulties *(43)*.

Table 3
Predicting Schizophrenia: Neuropsychological and Educational Factors in Population-Based Studies

Risk Factor	Effect Size	Sensitivity	Specificity	Positive Predictive Value	Negative Predictive Value
IQ at 4 years (51)[a]	OR 1.3[b]	30%	85%	2%	99%
IQ at 7 years (51)[a]	OR 1.6[b]	33%	83%	2%	99%
IQ at 11 and 15 years (43)[c]	OR 0.6 & 0.5[b]				
IQ at 16..17 years (57)[d]	OR 1.6	54%	53%		
IQ < 96 at 18 years (56)[e]	OR 3.5..8.6[f]	55%[f]	67%[f]	1%[f]	100%[f]
Class below age level or special education at 14 years (54)[g]	OR 2.8	17%	93%	3%	99%
Excellent school marks at 16 years (55)[g]	OR 3.8	11%	97%	4%	99%
Abnormal speech at 7 years (53)[a]	OR 12.7	14%	99%	17%	99%
Abnormal speech at 2.15 years (43)[c]	OR 2.8				
Expressive language ability at 7 years (53)[a]	OR 0.7				

OR = odds ratio.

[a]The Philadelphia birth cohort study (51,53) followed up over 90% (n = 9236) of all deliveries at two inner-city hospital obstetric wards in Philadelphia between 1959 and 1966. The psychiatric outcome was established between 19 and 36 years (72 subjects had developed schizophrenia), and the comparison group included 7941 nonpsychiatric controls.

[b]Odds ratio for linear trend, i.e., that associated with moving a category (e.g., tertile or quintile) of score distribution.

[c]Jones et al. (43) analyzed prospective data on a stratified random sample (n = 4746 alive at 16 years) of 13,687 births in Britain during the week March 3..9, 1946. The psychiatric outcome was established between 16 and 43 years (30 subjects had developed schizophrenia), and the comparison group (n = 4716) included the entire risk set after excluding those identified as cases of schizophrenia.

[d]Davidson et al. (57) compared a national sample of 16 to 17-year-old males who developed schizophrenia by the age of 26 (n = 509), with a national sample of 16- to 17-year-old males who did not appear in the national psychiatric registry by the same age (n = 9215).

[e]David et al. (56) studied a national sample of 49,968 male conscripts to the Swedish army, followed up until the age of 33..34 years (195 subjects had developed schizophrenia). The comparison group included psychiatrically normal individuals and cases with other psychotic outcomes (n = 49,773).

[f]Odds Ratios (unadjusted for confounders) were estimated separately for each IQ band (<74, 74.81, 82.89, 90..95) by David et al. (56); sensitivity, specificity, and positive/negative predictive values were estimated for all the IQ (<96) bands lumped together by the present authors.

[g]The Northern Finland birth cohort study (54,55) followed prospectively 96% of all births in Northern Finland in 1966 (n = 12,058 live-born children). The psychiatric outcome was established between 16 and 28 years (58 subjects had developed schizophrenia), and the comparison group included individuals with no hospital treatment for schizophrenia or other psychotic/nonpsychotic disorders (n = 5351).

Contrary to the prevailing view that schizophrenia risk increases linearly with decreasing intellectual capacity, findings from the Northern Finland 1966 birth cohort *(55)* failed to confirm linearity in the association between educational attainment and schizophrenia outcome, raising the possibility that it is distance from the cognitive norm   in either direction   that increases the odds for the disorder. Excellent school performance among 16-year-old males in the latter cohort was associated with nearly a fourfold increase in schizophrenia risk, with 11% of the preschizophrenic boys compared to only 3% of the comparison group (with no hospital-treated psychiatric outcome) obtaining excellent mean school marks. In accord with this finding, the proportion of preschizophrenia cases falling within the highest IQ category among the Israeli 16- to 17-year-old males was six times higher than that of the comparison subjects (with no hospital-treated psychiatric outcome) *(57)*.

Premorbid language dysfunction appears to be one of the most potent predictors of future schizophrenia. Abnormal summary ratings of speech intelligibility at age 7, based on an examination of receptive/expressive language ability and speech mechanism and production, were associated with a greater than 12-fold increase in risk for adult schizophrenia in the Philadelphia cohort *(53)*. Similarly, the evidence for abnormal speech development prior to schizophrenia is strong and complementary in the two British birth cohorts *(50)*. In the latter, the relevant abnormalities are more than reflections of developmental timing: oral ability and quality of speech at 7 and 11 years were rated as qualitatively abnormal in the preschizophrenic cases of the 1958 birth cohort; and speech defects (not owing to structural problems) persisted throughout childhood and adolescence in the 1946 cohort cases, being associated with a threefold increase in schizophrenia risk.

Although the large sample sizes (ranging from about 5000 to 50,000 individuals) in these epidemiological studies provide sufficient statistical evidence for the predictive potential of neuropsychological abnormalities, it would be misleading to conclude that the latter can be used as effective population screens for the identification of individuals at true risk for schizophrenia. A limitation in this regard is the extent to which premorbid neuropsychological deficits can distinguish between schizophrenia and other psychiatric disorders. Impairments in general ability have also been recorded in the early biographies of individuals with affective psychoses and anxiety or depressive disorders, with any distinction between the respective groups simply being one of magnitude: preschizophrenic cases usually perform worse than the other patient groups, which also perform below the norm *(50,56,57)*. Indeed, the association between receiving special education or repeating a school grade and the diagnostic category of "other psychoses" in the Finnish cohort was even stronger than that with schizophrenia *(54)*. A possible exception to this rather undifferentiated pattern of associations is the

one between speech difficulties and future schizophrenia: the only school-based assessment that distinguished the preschizophrenic children from the other patient groups in the British 1958 cohort, was the qualitative evaluation of "speech difficulties" at both 7 and 11 years (50).

A second problem is the significant impact on a population level of the false-negative properties carried by even highly sensitive and specific screens, when used for low-prevalence disorders, such as schizophrenia (58). Table 3 presents the odds ratios (all significant at the 0.05 level at least), sensitivity, specificity, and positive/negative predictive values of the neuropsychological and educational risk factors examined in the various studies. It should be borne in mind that these estimates are only indicative and not directly comparable: some authors have modeled the respective factors as continuous variables, whereas others have dichotomized the complex phenomena of interest into "normal" and "abnormal," using variable cutoff points for impairment; in addition, the reported odds ratios have been adjusted for different (albeit overlapping) sets of confounders, the follow-up intervals differ across studies, and the comparison groups have not uniformly included or excluded other psychiatric disorders (Table 3). A visual inspection of the table reveals that, although the proportion of true negatives (53...99%) detected by the predictor variables is moderate to excellent, the proportion of true positives (11.55%) is less satisfactory, and only a small proportion (1...17%) of individuals falling within the "impaired" range on the different measures eventually go on to develop schizophrenia. For example, receiving special education or repeating a school grade (mainly owing to low IQ) at 14 years of age in the Northern Finland cohort study (54) correctly predicted 10 of the 58 cases of schizophrenia (sensitivity: 17%) and 4986 of the 5351 noncases (specificity: 93%). However, of the 375 individuals repeating a class or receiving special education at age 14, only 10 went on to develop schizophrenia (positive predictive value: 3%). It is, therefore, unrealistic to target early identification and prevention programs for schizophrenia to individuals with deviant cognitive functioning or poor educational achievement, given the financial and ethical implications of such an approach. This observation applies to all the remaining risk factors identified in the population-based studies reviewed in this section (Table 3).

High-Risk Studies

A common method employed to reduce the chances of false positives in the face of low-prevalence disorders, is to increase the observed prevalence within the screened group, by utilizing the "high-risk" strategy (58). Children of one schizophrenic parent can be up to 15 times more likely to develop the disorder than members of the general population. Unlike population-based studies, which usually study general aspects of development rather than specifically seek effective

schizophrenia predictors, high-risk research is a longitudinal quest for variables that predict the disorder *(41)*. As such, the high-risk paradigm usually includes measurements of particular relevance to schizophrenia.

Among the most powerful and reliable neuroscience findings in the schizophrenia literature to date are deficits in attention and information processing, verbal memory, and intelligence *(22)*. With a growing body of evidence pointing to these impairments as sensitive, genetically mediated, candidate markers of the schizophrenic diathesis *(52,59–73)*, their ability to predict schizophrenia has formed an important focus of high-risk research.

Impaired attention is by far the most extensively investigated and validated neuropsychological predictor in the high-risk literature: preschizophrenic offspring of affected parents in the Copenhagen study have been reported to display poor concentration from infancy *(74)*, and childhood attentional deficits in the Israeli high-risk sample appear to successfully predict the development of schizophrenia-spectrum disorders *(75)*. In addition, findings from the New York High-Risk Project (NYHRP) have attested to both the predictive validity and the diagnostic specificity of attentional dysfunction: the relevant deficits appear to predict schizophrenia-related psychoses as opposed to other psychiatric outcomes *(41)*, to be more prevalent among children of schizophrenic parents than offspring of affectively ill patients *(41,76–78)*, and to display the greatest predictive power within the group at genetic risk for schizophrenia *(76,77)*.

Other cognitive functions have been less extensively investigated. However, emerging findings from the NYHRP suggest that measures of memory dysfunction, IQ change, and subtest scatter in standard intelligence tests, may provide sensitive indicators of the preschizophrenia state *(41,79)*; a combination of measures derived from the Wechsler Intelligence Scale for Children.Revised (WISC... R) or Wechsler Adult Intelligence Scale.Revised (WAIS.R) in the above study achieved one of the best predictive profiles reported to date, with a false-positive rate of just 2.5% (Table 4).

However, the focus on single neuropsychological constructs is less promising than using clusters of distinct cognitive and neurobehavioral variables. Combining an attentional screen with behavioral ratings in the NYHRP enhanced measurably the overall accuracy of the attentional model, reducing false positives by half *(80)* (Table 4). Similarly, combining deficits in attention, verbal memory, and gross motor skills in the above study achieved higher precision than any of the contributing variables alone *(41)*.

Table 4 presents the sensitivity, specificity, and positive/negative predictive values of selected neuropsychological predictors used (either in isolation or in combination with other neurobehavioral ratings) in high-risk studies. The predictive validity of the various models has been evaluated in samples of children at genetic risk for schizophrenia *(41,79)*, in mixed groups of offspring of schizo-

phrenic and psychiatrically normal parents *(81)*, and in mixed samples of children of schizophrenic, affectively ill, and psychiatrically healthy parents *(79,80)*. As expected from measures specifically selected for their relevance to schizophrenia, the examined predictors show moderate to high sensitivity, with 50... 89% of future spectrum cases being correctly identified by the predictor variables. The positive predictive values, although lower, are still substantially higher than those noted in population-based studies: of all subjects predicted to develop schizophrenia-related psychoses, 19..70% go on to develop the outcome of interest. The negative predictive values are more satisfactory: almost invariably, more than 90% of "nondeviant" performers do not develop schizophrenia or related psychoses. By contrast, the false-positive rates can sometimes be substantial: although in some models *(41,79)* only 2..10% of noncases are falsely predicted to develop spectrum disorders; about a third of noncases are false positives in others *(41,81)* (Table 4).

As only about 10..15% of future schizophrenia patients have an ill first-degree relative, the predictive performance of the reviewed models cannot as yet be extrapolated to the general population. Furthermore, the normal control samples in the existing studies are too small to test any indicator's capacity to predict schizophrenia in the general population *(41)*. Nevertheless, the investigated measures can provide useful aids in the identification of schizophrenia offspring who are most likely to carry the schizophrenia genotype. This is an important step toward formulating screening procedures for the early identification of truly vulnerable individuals within the high-risk population. Although the reported misclassification rates are still sufficiently high to prevent the implementation of invasive protocols for preventive intervention, this subgroup may potentially form a target for cognitive intervention treatments. The latter carry a lower risk for stigmatization, are considered relatively safe, and can be beneficial even for individuals who are falsely predicted to develop schizophrenia.

THE SOCIAL AND ENVIRONMENTAL ANTECEDENTS

The role of social and environmental factors in the development of schizophrenia was investigated enthusiastically until the late 1970s, when this field of study largely disappeared. However, epidemiological studies have recently reappraised the role of such factors, particularly living in a city or being an immigrant, which appear to operate at the group rather than individual level.

LIVING IN THE CITY

The prevalence of schizophrenia is higher in urban than in rural areas *(82)*. This was originally thought to be because of selective migration of preschizophrenic subjects from rural to urban areas before the onset of the illness. However, several studies have observed *(83,84)* that the risk is higher in people born

Table 4

Predicting Schizophrenia: Neuropsychological Deficits in High-Risk Studies

Risk Factor	Sensitivity	Specificity	Positive Predictive Value	Negative Predictive Value
Attention deficits at 12 years (80)[a]	67%	79%	19%	97%
Attention deficits at 12 years and behavior ratings at 12..17 years (80)[a]	83%	90%	38.5%	99%
Attention deviance at 7..12 years (41)[b]	58%	82%	37%	92%
Memory deficits at 7..12 years (41)[b]	83%	72%	34.5%	96%
Attention deviance, memory, and gross motor skills at 7..12 years (41)[b]	50%	90%	46%	91%
WISC.R or WAIS.R subtest scatter at 15 years, change in *Full Scale IQ* and *Vocabulary* between 9 and 15 years, *Picture Arrangement minus Vocabulary* score at 9 years and parental risk (79)[c]	54.85%[c]	95.98%[c]	61..70%[c]	96.99%[c]
WISC.R or WAIS.R subtest scatter at 15 years and *Picture Arrangement minus Vocabulary* score at 9 years (79)[d]	56%	90%	62.5%	87%
Deviance on a composite index of attentional, perceptual, and motor dysfunctioning at 8..15 years (81)[e]	89%	64%	22%	98%

[a]Cornblatt et al. (80) assessed sustained attention using the Continuous Performance Test, and behavior using the Behavioral Global Adjustment Scale. Predictive accuracy was established in a mixed sample of 21 offspring of schizophrenic parents, 26 children of affectively ill parents, and 40 offspring of psychiatrically normal parents ($N = 87$). Diagnostic outcome was last updated when the subjects were in their early 30s.

[b]Erlenmeyer-Kimling et al. (41) assessed attention as reflected in a global measure (Attention Deviance Index), memory using the Digit Span, Attention Span Task, and Visual Aural Digit Span Test, and motor skills using the Lincoln-Oseretsky Motor Development Scale. Predictive accuracy was established in a sample of 79 offspring of schizophrenic parents. The diagnostic outcome was established at a mean age of 30.7 years.

[c]Ott et al. (79) assessed the accuracy of a logistic regression model (including WISC.R/WAIS.R-derived variables) predicting schizophrenia-related psychoses (vs no diagnosis) in a mixed sample of 157 high- and low-risk children (offspring of schizophrenic, affectively ill, and psychiatrically normal parents). The diagnostic outcome was established at the mean ages of 30.17 years (sample A, recruited in 1971... 1972), and 22.09 years (sample B, recruited in 1977..1979). The range of sensitivity, specificity, and positive/negative predictive values resulted from varying the predicted cut-off probability.

[d]Ott et al. (79) assessed the predictive accuracy of WISC.R/WAIS.R-derived variables in a sample of 39 offspring of schizophrenic parents, derived from the sample described in Note[c].

[e]Marcus et al. (81) assessed neurobehavioral deviance using selected items from a broad neuropsychological battery, which were considered relevant to attention deficit disorder-like behavior. Predictive accuracy was established in 46 offspring of schizophrenic parents and 44 offspring of psychiatrically normal parents. The diagnostic outcome was established at 26..32 years of age.

241

or brought up in urban areas, independent of their place of residence. Being born or brought up in a city accounts for a sizable proportion of the attributable fraction (the proportion by which the incidence rate would be reduced if this "risk factor" were eliminated of schizophrenia), calculated at 34.6% by Mortensen and colleagues (84); this is largely because it is such a common exposure (Table 5). However, for the same reason, the predictive value of this factor is negligible. Presumably this variable is a proxy for one or more causal risk factors but it is not clear what these are.

BEING AN IMMIGRANT

The incidence of schizophrenia has long been reported as being increased in certain groups of immigrants (85). Recently, Eaton and his colleagues (86) reviewed 14 studies from the United Kingdom and 2 from the Netherlands, in an attempt to quantify the risk associated with ethnic status. They reported relative risks varying between 1.7 and 13.2 (Table 5). Thus, the effect of migration is too variable and unstable to be of much value in predictive studies.

Factors That Operate Nearer to the Onset of the Illness

ABUSE OF DRUGS

Comorbidity of schizophrenia and substance abuse is common, particularly with drugs that act as dopamine agonists, such as amphetamines and cocaine. There is also evidence that the heavy consumption of cannabis is associated with an increased risk of psychosis (87), and that cannabis can precipitate a psychotic illness in subjects genetically predisposed to the illness (88). Andreasson et al. (87) reported that using cannabis more than 50 times at age 18 was strongly associated with the subsequent development of schizophrenia, with a relative risk of 6 (Table 5). However, people who had smoked cannabis more than 50 times had only 3% probability of developing the illness. Thus, the likelihood of actually predicting schizophrenia on the basis of drug use alone remains poor.

SUFFERING LIFE EVENTS

An excess of stressful life events has been observed in schizophrenic subjects in the 3 months preceding the onset or a relapse of the illness, when compared to control subjects (89). In the study by Bebbington et al. (89), subjects with schizophrenia were 9.6 times more likely than healthy controls to have suffered a severe life event in the 3 months before the development of frank psychosis. However, the positive predictive value was only 56% (Table 5). The association between life events and onset of the illness is not specific to schizophrenia, and the effect sizes are greater for the affective disorders (89–91).

Some argue that the excess of life events in schizophrenia could constitute an effect of the illness rather than a cause of it (i.e., the event could be a consequence

Table 5
Predicting Schizophrenia: Social and Environmental Factors

Risk Factor	Effect Size	Sensitivity	Specificity	Positive Predictive Value	Negative Predictive Value
Capital vs rural area (84)[a]	RR 2.4				
Ethnic status (86)[b]	RR 1.7..13.2[b]				
Cannabis use (>50 times) at age 18 (87)[c]	RR 6	10%	98%	3%	99%
Life events (89)[d]	OR 9.6	52%	90%	56%	88%

OR = odds ratio, RR = relative risk.

[a]Mortensen et al. (84) identified 2669 cases of schizophrenia among the members of a population-based cohort of 1.75 million persons (whose mothers were born in Denmark between 1935 and 1978) and among their parents. The risk for schizophrenia was associated with the degree of urbanization of place of birth. Population attributable risk was 34.6%.

[b]Eaton et al. (86) reviewed 14 studies conducted in the United Kingdom, and 2 conducted in The Netherlands. The relative risk reported varied from 1.7 to 13.2.

[c]Andreasson et al. (87) investigated the association between level of cannabis consumption (expressed as number of occasions: 0, 1..10, 11..50, >50) and development of schizophrenia in a cohort of 45,570 Swedish conscripts, who were followed up for 15 years.

[d]Bebbington et al. (89) investigated life events in the 6 months preceding the onset of psychosis in 97 patients from the Camberwell Collaborative Psychosis study, in comparison to 207 healthy controls. Schizophrenia patients (n = 52) experienced a significant excess of severe life events during the 3 months preceding the onset of psychosis compared to the control group.

243

of the abnormal behavior exhibited in a prodromal phase of the illness) and, therefore, may not be particularly informative as a schizophrenia predictor. In our view, it is difficult to use life events alone as schizophrenia predictors since they are an almost universal experience, but they may be modestly informative if analyzed in association with other factors discussed earlier. Some *preschizophrenic* individuals may proceed on a course of increasing deviance with an accumulation of risk factors pushing them toward the threshold for the development of frank psychosis; among these risk factors, social adversity might precipitate psychosis in these already predisposed individuals.

PRESCHIZOPHRENIC SYMPTOMS?

It is also important to consider whether some of the symptoms that characterize schizophrenia are actually present, to a lesser extent and in a more moderate form, before the onset of the illness. Mrazek and Haggerty *(92)* use the term "indicated prevention" for the ability to target a population of subjects at high risk of psychosis on the basis of the identification of subthreshold symptoms. Eaton et al. *(93)* have suggested a differentiation between the "precursor signs," which would confer an increased risk to the individual, and the "prodrome," in which some signs, present before the onset of the disorder, are identified as salient to the disorder.

So, can specific prodromal symptoms help to identify individuals who will develop schizophrenia? Klosterkotter and colleagues *(94)* followed up a sample of nonpsychotic psychiatric outpatients for 9.6 years, after having carried out an assessment using the Bonn Scale for the Assessment of Basic Symptoms *(95)*; this scale rates early schizophrenia symptoms that are claimed to represent the subjective experience of the neurophysiological changes that subjects undergo before developing schizophrenia. Approximately half of the sample had developed schizophrenia after 9.6 years; the presence of prodromal symptoms predicted the disorder with a probability of 70% (Table 6). The best prediction for the transition to schizophrenia resulted from a cluster of symptoms including thought, language, perception, and motor disturbances. When at least 15% of the symptoms listed in this cluster were present, the specificity was 84% and the positive predictive value 77%. Of course, the sample used in this study was selected; therefore, the predictive power of the "basic" symptoms is likely to be less impressive when applied in a general-population setting.

McGorry et al. *(96)* evaluated the diagnostic efficiency and the predictive power of a number of prodromal signs in relation to a diagnosis of schizophrenia. Again, it was the combination of items that showed the highest predictive power. In fact, the key factor for the prediction of later schizophrenia was the presence of prodromal symptoms evaluated in conjunction with variables concerning duration

Table 6
Predicting Schizophrenia: Prodromal Symptoms

Risk Factor	Effect Size	Sensitivity	Specificity	Positive Predictive Value	Negative Predictive Value
General prodromal symptoms (at least one symptom) (94)[a]	OR 56	98%	59%	70%	96%
Thought, language, perception, and motor disturbances (94)[a]		56%	84%	77%	66%
Duration of prodrome and premorbid deterioration (96)[b]		64%	90%	74%	85%
Psychotic symptoms at age 11 (104)[c]	OR 16.4	19%	99%	25%	98%

OR = odds ratio.

[a]Klosterkotter et al. (94) investigated prodromal symptoms in 385 outpatients of psychiatric services in Germany, using the Bonn Scale for the Assessment of Basic Symptoms Clusters (BSABS). Of the 160 subjects who were followed up for 9.6 years, 79 (49.4%) had developed schizophrenia. The table reports on the odds ratio obtained for the dichotomization of subjects with "at least 1 BSABS present," vs subjects with "no BSABS symptom present" at the time of baseline assessment. The authors then analyzed the predictive accuracy of the different clusters of symptoms composing the BSABS. They introduced a general cut-off point when 15% of symptoms were present (for the cluster investigating thought, language, perception, and motor disturbances, the cut-off was reached when any 5 of the 35 symptoms in this cluster were present).

[b]McGorry et al. (96) investigated the presence of prodromal symptoms in 122 first-episode psychosis subjects. The prediction of schizophrenia diagnosis was evaluated using the DSM–III–R prodromal symptom checklist in conjunction with duration- and premorbid adjustment variables. The best predicting decision rule was: Premorbid adjustment defined as: duration of DSM–III–R prodromal symptoms for at least 185 days and social isolation/withdrawal, or poor premorbid social adjustment/work history and poor premorbid adjustment (total PAS score >51.6).

[c]Poulton et al. (104) analyzed prospective data from a (birth) cohort of 761 11-year-old children, who were investigated for delusional beliefs and hallucinatory experiences with the Diagnostic Interview Schedule for Children. Computerized (DISC .C). Subjects were reassessed at age 26, and 25 had developed a schizophreniform disorder.

and premorbid adjustment (Table 6). This model showed good specificity (90%) and positive predictive value (74%).

It is, of course, much easier to predict schizophrenia in individuals who have already come to the notice of psychiatrists than in the general population. Much evidence suggests that phenomena such as delusions and hallucinations are more common in the general population than previously thought *(97–99)*. McGorry et al. *(100)*, for example, reported that *DSM–III–R* prodromal symptoms for schizophrenia were present in 15.50% of high school students. However, these signs could be neutral as indicators of psychopathology, and the way the single individual reacts to them could be what determines whether they come to psychiatric attention *(101)*. Indeed, this is suggested in studies by Van Os and colleagues *(102,103)*, who reported that copying styles associated with particular personality traits may increase (e.g., neuroticism) or decrease (e.g., extraversion) the risk that isolated symptoms progress to the full-blown disorder. Nevertheless, in an extensive follow-up of a population-based group of 761 children (seen at regular intervals from birth to age 26) in Dunedin (New Zealand), Poulton et al. *(104)* described continuity between unusual childhood experiences and beliefs, and the much later development of psychosis. In their study, reporting experiences such as possibly being followed or hearing voices carried a 16.4-fold increase in risk for schizophreniform disorder at age 26, with a specificity of 99% (Table 6).

We can see from these studies that a considerable number of individuals in the general population score positively for symptoms that psychiatrists consider as quasi-psychotic. Nevertheless, the majority of these individuals will not develop schizophrenia. Symptoms present in a high-risk population have to be treated more seriously, but nevertheless, one should be very cautious before informing an individual or their family that such symptoms are associated with an increased risk for the disorder. If such caution is warranted in high-risk subjects, who are already genetically vulnerable or symptomatic, it is even truer for the general population.

CONCLUSION

So far, research has not identified a "single predictor" of schizophrenia. The preceding sections have demonstrated that the positive predictive value of any predictor in isolation remains low, even when applied to high-risk groups. Rather, a number of weak risk factors have been identified that seem to act together, some reflecting a vulnerability to the illness (e.g., familial risk), some being the early manifestations of the disorder (strange ideas), and some appearing to contribute to triggering the onset of the illness (drug abuse). At present, the best way to predict schizophrenia is to combine several of these factors; among these, attentional deficits, neurobehavioral and social variables, and quasi-psychotic symptoms,

appear to confer the best predictive power. Further work is needed to establish which combination of the least number of factors will have the highest predictive power.

The major issue confronting those seeking predictive signs is that although it has been established that neurological, cognitive, and social abnormalities are already present in many children destined to develop schizophrenia, these deficits do not appear to be specific to the disorder, and at least some of them are also present in children who develop other psychiatric disorders in adult life. Indeed, Van Os and colleagues (105) suggest that "there is little evidence that any risk factor is specific to any diagnostic category within the functional psychosis." These authors also observe that there is a considerable overlap between schizophrenic and affective symptoms. It could then be the magnitude of the effect of some risk factors, rather than their qualitative difference that projects an individual on a trajectory toward a schizophrenic rather than an affective psychosis.

Instead of searching for specific precursors that can identify those destined to develop schizophrenia rather than other psychiatric conditions, perhaps it is now time to move toward evaluating the distribution of these factors in those who will develop schizophrenia and other disorders, and then gain a better understanding of what determines the diagnostic outcome. By changing our approach, the lack of specificity of prodromal symptoms could potentially become an advantage for primary intervention (106). For example, if a preventive intervention successfully ameliorates a particular characteristic or symptom, and this characteristic is known to be a predictor not only of schizophrenia but also of another psychiatric disorder, intervention might improve the outcome not only in relation to schizophrenia, but also in relation to other disorders.

REFERENCES

1. Bleuler E. Dementia Praecox or the Group of Schizophrenias. New York: International Universities, 1911.
2. McNeil TF, Cantor-Graae E. Neuromotor markers of risk for schizophrenia. Aust N Z J Psychiatry 2000; 34(Suppl):S86..S90.
3. Gottesman II, Shields J. Schizophrenia: The Epigenetic Puzzle. New York: Cambridge University Press, 1982.
4. Cardno AG, Marshall EJ, Coid B, et al. Heritability estimates for psychotic disorders: the Maudsley twin psychosis series. Arch Gen Psychiatry 1999; 56:162..168.
5. Sham PC, Jones P, Russell A, et al. Age at onset, sex, and familial psychiatric morbidity in schizophrenia. Camberwell Collaborative Psychosis Study. Br J Psychiatry 1994; 165:466.473.
6. McNeil TF. Perinatal risk factors and schizophrenia: selective review and methodological concerns. Epidemiol Rev 1995; 17:107..112.
7. McGrath J, Murray RM. Risk factors for schizophrenia: from conception to birth. In: Hirsh S, Weinberger D, eds. Schizophrenia. Oxford, England: Blackwell, 1995:187.205.
8. Geddes JR, Lawrie SM. Obstetric complications and schizophrenia: a meta-analysis. Br J Psychiatry 1995; 167:786..793.

9. Verdoux H, Geddes JR, Takei N, et al. Obstetric complications and age at onset in schizophrenia: an international collaborative meta-analysis of individual patient data. Am J Psychiatry 1997; 154:1220..1227.

10. Cannon TD, Rosso IM, Hollister JM, Bearden CE, Sanchez LE, Hadley T. A prospective cohort study of genetic and perinatal influences in the etiology of schizophrenia. Schizophr Bull 2000; 26:351..366.

11. Rosso IM, Cannon TD, Huttunen T, Huttunen MO, Lonnqvist J, Gasperoni TL. Obstetric risk factors for early-onset schizophrenia in a Finnish birth cohort. Am J Psychiatry 2000; 157:801..807.

12. Castle DJ, Murray RM. The neurodevelopmental basis of sex differences in schizophrenia. Psychol Med 1991; 21:565..575.

13. Hultman CM, Sparen P, Takei N, Murray RM, Cnattingius S. Prenatal and perinatal risk factors for schizophrenia, affective psychosis, and reactive psychosis of early onset: case-control study. Br Med J 1999; 318:421..426.

14. Byrne M, Browne R, Mulryan N, et al. Labour and delivery complications and schizophrenia. Case-control study using contemporaneous labour ward records. Br J Psychiatry 2000; 176:531..536.

15. Murray RM, Lewis SW, Reveley AM. Towards an aetiological classification of schizophrenia. Lancet 1985; 1:1023..1026.

16. McDonald C, O'Callaghan E, Keogh F, et al. Number of older siblings of individuals diagnosed with schizophrenia. Schizophr Res 2001; 47:275..280.

17. Stefanis N, Frangou S, Yakeley J, et al. Hippocampal volume reduction in schizophrenia: effects of genetic risk and pregnancy and birth complications. Biol Psychiatry 1999; 46: 697..702.

18. Suddath RL, Christison GW, Torrey EF, Casanova MF, Weinberger DR. Anatomical abnormalities in the brains of monozygotic twins discordant for schizophrenia. N Engl J Med 1990; 322:789..794.

19. Jones PB, Rantakallio P, Hartikainen A-L, Isohanni M, Sipila P. Schizophrenia as a long-term outcome of pregnancy, delivery, and perinatal complications: a 28-year follow-up of the 1966 North Finland general population birth cohort. Am J Psychiatry 1998; 155:355..364.

20. Sham PC, O'Callaghan E, Takei N, Murray GK, Hare EH, Murray RM. Schizophrenia following pre-natal exposure to influenza epidemics between 1939 and 1960. Br J Psychiatry 1992; 160:461..466.

21. Kunugi H, Nanko S, Takei N, Saito K, Hayashi N, Kazamatsuri H. Schizophrenia following in utero exposure to the 1957 influenza epidemics in Japan. Am J Psychiatry 1995; 152: 450..452.

22. Heinrichs RW. In Search of Madness. New York: Oxford University Press, 2001.

23. Clouston T. The Neuroses of Development. Edinburgh, Scotland: Oliver & Boyd, 1891.

24. McGrath JJ, Van Os J, Hoyos C, Jones PB, Harvey I, Murray RM. Minor physical anomalies in psychoses: associations with clinical and putative aetiological variables. Schizophr Res 1995; 18:9..20.

25. Fearon P, Lane A, Airie M, et al. Is reduced dermatoglyphic a-b ridge count a reliable marker of developmental impairment in schizophrenia? Schizophr Res 2001; 50:151..157.

26. Fananas L, Van Os J, Hoyos C, McGrath J, Mellor CS, Murray R. Dermatoglyphic a-b ridge count as a possible marker for developmental disturbance in schizophrenia: replication in two samples. Schizophr Res 1996; 20:307..314.

27. Lane A, Kinsella A, Murphy P, et al. The anthropometric assessment of dysmorphic features in schizophrenia as an index of its developmental origins. Psychol Med 1997; 27:1155..1164.

28. Ismail B, Cantor-Graae E, McNeil TF. Minor physical anomalies in schizophrenic patients and their siblings. Am J Psychiatry 1998; 155:1695..1702.
29. David AS, Wacharasindhu A, Lishman WA. Severe psychiatric disturbance and abnormalities of the corpus callosum: review and case series. J Neurol Neurosurg Psychiatry 1993; 56: 85..93.
30. Lewis SW, Mezey GC. Clinical correlates of septum pellucidum cavities: an unusual association with psychosis. Psychol Med 1985; 15:43..54.
31. O'Flaithbheartaigh S, Williams PA, Jones GH. Schizophrenic psychosis and associated aqueduct stenosis. Br J Psychiatry 1994; 164:684..686.
32. Wright IC, Rabe-Hesketh S, Woodruff PW, David AS, Murray RM, Bullmore ET. Meta-analysis of regional brain volumes in schizophrenia. Am J Psychiatry 2000; 157:16..25.
33. Lawrie SM, Whalley H, Kestelman JN, et al. Magnetic resonance imaging of brain in people at high risk of developing schizophrenia. Lancet 1999; 353:30..33.
34. Sharma T, Lancaster E, Sigmundsson T, et al. Lack of normal pattern of cerebral asymmetry in familial schizophrenic patients and their relatives   the Maudsley Family Study. Schizophr Res 1999; 40:111..120.
35. Andreasen NC, Swayze V, Flaum M, Alliger R, Cohen G. Ventricular abnormalities in affective disorder: clinical and demographic correlates. Am J Psychiatry 1990; 147:893..900.
36. Weinberger DR, DeLisi LE, Perman GP, Targum S, Wyatt RJ. Computed tomography in schizophreniform disorder and other acute psychiatric disorders. Arch Gen Psychiatry 1982; 39:778..783.
37. Elkis H, Friedman L, Wise A, Meltzer HY. Meta-analyses of studies of ventricular enlargement and cortical sulcal prominence in mood disorders. Comparisons with controls or patients with schizophrenia. Arch Gen Psychiatry 1995; 52:735..746.
38. Fish B, Marcus J, Hans SL, Auerbach JG, Perdue S. Infants at risk for schizophrenia: sequelae of a genetic neurointegrative defect: a review and replication analysis of pandysmaturation in the Jerusalem infant development study. Arch Gen Psychiatry 1992; 49:221..235.
39. Marcus J, Hans SL, Auerbach JG, Auerbach AG. Children at risk for schizophrenia: the Jerusalem Infant Development Study: II. Neurobehavioral deficits at school age. Arch Gen Psychiatry 1993; 50:797..809.
40. Rieder RO, Nichols PL. Offspring of schizophrenics III. Hyperactivity and neurological soft signs. Arch Gen Psychiatry 1979; 36:665..674.
41. Erlenmeyer-Kimling L, Rock D, Roberts SA, et al. Attention, memory, and motor skills as childhood predictors of schizophrenia-related psychoses: the New York High-Risk Project. Am J Psychiatry 2000; 157:1416..1422.
42. Crow TJ, Done DJ, Sacker A. Childhood precursors of psychosis as clues to its evolutionary origins. Eur Arch Psychiatry Clin Neurosci 1995; 245:61..69.
43. Jones P, Rodgers B, Murray R, Marmot M. Child developmental risk factors for adult schizophrenia in the British 1946 birth cohort. Lancet 1994; 344:1398..1402.
44. Cannon M, Jones P, Huttunen MO, Tanskanen A, Murray RM. Motor co-ordination deficits as predictors of schizophrenia among Finnish school children. Hum Psychopharmacol Clin Exp 1999; 14:491..497.
45. Walker E, Lewine RJ. Prediction of adult-onset schizophrenia from childhood home movies of the patients. Am J Psychiatry 1990; 147:1052..1056.
46. Buchanan RW, Heinrichs DW. The neurological evaluation scale (NES): a structured instrument for the assessment of neurological signs in schizophrenia. Psychiatry Res 1989; 27:335..350.
47. Boks MP, Russo S, Knegtering R, Van Den Bosch RJ. The specificity of neurological signs in schizophrenia: a review. Schizophr Res 2000; 43:109..116.

48. Nasrallah HA, Tippin J, McCalley-Whitters M. Neurological soft signs in manic patients. A comparison with schizophrenic and control groups. J Affect Disord 1983; 5:45..50.
49. Manschreck TC, Ames D. Neurologic features and psychopathology in schizophrenic disorders. Biol Psychiatry 1984; 19:703..719.
50. Jones P, Done DJ. From birth to onset: a developmental perspective of schizophrenia in two national birth cohorts. In: Keshavan MS, Murray RM, eds. Neurodevelopment & Adult Psychopathology. Cambridge, England: University Press, 1997:119..136.
51. Cannon TD, Rosso IM, Bearden CE, Sanchez LE, Hadley T. A prospective cohort study of neurodevelopmental processes in the genesis and epigenesis of schizophrenia. Dev Psychopathol 1999; 11:467..485.
52. Cannon TD, Bearden CE, Hollister JM, Rosso IM, Sanchez LE, Hadley T. Childhood cognitive functioning in schizophrenia patients and their unaffected siblings: a prospective cohort study. Schizophr Bull 2000; 26:379..393.
53. Bearden CE, Rosso IM, Hollister JM, Sanchez LE, Hadley T, Cannon TD. A prospective cohort study of childhood behavioral deviance and language abnormalities as predictors of adult schizophrenia. Schizophr Bull 2000; 26:395..410.
54. Isohanni I, Jarvelin M-R, Nieminen P, et al. School performance as a predictor of psychiatric hospitalization in adult life. A 28-year follow-up in the Northern Finland 1966 birth cohort. Psychol Med 1998; 28:967..974.
55. Isohanni I, Jarvelin MR, Jones P, Jokelainen J, Isohanni M. Can excellent school performance be a precursor of schizophrenia? A 28-year follow-up in the Northern Finland 1966 birth cohort. Acta Psychiatr Scand 1999; 100:17..26.
56. David AS, Malmberg A, Brandt L, Allebeck P, Lewis G. IQ and risk for schizophrenia: a population-based cohort study. Psychol Med 1997; 27:1311..1323.
57. Davidson M, Reichenberg A, Rabinowitz J, Weiser M, Kaplan Z, Mark M. Behavioral and intellectual markers for schizophrenia in apparently healthy male adolescents. Am J Psychiatry 1999; 156:1328..1335.
58. O'Toole BI. Screening for low prevalence disorders. Aust N Z J Psychiatry 2000; 34(Suppl): S39..S46.
59. Aylward E, Walker E, Bettes B. Intelligence in schizophrenia: meta-analysis of the research. Schizophr Bull 1984; 10:430..459.
60. Nuechterlein KH, Dawson ME. Information processing and attentional functioning in the developmental course of schizophrenic disorders. Schizophr Bull 1984; 10:160..203.
61. Cannon TD, Zorrilla LE, Shtasel D, et al. Neuropsychological functioning in siblings discordant for schizophrenia and healthy volunteers. Arch Gen Psychiatry 1994; 51:651..661.
62. Cornblatt BA, Keilp JG. Impaired attention, genetics, and the pathophysiology of schizophrenia. Schizophr Bull 1994; 20:31..46.
63. Faraone SV, Seidman LJ, Kremen WS, Pepple JR, Lyons MJ, Tsuang MT. Neuropsychological functioning among the nonpsychotic relatives of schizophrenic patients: a diagnostic efficiency analysis. J Abnorm Psychol 1995; 104:286..304.
64. Goldberg TE, Torrey EF, Gold JM, et al. Genetic risk of neuropsychological impairment in schizophrenia: a study of monozygotic twins discordant and concordant for the disorder. Schizophr Res 1995; 17:77..84.
65. Lyons MJ, Toomey R, Seidman LJ, Kremen WS, Faraone SV, Tsuang MT. Verbal learning and memory in relatives of schizophrenics: preliminary findings. Biol Psychiatry 1995; 37: 750..753.
66. Chen WJ, Liu SK, Chang CJ, Lien YJ, Chang YH, Hwu HG. Sustained attention deficit and schizotypal personality features in nonpsychotic relatives of schizophrenic patients. Am J Psychiatry 1998; 155:1214..1220.

67. Kremen WS, Faraone SV, Seidman LJ, Pepple JR, Tsuang MT. Neuropsychological risk indicators for schizophrenia: a preliminary study of female relatives of schizophrenic and bipolar probands. Psychiatry Res 1998; 79:227..240.
68. Toomey R, Faraone SV, Seidman LJ, Kremen WS, Pepple JR, Tsuang MT. Association of neuropsychological vulnerability markers in relatives of schizophrenic patients. Schizophr Res 1998; 31:89..98.
69. Byrne M, Hodges A, Grant E, Owens DC, Johnstone EC. Neuropsychological assessment of young people at high genetic risk for developing schizophrenia compared with controls: preliminary findings of the Edinburgh High Risk Study (EHRS). Psychol Med 1999; 29: 1161..1173.
70. Faraone SV, Seidman LJ, Kremen WS, Toomey R, Pepple JR, Tsuang MT. Neuropsychological functioning among the nonpsychotic relatives of schizophrenic patients: a 4-year follow-up study. J Abnorm Psychol 1999; 108:176..181.
71. Laurent A, Moreaud O, Bosson JL, et al. Neuropsychological functioning among non-psychotic siblings and parents of schizophrenic patients. Psychiatry Res 1999; 87:147..157.
72. Cosway R, Byrne M, Clafferty R, et al. Neuropsychological change in young people at high risk for schizophrenia: results from the first two neuropsychological assessments of the Edinburgh high risk study. Psychol Med 2000; 30:1111..1121.
73. Michie PT, Kent A, Stienstra R, et al. Phenotypic markers as risk factors in schizophrenia: neurocognitive functions. Aust N Z J Psychiatry 2000; 34(Suppl):S74..S85.
74. Parnas J, Schulsinger F, Schulsinger H, Mednick SA, Teasdale TW. Behavioral precursors of schizophrenia spectrum. A prospective study. Arch Gen Psychiatry 1982; 39:658..664.
75. Mirsky AF, Ingraham LJ, Kugelmass S. Neuropsychological assessment of attention and its pathology in the Israeli cohort. Schizophr Bull 1995; 21:193..204.
76. Cornblatt BA, Erlenmeyer-Kimling L. Global attentional deviance as a marker of risk for schizophrenia: specificity and predictive validity. J Abnorm Psychol 1985; 94:470..486.
77. Cornblatt BA, Lenzenweger MF, Dworkin RH, Erlenmeyer-Kimling L. Childhood attentional dysfunctions predict social deficits in unaffected adults at risk for schizophrenia. Br J Psychiatry Suppl 1992;59..64.
78. Freedman LR, Rock D, Roberts SA, Cornblatt BA, Erlenmeyer-Kimling L. The New York High-Risk Project: attention, anhedonia and social outcome. Schizophr Res 1998; 30:1..9.
79. Ott SL, Spinelli S, Rock D, Roberts S, Amminger GP, Erlenmeyer-Kimling L. The New York High-Risk Project: social and general intelligence in children at risk for schizophrenia. Schizophr Res 1998; 31:1..11.
80. Cornblatt B, Obuchowski M, Roberts S, Pollack S, Erlenmeyer-Kimling L. Cognitive and behavioral precursors of schizophrenia. Dev Psychopathol 1999; 11:487..508.
81. Marcus J, Hans SL, Nagler S, Auerbach JG, Mirsky AF, Aubrey A. Review of the NIMH Israeli Kibbutz-City Study and the Jerusalem Infant Development Study. Schizophr Bull 1987; 13:425..438.
82. Torrey EF, Bowler A. Geographical distribution of insanity in America: evidence for an urban factor. Schizophr Bull 1990; 16:591..604.
83. Lewis G, David A, Andreasson S, Allebeck P. Schizophrenia and city life. Lancet 1992; 340: 137..140.
84. Mortensen PB, Pedersen CB, Westergaard T et al. Effects of family history and place and season of birth on the risk of schizophrenia. N Engl J Med 1999; 340:603..608.
85. Odegaard O. Emigration and insanity: a study of mental disease among Norwegian born population in Minnesota. Acta Psychiatrica and Neurologica Scandinavica 1932; (Suppl 4):1..206.
86. Eaton W, Harrison G. Life chances, life planning, and schizophrenia. A review and interpretation of research on social deprivation. Int J Ment Health 2001; 30:58..81.

87. Andreasson S, Allebeck P, Engstrom A, Rydberg U. Cannabis and schizophrenia. A longitudinal study of Swedish conscripts. Lancet 1987; 2:1483..1486.
88. McGuire PK, Jones P, Harvey I, et al. Cannabis and acute psychosis. Schizophr Res 1994; 13:161..167.
89. Bebbington P, Wilkins S, Jones P, et al. Life events and psychosis. Initial results from the Camberwell Collaborative Psychosis Study. Br J Psychiatry 1993; 162:72..79.
90. Brown GW, Harris TO, Peto J. Life events and psychiatric disorders. 2. Nature of causal link. Psychol Med 1973; 3:159..176.
91. Paykel ES. Contribution of life events to causation of psychiatric illness. Psychol Med 1978; 8:245..253.
92. Mrazek PJ, Haggerty RJ. Reducing Risks for Mental Disorders: Frontiers for Preventive Intervention Research. Washington, DC, National Academy, 1994.
93. Eaton WW, Badawi M, Melton B. Prodromes and precursors: epidemiologic data for primary prevention of disorders with slow onset. Am J Psychiatry 1995; 152:967..972.
94. Klosterkotter J, Hellmich M, Steinmeyer EM, Schultze-Lutter F. Diagnosing schizophrenia in the initial prodromal phase. Arch Gen Psychiatry 2001; 58:158..164.
95. Gross G, Huber G, Klosterkotter J, Linz M. Bonner Skala fur die Beurteilung von Basissymptomen. Berlin, Hedelberg, New York: Springer-Verlag, 1987.
96. McGorry PD, McKenzie D, Jackson HJ, Waddell F, Curry C. Can we improve the diagnostic efficiency and predictive power of prodromal symptoms for schizophrenia? Schizophr Res 2000; 42:91..100.
97. Van Os J, Hanssen M, Bijl RV, Ravelli A. Strauss (1969) revisited: a psychosis continuum in the general population? Schizophr Res 2000; 45:11.20.
98. Eaton WW, Romanoski A, Anthony JC, Nestadt G. Screening for psychosis in the general population with a self-report interview. J Nerv Ment Dis 1991; 179:689.693.
99. Verdoux H, Van Os J, Maurice-Tison S, Gay B, Salamon R, Bourgeois M. Is early adulthood a critical developmental stage for psychosis proneness? A survey of delusional ideation in normal subjects. Schizophr Res 1998; 29:247.254.
100. McGorry PD, McFarlane C, Patton GC, et al. The prevalence of prodromal features of schizophrenia in adolescence: a preliminary survey. Acta Psychiatr Scand 1995; 92:241.249.
101. Claridge G. Final remarks and future directions. In: Claridge G, ed. Schizotypy. Implications for Illness and Health. Oxford, England: Oxford University Press, 1997:301.313.
102. Van Os J, Driessen G, Gunther N, Delespaul P. Neighbourhood variation in incidence of schizophrenia. Evidence for person-environment interaction. Br J Psychiatry 2000; 176:243.248.
103. Van Os J, Jones PB. Neuroticism as a risk factor for schizophrenia. Psychol Med 2001; 31:1129..1134.
104. Poulton R, Caspi A, Moffitt TE, Cannon M, Murray R, Harrington H. Children's self-reported psychotic symptoms and adult schizophreniform disorder: a 15-year longitudinal study. Arch Gen Psychiatry 2000; 57:1053..1058.
105. Van Os J, Jones P, Sham P, Bebbington P, Murray RM. Risk factors for onset and persistence of psychosis. Soc Psychiatry Psychiatr Epidemiol 1998; 33:596.605.
106. Jones PB, Tarrant CJ. Developmental precursors and biological markers for schizophrenia and affective disorders: specificity and public health implications. Eur Arch Psychiatry Clin Neurosci 2000; 250:286.291.
107. Geddes JR, Verdoux H, Takei N, et al. Schizophrenia and complications of pregnancy and labor: an individual patient data meta-analysis. Schizophr Bull 1999; 25:413..412.

III

EARLY INTERVENTION AND PREVENTION OF SCHIZOPHRENIA

12 Prevention of Schizophrenia and Psychotic Behavior

Definitions and Methodological Issues

C. Hendricks Brown, PhD
and Stephen V. Faraone, PhD

In this chapter we provide a framework for designing primary and very early screening (secondary-prevention) programs for schizophrenia and other psychotic disorders. We also show how a number of alternative approaches can be applied to achieve the goal of reducing the incidence of schizophrenia. The approaches of a broadly population-based vs more targeted prevention program for schizophrenia are contrasted based on current knowledge.

A unique feature of schizophrenia is that compared with many other targets of current prevention programs, such as those focusing on drug abuse (1) aggression, conduct disorder and delinquency (2–4), depression (5,6), and child abuse (7), schizophrenia has a low incidence rate, about 1%. Because it has such a low baserate, the design of any study to test a prevention strategy will need to deal with the low incidence, as well as the predictive ability of risk factors and the efficacy of interventions across different subgroups. Without such attention, one is likely to design a prevention trial that has minimal power to detect preventive impact. We also show how three epidemiologic terms, indicating in turn the predictive ability of a risk factor, the frequency of that risk factor in the population, and the effectiveness of a preventive intervention targeting that risk factor, all work together to determine the effect of intervention strategy would have on preventing a target outcome in the population.

To realize the full potential for preventing schizophrenia, we demonstrate the efficacy or effectiveness of intervention programs based on the results of carefully designed randomized trials. The scientific community generally considers

From: *Early Clinical Intervention and Prevention in Schizophrenia*
Edited by: W. S. Stone, S. V. Faraone, and M. T. Tsuang © Humana Press Inc., Totowa, NJ

single and multiple randomized controlled field trials as the gold standard design for testing an intervention's effect *(8)*. Among other qualities, carefully designed and implemented randomized preventive trials have low attrition and selection bias, use valid and reliable measures, conduct assessments blindly, and have sufficient statistical power to detect a meaningful intervention effect *(9,10)*. Standard methods of clinical trials, originally designed for treatment trials *(11)*, are now being used across a diverse set of prevention programs. Eventually, we will need to rely on such preventive trials to identify which interventions have the best opportunity for preventing schizophrenia. Throughout this chapter, we illustrate whenever possible the terms and concepts by examining the prevention of schizophrenia and other psychotic disorders. However, scientific prevention efforts have been applied much less frequently to schizophrenia than they have to other areas, so we liberally use examples from other health outcomes for illustrative purposes. These examples from other fields of prevention will hopefully stimulate related applications to schizophrenia.

RISK AND PROTECTIVE FACTORS, TARGET POPULATION

Modern prevention science is based on the concept of targeting or altering known risk factors or enhancing known protective factors that appear before the onset of a disorder *(12,13)*. A risk factor is a condition that, when present, leads to a larger probability of later disorder than that experienced by the population without such a condition. A protective factor is one that leads to lower risk. Rather than simply being the converse of a risk factor, a protective factor is one that protects against a known risk factor but has no effect on illness if that known risk factor is not present. For example, estrogens may delay the onset of schizophrenia among genetically vulnerable people but they are not believed to modify the risk for schizophrenia among people not already at risk for the disorder *(14)*.

Risk and protective factors must be antecedent to the outcome of interest; they may be very distant in time or proximal to onset. For example, genes and obstetric complications (OCs) are distal risk factors for schizophrenia *(15)*, drug use is a proximal risk factor. Risk and protective factors can be classified as modifiable or nonmodifiable. The presence of a relative diagnosed with schizophrenia is an example of a nonmodifiable risk factor whereas OCs could be modified by good pre-, peri-, and postnatal care. Risk and protective factors can be measured at the individual level, such as season of birth; they can be specific to the subject's behavior or interactions within specific social fields, such as peer relations; or they may be ecologically based factors, such as the urbanicity of the subject's community of residence *(16)*. Notably, twin studies suggest that most environmental risk factors for psychiatric disorders are those that are not shared by siblings *(17)*.

Inherent in these definitions of risk and protective factors are two character-istics. First, the relationship between a measured risk factor and a later disorder is statistical in nature, not necessarily causal. Second, the risk or protective factor must be antecedent to the onset of the disorder. By this definition, a family history is a risk factor for schizophrenia, because it increases the probability that the rela-tive will develop schizophrenia. Estrogen is believed to be a protective factor, because female sex predicts a delayed onset and reduced prevalence of schizo-phrenia *(18)*.

Both modifiable and nonmodifiable risk and protective factors, as well as individuals and group-level factors are important to consider in prevention. We take as examples the prevention of two diseases   pellagra and syphilis   that in the past were responsible for a large portion of mental disorders, including psy-choses, worldwide. By classifying effective prevention strategies for these known causes of mental disorders, we can compare alternative prevention strategies aimed at those processes where the etiology is not fully known. The first preven-tion strategy, illustrated on the prevention of psychosis caused by pellagra, involves direct targeting of modifiable risk factors. In the southern United States, the dis-ease pellagra was responsible for a large percentage of hospitalizations for mental disorders in the early part of the 20th century. After the discovery of the major cause of pellagra, a dietary deficiency in niacin, direct targeting of this risk factor by improving diet virtually eliminated this disease and its consequent psychosis in many parts of the world. This dietary strategy reaches a large segment of the population and therefore we can refer to it as broadly population based.

Identification of risk factors can also lead one to develop interventions that target a specific group of subjects who share that risk factor. Here we use syphilis as an example. Untreated syphilis can lead to neurosyphilis with symptoms of grandiosity and psychotic behavior as well as dementia and depression. Although the disease itself is far from being eliminated, the availability of antibiotic treat-ment has virtually eliminated the most serious mental conditions associated with the later stages of this disease. Two of the common screening strategies are tar-geted: screening of couples before marriage and screening of commercial sex workers for this disease. These screenings involve targeting groups that are at risk for transmission. Appropriate treatment is then provided to those with positive serological tests. The distribution of syphilis cases is also not random. Impov-erished communities living with limited clinic access and closeness to trucking thoroughfares are at elevated risk *(19)*. Thus a broad-based campaign involving screening and education in such a community represents a prevention strategy that is based on risk factors commonly considered to be nonmodifiable, that is, geographic and community economic health.

In these examples, we target a group of individuals based on a risk character-istic (e.g., sex worker) but the intervention is directed at another factor that is

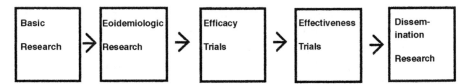

Fig. 1. Preventive intervention research cycle.

thought to be causal in the development of the disorder (syphilis infection). It is also possible to select a group based on a modifiable risk factor and then eliminate that risk factor. For example, it is possible to screen individuals for niacin deficiency and then provide direct supplements. Such a general strategy may be useful in the prevention of schizophrenia. For example, improving the care of pregnant schizophrenic women or pregnant women known to have schizophrenic partners could reduce OCs and the risk for schizophrenia. Providing supportive therapy and family education could reduce stress levels in the homes of adolescents known to be at risk for schizophrenia because they have a schizophrenic parent or sibling.

The successful elimination of pellagra and reduction in syphilis required the use of traditional epidemiologic methods of case identification and surveillance and prevention/treatment orientations relevant to person, place, and time, as well as host, agent, and environment. This epidemiologic investigation is a key component to the preventive intervention research cycle adopted by the National Institutes of Health and shown in Fig. 1 *(8)*. The epidemiologic research needs to stand on findings from basic research that identifies potential biological, genetic, behavioral, and societal factors leading to schizophrenia. Once interesting regions of abnormal brain functioning, attention, genetic abnormalities, behavioral patterns, and the like are identified from basic research, epidemiologic research can determine the overall risk of these conditions at different stages of life and across different populations. The findings of epidemiologic studies, which comprise identifiable risk and protective factors, then can be tested in small carefully controlled efficacy studies, the third stage of the prevention research cycle. This is followed by effectiveness trials, which examine a preventive intervention's impact in real-world settings where program implementation and adherence are much more like they would be in real-world settings. A last stage involves the dissemination of an effective prevention program into different communities, examining its adoption, adherence, or reinvention, and its sustainability. Each of these stages can not only inform the latter stages, but deliberate steps are taken to cycle back to previous steps in order to improve the impact of the preventive interven-

tion. We refer the reader to other chapters in the book for basic research on schizophrenia and specific epidemiologic findings. Further advances in the prevention of psychosis will depend heavily on these basic science and epidemiologic approaches to understanding the complex interactions between host factors of genetics, and person. environment interactions. Our attention will be on applying the epidemiologic information to develop useful prevention approaches that can be tested in randomized trials for efficacy and effectiveness.

We next point out both the advantages and disadvantages of the terms primary, secondary, and tertiary prevention, somewhat older terms that have been replaced by other terms described here. The classification of primary, secondary, and tertiary prevention is based on the intended outcome: prevent new cases, reduce duration, or reduce consequent disability once diagnosed. Primary prevention of psychosis owing to pellagra can be accomplished by supplementing niacin in the diet. All primary-prevention strategies focus on unaffected individuals. Screening for syphilis or other sexually transmitted diseases is an example of secondary prevention. Here a clear sign for the disease can be detected even if not symptoms are present. For those who already have developed primary or secondary syphilis, antibiotic treatment halts the progression to greater mental disability and can therefore be considered a tertiary preventive strategy for syphilitic patients. This classification into primary, secondary, and tertiary prevention is not sufficient since this focuses on intended outcome rather than target population or prevention strategy. For example, improved diet not only reduces new cases (primary prevention) but also treats those in the population who already have pellagra (secondary and tertiary prevention). This population-based dietary approach thus extends beyond pure primary prevention. Also, tertiary prevention is less clearly defined when there is comorbidity or multiple disorders; syphilis treatment is a primary preventive strategy for HIV, for example. A more recent classification of preventive interventions is discussed here.

EPIDEMIOLOGIC TERMS
INVOLVING RISK AND PROTECTIVE FACTORS

The incidence rate is defined to be the proportion of the unexposed population that experiences the disorder within a specified time period. By common convention, we use the same terms of risk and protective factors for those characteristics that merely delay the onset of a disorder, even though the lifetime incidence could be the same. For example, there is suggestive evidence that taking a nonsteroidal anti-inflammatory drug (NSAID) could delay the onset of Alzheimer's disease; because Alzheimer's disease most often strikes so late in life, its preventive effect may be to delay onset rather than reduce the lifetime risk of Alzheimer's

disease. In measuring the delay of onset of a diagnosis, we often compare the distribution of event times, rather than probabilities of an onset by a certain time. Terms of survival analysis such as hazard rate or median time of onset, as well as the direct modeling of the delay of onset using accelerated failure times *(20)* can be used to assess risk and protective factors as well as preventive intervention effects themselves. For low-base rate disorders such as schizophrenia, there can be significant improvements in statistical power when survival analysis is used rather than the presence or absence of the disorder during a specified time period *(20)*.

For risk and protective factors that are dichotomous, their strength is generally measured by the relative risk (RR) or odds ratio (OR). The relative risk is simply the ratio of the probability of a later diagnosis in the subpopulation that shares this attribute compared to the probability of a later diagnosis in the subpopulation without such an attribute. Letting D represent a later diagnosis and X represent a potential risk factor, and X^c the absence of such a factor, then

$$RR = \Pr\{D \mid X\} / \Pr\{D \mid X^c\}.$$

Here we let $\Pr\{\ \}$ represent the probability of an event, and we use $\Pr\{D \mid X\}$ to represent the conditional probability of a diagnosis occurring to individuals having characteristic X. When the relative risk is larger than one, the factor places the person at excess risk; when it is smaller than one, the factor is protective. Another common measure of the strength of relationship is the odds ratio. Since the odds of a disorder given X is defined as the ratio of the probability of the disorder given X divided by the probability of not having the disorder (D^c) given X,

$$Odds = \Pr\{D \mid X\} / \Pr\{D^c \mid X\}, \tag{1}$$

the odds ratio is the ratio of this odds for factor X divided by the odds for the absence of factor X,

$$OR = \Pr\{D \mid X\} * \Pr\{D^c \mid X^c\} / (\Pr\{D^c \mid X\} * \Pr\{D \mid X^c\}). \tag{2}$$

Note that when the disorder is rare, as in the case of schizophrenia, the two conditional probabilities of no disorder in the above expression (second and third factors) are both very close to one, so the odds ratio and relative risk are virtually identical.

We gain nearly all of our knowledge of risk and protective factors in schizophrenia by conducting case-control studies or prospective epidemiologic studies *(21)*. Case-control studies begin with a sample of individuals who have the disorder and then construct a sample of nondisordered individuals who are matched on demographic characteristics of interest. By collecting retrospective data, either through interviews or through record retrieval, one can examine the strength of association between the disorder and antecedent factors. The odds ratio obtained

from a satisfactorily designed case-control study is also a completely appropriate estimate of the odds ratio mentioned above, provided there are no selection biases in either the cases or controls and the exposure or risk status is also measured without bias. And since schizophrenia is a rare disorder, this odds ratio will be very close to the relative risk that would have been estimated from a much more expensive population-based study. Case-control studies are relatively inexpensive, and when multiple studies are combined in meta-analyses, various checks can be made to examine potential sources of bias *(22)*. Case-control studies have indicated, for example, that an obstetric complication at birth is associated with a twofold increase in risk for schizophrenia *(23)*.

Prospective cohort studies, on the other hand, generate a set of measures on a sample of subjects at one point in time and follow these same subjects over time to determine onset of a disorder. Odds ratios or relative risks can be computed directly from prospective studies by forming the relevant 2-by-2 contingency tables of disease status by exposure status (although many odds ratios require adjustment for potential confounders). The odds ratios or relative risks based on prospective data provide direct estimates of Eq. 1 and Eq. 2, and are appropriate when there are no selection or follow-up biases.

Ordinarily such prospective or longitudinal studies start with a nonaffected population so that we can infer the antecedence of a condition relative to the disorder. This condition is made because subjects who are known to have a diagnosis at the start of the study provide no information on the incidence of that disorder. For low base rate disorders such as schizophrenia, improper inclusion of so-called prevalent cases at baseline can lead to substantial biases when trying to identify risk factors   a factor may be a consequent event to schizophrenia rather than antecedent, and inclusion of even a low number of prevalent cases may lead to the erroneous conclusion that a factor is antecedent when it is actually co-occurring or consequent. The potential for including affected subjects in a cohort study drops precipitously if the study focuses on an age group younger than the age where the incidence curve begins to rise. Notably, birth cohort studies have confirmed that obstetric complications, especially those leading to hypoxia, are risk factors for schizophrenia Buka et al. *(24)*.

Prospective studies are not subject to the risk of retrospective recall bias the way case-control studies are, and as well are not susceptible to the unknown biases that may be inadvertently introduced in case-control studies through the selection of the controls. Usually the relative risk or odds ratio calculated from prospective longitudinal studies generates less bias than those from case-control studies. The main disadvantages of prospective studies relative to case-control studies are their cost and lengths of follow-up, so prospective longitudinal studies are less common than case-control studies. In addition, prospective longitudinal studies may be affected by differential follow-up bias. For example, in studying

whether the family's social class during childhood is a risk factor for schizophrenia, one could easily introduce biases in the relative risk if disorder status were limited only to hospitalizations since some affected individuals never get treated *(25)*. If the chance of being hospitalized given the same set of schizophrenia symptoms varies by social class, then odds ratios and relative risks based on hospitalization status may be incorrect measures for schizophrenia.

POPULATION ATTRIBUTABLE RISK

By itself, the strength of a risk factor, indicated by the relative risk, does not provide sufficient information on how strongly it affects the incidence within a population. A strong risk factor that is extremely rare usually contributes to fewer cases in the population than does a weaker risk factor that is much more common. Whenever considering the effects of a prevention program on a population, one must consider not only the strength of the risk factor but also its prevalence, or $Pr\{X\}$ for a dichotomous risk factor X. (When X is a continuous measure, for example, severity of psychiatric symptoms in the parents, we require information about the full distribution of X, as well as the conditional probability of $Pr\{D \mid X\}$, to compute its risk at the population level.) These two quantities of the strength and prevalence of a risk factor are traditionally combined into a measure called the population attributable risk (PAR). PAR measures the relative reduction in the disorder for the entire population that would be achieved if the effects of the risk factor were to be completely removed. In such a hypothetical case, those exposed to the risk factor would suffer the same rate of disorder as those without the risk factor. Thus, PAR is calculated by replacing the probability of disorder for those exposed to X with the probability of disorder for those not exposed to X.

$$PAR = - \text{ Reduction in Disorder}$$
$$\text{if X is Removed / Frequency of Disorder in Population}$$

$$= Pr\{X\} * (Pr\{D \mid X\} - Pr\{D \mid X^c\}) / Pr\{D\}$$

$$= \frac{Pr\{X\} (RR - 1)}{1 + Pr\{X\} (RR - 1)} \sim \frac{Pr\{X \mid D\} (OR - 1)}{OR}$$

The two latter expressions are virtually equivalent for low baserate disorders; the first is best suited for prospective studies, which directly measure $Pr\{X\}$ and relative risk, whereas the latter is more suited for case-control studies, which directly measure $Pr\{X \mid D\}$ and odds ratio. Thus the potential effect of an intervention that targets a particular risk factor X depends on its prevalence times the added risk above that in the population not at risk. PAR is always smaller than one; it allows comparison of the relative benefit of targeting different risk factors in the population.

For later work, we introduce the odds of risk factor X using the symbol $Odds_x$ = $Pr\{X\}$ / $Pr\{X^c\}$ since this is more convenient than prevalence.

OUR CURRENT KNOWLEDGE OF RISK AND PROTECTIVE FACTORS FOR SCHIZOPHRENIA

In this section we briefly review current knowledge about risk and protective factors for schizophrenia. This review focuses on factors believed to be causally linked to schizophrenia. Factors associated with "schizotaxia," the predisposition to schizophrenia, are also predictive of subsequent schizophrenia but are reviewed in another chapter. The epidemiologic terms we have just described, particularly PAR, are not generally available in the literature. We report known odds ratios when they are available from existing publications.

Genes

The cumulative evidence from more than a century of research overwhelmingly implicates genes in the etiology of schizophrenia (26,27). Twin studies consistently find higher rates of schizophrenia among co-twins of monozygotic (MZ) compared with dizygotic twins (28) and adoption studies show that familial transmission is mediated by genetic, not adoptive relationships (29,30). Although no schizophrenia gene has yet been discovered (31), mathematical analyses suggest that many genes are involved (32) and that the effect of any one gene is likely to be small (33), with the odds ratio not exceeding 2. Because of this modest odds ratio and small prevalence for each gene in the general population, the PAR for single genes will be quite small. Targeting individuals in families with single genes can have a dramatic benefit for those family members but will not substantially reduce the overall population incidence of schizophrenia.

Eventually, the discovery of schizophrenia susceptibility genes may yield useful predictors of subsequent schizophrenia. Until then, we must predict genetic risk based on the presence of schizophrenia in relatives. A review of 40 European studies, selected for similarities in diagnostic and ascertainment procedures, and performed between 1920 and 1987 (26) showed the following approximate lifetime risks for schizophrenia to relatives of schizophrenic patients: parents, 6%; siblings, 9%; offspring (of one parent with schizophrenia), 13%; and offspring of two schizophrenic parents, 46%. Note that the risk to offspring exceeds the risk to parents, which is unexpected because similar risks to first-degree biological relatives would be anticipated in a standard genetic model. The difference occurs because schizophrenia has an adverse affect on the probability of reproducing, whereby parents, by definition, have already reproduced. Parents are thus a more selective   and less vulnerable   group, on average, than are offspring. The risks to second-degree relatives ranged from 6% for half-siblings to 2% for uncles and aunts. First cousins,

a type of third-degree relative, had an average risk of 2%. Modern family studies, using more stringent diagnostic criteria, have essentially confirmed both the pattern of risk in families, and the approximate rates at which they occur *(34)*.

Psychosocial Factors

Kinney et al. *(35)* found elevations of the Thought Disorder Index (TDI) in biological relatives of schizophrenic patients, compared to normal controls. In contrast, elevations of the TDI were not evident in the adoptive relatives of either schizophrenic or control subjects. Consistent findings were reported by others *(36–38)*. Wahlberg et al. *(38)* showed that young-adult offspring of schizophrenic mothers were more likely to be thought disordered when raised by adoptive mothers who showed "communication deviance." But adoptees raised by adoptive parents with low communication deviance were less likely to show thought disorder. In contrast, control adoptees showed no relationship between adoptee thought disorder and communication deviance in the adoptive parents. Thus, communication deviance appears to be a risk factor only for people with a genetic vulnerability to schizophrenia.

Obstetric Complications

Many studies have found increased rates of OCs in the births of children who eventually become schizophrenic. For example, schizophrenic patients are more likely to have been born prematurely and to have had relatively low birthweights *(39,40)*. The finding that OCs are predictive of subsequent schizophrenia has been confirmed in other studies *(41,42)* and a review by McNeil *(43)* suggested that complications leading to oxygen deprivation or trauma appear to be most relevant to the subsequent development of schizophrenia, a finding that has been confirmed by subsequent studies *(24,44–46)*.

Several studies have found that OCs tend to be more common in sporadic schizophrenic patients (those having no affected close relatives) compared with familial cases of schizophrenia *(47–50)*. McNeil et al. *(51)* found that OCs among identical twin pairs were more common among those discordant for schizophrenia than those concordant for schizophrenia. A similar trend had been reported by Onstad et al. *(52)*. Also, among MZ twins discordant for schizophrenia, OCs were more likely to involve the schizophrenic twin than the co-twin *(53)*. However, birthweight differences were not found between schizophrenic and well MZ co-twins in a review of six systematically ascertained twin samples *(54)*.

It is also possible that the effect of OCs is to activate the genetic predisposition to schizophrenia. For example, DeLisi et al. *(55)* found more OCs among schizophrenic compared with nonschizophrenic siblings in families having at least two siblings with schizophrenia. This suggested that OCs work in combination with

familial factors. Similary, among children of schizophrenic mothers, OCs are predictive of subsequent psychiatric abnormality *(56)*. Among these high-risk children, the children who became schizophrenic were exposed to more OCs *(57)*. Those with the least complicated births had milder schizophrenia-like conditions. The investigators suggested that children with the schizophrenic genotype would not develop schizophrenia if they had uncomplicated births.

Viruses and Schizophrenia

The idea that schizophrenia is caused by a virus is consistent with epidemiological and clinical observations *(58)*. The births of schizophrenic patients are more likely to occur during the late winter and spring months when the fetus is at increased risk for exposure to viruses *(59–61)*. Studies of immunological parameters have found in the serum and cerebral spinal fluid of schizophrenic patients excess levels of herpes antibody titer, immunoglobulins, cytomegtalovirus antibody titer, interleukin-2 receptors, α-interferon, and autoantibodies *(62–68)*. And some studies report an association between schizophrenia and the human leukocyte antigen (HLA) A9 locus *(69)*. Since the HLA loci are known to be associated with autoimmune diseases, these data led Wright et al. *(70)* to suggest that some cases of schizophrenia may have an autoimmune basis.

Mednick et al. *(71)* studied a Finnish cohort who had been fetuses during a 1957 influenza epidemic. Those exposed to the epidemic during their second trimester of development were at increased risk for subsequent schizophrenia. However, a Scottish study failed to find an increased risk for schizophrenia associated with influenza epidemics in 1918, 1919, and 1957. Analyses limited to the city of Edinburgh in 1957 supported the viral hypothesis, but the nationwide data did not *(72)*. Also, only limited evidence of an association between viral epidemics and schizophrenia was found in a U.S. study *(73)*.

Barr et al. *(74)* criticized the negative studies on methodological grounds and replicated the Finnish results in a Danish sample. Sham et al. *(75)* showed a link between schizophrenia and maternal influenza but suggested that it would account for less than 2% of schizophrenia cases. In contrast, Crow and Done *(76)* did not support the hypothesis that maternal influenza was a risk factor for schizophrenia. Takei et al. *(77)*, found that females-but not males-exposed to influenza epidemics 5 months prior to birth had an increased rate of schizophrenia in adulthood.

Several studies show that nonfamilial schizophrenic patients are more likely to be born during winter months (and hence are more likely to have been exposed to viruses) compared with familial schizophrenic patients *(78–81)*. For example, Roy et al. *(79)* reported that 32% of sporadic schizophrenic patients were born between December 21 and March 21 compared with 18% of familial patients. Goldstein et al. *(78)* delineated a cluster of schizophrenic patients characterized

by poor premorbid history, flat affect, winter birth, and no family history of schizophrenia. This cluster was more common in male sporadic cases.

Other studies have implicated winter. spring births as a risk factor for familial schizophrenia. For example, Pulver et al. *(82)* found the highest rates of schizophrenia among relatives when the proband had been born between February and May. The lowest rates occurred when the proband's birth was between October and January. This effect was observed for all female probands and for male probands for relatives younger than 30 years of age. The older relatives of male probands were *less* likely to have schizophrenia if the proband had been born between February and May.

STRENGTH OF INTERVENTION EFFECT

The strength of an intervention   along with the two terms we introduced earlier, risk factor prevalence and the strength of the risk factor on later outcomes together provide a full measure of an intervention's effectiveness at the population level. We define the strength of an intervention effect in terms of the relative risk of an outcome for an individual who is provided an intervention compared to the response without intervention. We call an intervention's strength its preventive intervention effectiveness (IE). Specifically, IE is the fractional reduction in disorder when the intervention is available compared to when it is not. In terms of probabilities,

$$IE = 1 - \frac{Pr\{D \mid I\}}{Pr\{D \mid I^c\}}$$

where I refers to assignment to preventive intervention and I^c is nonassignment, or general condition in the population. The stronger the intervention effect the closer IE is to one. IE can vary based on risk factors or other conditions; that is, other conditions may moderate the relationship between the intervention and outcome. In such a situation we estimate its effect as a function of relevant covariates. Below we use the generic term Z to refer all the covariates and z the value for a particular individual.

$$IE(z) = 1 - \frac{Pr\{D \mid I, Z = z\}}{Pr\{D \mid I^c, Z = z\}}$$

Well-conducted randomized trials that are analyzed using so-called intent-to-treat analyses provide model specific estimates that can be used to calculate IE and IE(z). Different classes of covariate analyses of various types can be used to measure how IE(z) and related measures of iintervention effect depend on z *(82a,82b)*.

A THREE-FACTOR MODEL OF PREVENTIVE INTERVENTION EFFECT ON A POPULATION

One can combine the three factors to assess the potential impact of a preventive intervention strategy on a defined population. We use the term population preventive effect (PPE) to refer to the proportional reduction in the incidence of a disorder that would occur if an intervention were offered to the full target group. This quantity is bounded between zero and one; higher numbers refer to stronger intervention effects. An expression for PPE can be obtained using the quantities we have just defined and breaking apart the impact of the intervention for those who have a risk factor X and those without (X^c),

$$PPE = \frac{Odds_x \; RR \; IE(X) + IE(X^c)}{Odds_x \; RR + 1}$$

There are thus four factors that determine a prevention program's effect on a population: the odds of a risk factor, the relative risk of that risk factor leading to a diagnosis in the absences of intervention, and the intervention's effectiveness when the risk factor is present and when it is absent. If an intervention is applied only to those with risk factor X, then $IE(X^c)$ is necessarily zero; PPE is then proportionally reduced in effect compared to $IE(X)$ by the factor $Odds_x \; RR/(Odds_x \; RR + 1)$. The latter factor is only large when both the prevalence of X and its influence on disorder are relatively large. At the other extreme are interventions that target the entire population. When the odds of X and relative risk are small, the overall population effect will depend more on the impact of the intervention in the more common low-risk group than the high-risk group. In fact based on our current knowledge, there are many more cases of schizophrenia coming from low-risk groups without affected relatives than from families with affected relatives. Substantial reduction in incidence will likely require a combination of prevention strategies that reach low-risk as well as high-risk individuals.

A TYPOLOGY OF PREVENTION APPROACHES BASED ON TARGET POPULATION

The terms universal, selective, and indicated provide a valuable way to distinguish preventive interventions. All three of these preventive intervention strategies refer to the target population. Universal preventive interventions are applied to whole populations. A childhood vaccination program, a fluoride treatment of the water supply, and a state-mandated health education course are all examples of universal preventive interventions. Universal intervention programs still need to aim at reducing risk and promoting protective factors. There are now a number of successful universal intervention programs aimed at preventing conduct disorder,

for example, by classroom, peer, school, and family interventions for children as young as first grade *(2,3,83)*. All of these programs are designed to deliver interventions to all children, even though some components may be delivered in the classroom, some on the playground, and some at parent-family meetings. Components would focus on such areas as classroom management of behavior by the teacher, parental monitoring and supervision, and positive peer relations, all known to be protective for later conduct disorder. One universal intervention strategy of potential benefit to schizophrenia would focus on lowering the overall prevalence of OCs through improved pre-, peri-, and postnatal care.

In contrast, selective and indicated interventions target specific subgroups for intervention. Selective interventions target those who are at elevated risk based on group-level characteristics that are not directly related to etiology. For example, children raised in families where there is a recent divorce are at higher risk for internalizing and externalizing problems *(84)*. An intervention that provides parenting skills to divorcing parents during this critical time is selective because it targets an entire subpopulation at risk, even though there are certainly cases where some children fare much better after the divorce *(85)*. Other examples of selective interventions include a program to prevent depression when an adult becomes unemployed *(86)*, a family program also aimed at reducing depression in children whose parents have a depressive disorder *(5)*, and a drug prevention program for children of heroin users *(87)*. In schizophrenia research, a selective prevention program could focus on asymptomatic children with first-degree affected relatives. There may well be individuals in this group with genetic risk factors, but there will certainly be individuals without such genetic risks as well.

Finally, an indicated intervention involves targeting individuals who either have signs but are currently asymptomatic for a disorder or are in an early stage of a progressive disorder. It should be noted that in its original usage pertaining to heart disease, the term *indicated intervention* referred only to those who were asymptomatic, i.e., those with hypertension. Because there are few signs of mental disorder that are currently available, indicated interventions for mental disorders has a somewhat broader definition than that used in other health fields where clear signs are available, such as high blood pressure for heart disease *(8)*.

There have been two lines of research that may lead to indicated interventions for schizophrenia. Both of these are described in detail in other chapters of this book. Briefly, the first method identifies people who have prodromal signs of schizophrenia (e.g., social withdrawal, or subtle changes in thinking or affect) *(88–92)*. McGorry et al. *(91)* showed that prodromal symptoms for schizophrenia occurred in 15.50% of high school students. Thus, more work is needed to develop sensitive and specific prodromal indicators.

A second line of schizophrenia research focuses on schizotaxia, the underlying predisposition to schizophrenia that may or may not be expressed in prodro-

mal symptoms *(93,94)*. Studies of schizotaxia focus on clinical features such as negative symptoms. But they also use as indicators neurobiologic measures known to be sensitive to schizophrenia's genetic predisposition. Examples include eye-tracking dysfunction *(95–97)*, neurologic signs and motor skill deficits *(98)*, characteristic auditory evoked potentials *(99)*, neuroimaging-assessed brain abnormalities *(100,101)* and neuropsychological impairment *(102,103)*.

Prevention programs in areas other than psychotic behavior have begun to combine these different approaches. For example, a universal intervention in first-grade schools that aims at reducing aggressive behavior can be followed by a more targeted intervention on a high-risk subset *(4)*. Such a strategy is also common in school-based suicide prevention programs *(104)*. Because everyone receives the universal intervention, there are opportunities to change norms and reduce stigma that are commonly associated with the more targeted interventions. Unified interventions, comprising multiple target groups, can be based either sequentially so that nonresponders to broader interventions receive additional support, or non-sequentially so that components can work synergistically *(105)*. For example, a universal alcohol prevention program can target the supply side of underage drinking at alcohol outlets whereas a selective program in the same community can address specific needs of children from alcoholic families. Regarding the prevention of psychosis, an indicated program involving low-dose resperidone, such as that being tested by the Pace Clinic in Melbourne, may vary from community to community in its successful recruitment of at-risk adolescents. Some communities may increase early recruitment by implementing broad-based programs to reduce the stigma of mental disorders and enhance gatekeeper training to refer high-risk youth *(106)*.

It should be noted that the terms *universal, selective,* and *indicated* are helpful in assessing the intended audience and comparing different approaches. The terms are generally clear, but there are some differences in the usage of these terms within the scientific community. Is an intervention that is delivered to impoverished families necessarily selective, even if it could be used on all communities but has not been implemented as yet? Similar confusions exist when one attempts to distinguish selective and indicated interventions *(9,105)*. It is sometimes convenient to emphasize the alternatives of broad population-based prevention, for which a 100% universal intervention is an extreme case, and a more targeted intervention, which include those that are clearly selective and indicated preventive interventions. We refer to this polarity between broad population-based prevention and targeted prevention in the following discussion.

One might at first impression conclude that for low baserate disorders such as schizophrenia, broad population-based programs, and especially universal programs would not be as effective as targeted ones based on very high-risk subgroups. After all, targeting a large group of subjects, most of whom have very low

risk for schizophrenia, seems inefficient compared to focusing more intense resources on a smaller number of subjects with higher risk. There are a number of reasons that this might not be so. First, PAR may be smaller with a rare high-risk sample compared to a larger group with more moderate risk. Recall that PAR depends on both the prevalence of the risk factor in schizophrenics as well as the odds ratio. Although good quantitative data on risk are not readily available, it is believed that two factors that have low PARs involve targeting those at very high risk for early psychosis that are picked up in the PACE clinics (106), and season of birth. Both of these are much lower than that for OCs.

Second, even though a universal intervention targets the entire population, we do not expect that its impact would be the same throughout. There are many situations where an intervention that is delivered to everyone has greater effect than that given to a smaller group even though they have higher risk. Vaccinations, for example, count on reducing the infectivity rate by reducing the pool without inoculation. Similarly, universal interventions can often reduce the negative effects of labeling, thereby improving the outcome even among the highest risk group. Finally, behaviorally based interventions can be highly effective when peers, classmates, or neighborhood families participate together (3) rather than individually.

DETERMINING OTHER CHARACTERISTICS OF PREVENTION PROGRAMS BASED ON DEVELOPMENTAL EPIDEMIOLOGIC DATA

We have described how the dimensional aspect of broadly population-based and targeted risk groups helps identify the target group for a prevention program. Other criteria are also important, such as the timing and duration of the intervention, who the intervenor should be, and the social context under which it is delivered. A complete mapping of the combination of risk and protective factors at the individual or contextual level over the life course would provide valuable knowledge for the design of prevention programs. Even incomplete mapping, or mappings generated by combining findings across different samples can be useful as well. This is the perspective of developmental epidemiology (107), which guides our understanding of the development as well as formation of and interactions of individuals within their environments within a defined population.

Key elements of this theory include developmental psychopathology (107), which compares non-normative and normative pathways, life course social field theory (108), which emphasizes the interplay between symptomatology, social adaptation, and social adjudication in relevant social fields across different stages of life, and Bronfenbrenner's ecological systems model (109,110), which examines the nested levels of influence on development over time. Recent advances in statistical modeling allow for models that incorporate time and development

either as single *(111,112)* or multiple trajectories *(113–116)*. New findings in randomized trial designs using the developmental epidemiology approach are also available *(105)*.

A developmental perspective on schizophrenia suggests that we should consider not the predictive ability of risk factors across age groups but their predictive ability when measured within and across different stages of development. It seems likely that schizophrenia genes will express themselves differently at different stages of development. For example, current neurobiological theories of schizophrenia implicate dysfunction of the frontal cortex and of circuits connecting to that region. Because frontal cortex is developing through childhood, it would be reasonable to suspect age-related changes in the expression of premorbid predictors of schizophrenia.

PREVENTION TIMING

Prevention programs for schizophrenia can aim to improve host resistance (i.e., providing neuroleptics prophylactically), behavioral change (i.e., improved attention and processing), or environmental change (i.e., peer relationships). In each of these categories we can aim at immediate reduction in risk or may use an early inoculation model, sometimes with boosters, that seeks to influence host resistance prior to or during major periods of risk. In the broad field of prevention of mental disorders and substance abuse, there have been successful prevention programs in both of these general categories of immediate reduction or early inoculation, and both are potentially useful for the prevention of schizophrenia as well. Timing of an intervention will depend on the strength of risk factors across time and on the theory of change underlying the target mediators.

Preventive Intervention Near the Period of High Incidence

Strategies that focus on age groups just entering or within a high-risk period all presume that the intervention will achieve a larger effect when it is delivered close in time to the outcome of interest. Such a strategy has dominated the field of HIV prevention, for example, where programs for adolescents *(117)* and attendees at gay bars *(118)* are all exposed to programs designed to change immediate behavior. Timing of intervention can also be linked to the occurrence of specific stressful events, such as job loss for depression *(86)* or infection with a sexually transmitted disease for preventing HIV *(119)*. For delinquency prevention, a program such as lighting streets in high-crime areas is called a situational prevention program because it is designed to be effective only in particular circumstances. These types of programs need not target select populations nor limit their focus on short-term outcomes. Indeed some broad population-based and school-based drug prevention programs that target children when drug use just begins to

increase in incidence have been shown to have both immediate and long-lasting effects (1). What these prevention approaches share is an attempt to make immediate improvement on a set of mediators, e.g., self-efficacy for drug resistance and HIV (120), which is thought to be causally linked to outcome of interest. Change on hypothesized mediators is a necessary but not necessarily sufficient indicator of program effectiveness (121,122).

Preventive Intervention Based on Early Risk Factors

Often the epidemiological evidence indicates risk factors exist much earlier than the period where incidence of a disorder arises. A population-based approach that takes into account developmental notions leads us to examine prevention approaches that target these early risk factors. For preventing conduct disorder, drug use, violence, and other externalizing behaviors, this early preventive intervention model, called a developmental epidemiologic approach, is a leading model for the field (123). It is also a familiar approach in heart disease, where it goes by the name of primordial prevention (124). In both of these examples, early risk factors are known, i.e., aggression, poor peer relations, parenting, hostile attributions, and low achievement for conduct disorder, and smoking and diet for heart disease. Cognitive and behavioral changes that target these early factors are also much easier to achieve than corresponding changes on more immediate risk factors. In addition, because even modest behavior changes learned early, e.g., diet or self-regulation of aggressive behaviors in our two examples, can continue across time, targeting early risk and protective factors can lead to long-term benefits.

There is an ongoing interplay between psychiatric symptoms and adaptational status-or ratings by natural raters within social fields (125) across the life span, and this relationship is likely to be influenced by as yet unknown genetic factors as well. For example, in the Israeli High Risk Study of offspring of schizophrenic parents, there was a dramatic difference in risk based on social adaptional status. Only those who performed poorly in each important stage of life from preschool, early school, and adolescence were at risk for schizophrenia; none of those who made successful transitions through most of these stages received a diagnosis of schizophrenia (126). Thus poor social adaptation throughout the life course among offspring of schizophrenic parents constitutes a particularly high-risk developmental process toward schizophrenia.

It should be noted that low neighborhood socioeconomic status (SES), as well as family's poverty status, both have direct impact on a child's aggressive behavior ratings from elementary school to early adolescence (127). (Poverty is also a risk factor for schizophrenia; see ref. 25). Aggressiveness, particularly when accompanied by shy/withdrawn behavior, is strongly associated with poor peer and parent relations, and low academic performance. This cluster of multiple problems con-

centrated in a genetically vulnerable group of children may also be an important developmental pathway toward later psychopathology.

For example, in two independent studies of children of schizophrenic patients, Fish *(128)*, described a syndrome of motor abnormalities that predicted subsequent schizophrenia or related disorders. Similarly, in both the Copenhagen and New York high-risk projects, neuromotor impairment predicted the onset of schizophrenia *(129,130)*. These findings are consistent with Walker and Lewine's *(131)* finding of poorer fine and gross motor coordination in videotapes of children who subsequently became schizophrenic. In addition to neuromotor impairment, attentional deficits have also been found to predict subsequent schizophrenia and related disorders, e.g., ref. *130)*.

VARIATION IN INTERVENTION IMPACT

To test these developmental epidemiologic or early-prevention approaches, we will need to compare the growth trajectories of these risk behaviors across time. Change on these proximal risk targets should theoretically carry forward to changes on the more distal outcome. We thus construct models that link repeated measures of early target behavior with that of a long-term outcome. Thus, statistical growth-modeling techniques used to chart changes in proximal risk behaviors are combined with the analysis of a binary outcome-diagnosis or not-or a survival analysis   time to diagnosis. Both theoretical and empirical work indicate that the intervention effect is likely to differ by early risk status, so recent evaluations examine the intervention's effect on different subgroups of the population, often divided based on their early risk status *(113,114)*. In epidemiology, this variation in intervention impact is called moderation, as opposed to mediation where the intervention produces the same effect across subgroups. Thus, even though the overall impact on a population is reported in these developmental epidemiologic trials, one also searches for specific variations in impact as predicted by theory.

In schizophrenia research, one would logically attempt to examine (based on sample size limitations) whether an intervention varies in effectiveness among those who have a family risk, including a history of schizophrenia, whether there were OCs, or early attention problems. Recent work using the General Growth Mixture Model (GMMM) *(132)* allows for multiple pathways and tests of differential intervention impact, even when the risk group is measured with error, as is currently the case with genetic factors. This approach was taken by Muthen and Muthen *(132)* regarding familial factors related to alcohol use and later dependence.

A consistent finding across a number of broad population-based preventive interventions is that their impact can be highest among the highest risk group even

though they target a group that varies considerably in risk *(105)*. Because high-risk groups tend also to have few protective factors *(133)*, there may be more opportunity for improved outcomes should the intervention focus on building the right protective factors *(133)*. It is not necessarily true, however, that a more targeted intervention, focused on just the highest risk group, would be just as successful. Risk status on measures such as attention processing can vary across time *(134)*; a targeted intervention at one point in time would miss those who may develop the risk shortly afterward *(135)*. This is not the case for a universal intervention because everyone would be exposed to the intervention.

If we vary the timing of an intervention, its effect may also vary. Timing should take into account not only the incidence but also the influence of time and life transitions on intervention effectiveness. Poor adaptational status during times of major transition, such as entry into elementary and middle school, is associated with elevated risk for mental disorders *(125)*, and thus these key transition points are potentially beneficial times to intervene with universal or broad-based preventive programs.

ADHERENCE, IMPLEMENTATION, AND PARTICIPATION

Preventive intervention effectiveness can diminish considerably when the intervention is not delivered at full strength, that is, decreased implementation or fidelity, or when participation by subjects is limited. Likewise in the treatment field, both implementation and participation are important. Depression is underdiagnosed particularly in the aged, for example, and many physicians do not prescribe antidepressant medication or referrals for psychotherapy *(136)*. These factors contribute to low implementation. In contrast, patients may choose not to take medication or pursue psychotherapy, two contributing factors to low participation. Conceptually, these factors of implementation and participation that focus on health behaviors of intervenors and subjects are interrelated; the term adherence appropriately captures this interdependence and is especially useful for subjects with HIV or AIDS *(137)*.

In preventive interventions, implementation can refer to behavioral, systemic, or prescription practices. Currently, there is no uniformly accepted pharmacologic approach for high-risk adolescent population at risk for schizophrenia, such as that being studied in a natural setting by Cornblatt et al. *(138)*. About half of such adolescents are now being given selective serotonin reuptake inhibitors (SSRIs), with higher levels being given to those with more severe symptoms. Although there is no definitive evidence of benefit or harm from such medication, the overall benefit-or potential harm-is attenuated by this lack of implementation standard for the field. For broad-based preventive interventions where intervention involves the delivery of multiple components, there is ample evi-

dence that preventive effectiveness varies with level of implementation *(2)*, and for a multiyear intervention preventive effectiveness varies by level of exposure caused by entrances and exits to a school system *(1)*.

The findings on participation in preventive interventions are somewhat less generalizable. Participation can vary from nearly 100% for interventions within classroom settings *(3)* to less than 50% when individuals are asked to attend group sessions *(86)*. Usually, the level of participation is not related in a strong systematic way to risk; sometimes higher levels of participation occur in low-risk groups and sometimes in higher-risk groups. Nevertheless, because no intervention impact can occur for those subjects who choose not to participate, the overall level of participation strongly affects the population preventive effectiveness. That is, if half of the eligible subjects participate in a preventive intervention, we can anticipate roughly half the effect of a preventive intervention if delivered to the entire population. Because participants self-select, they may differ from nonparticipants on both risk profiles and their potential to benefit from a specific intervention. Thus increasing the percent participation by 10% may not change preventive effectiveness by a corresponding 10%. Generally a randomized experiment needs to be used to deliberately manipulate the level of participation using known technologies for increasing participation rates. Several prevention programs have used a second level of randomization to test for the benefit of these methods in the invitation and recruitment period.

TESTING PREVENTION PROGRAMS
AND SAMPLE SIZE CONSIDERATIONS

There are now literally thousands of preventive trials that have been used to evaluate programs to prevent behavioral and emotional disorders such as conduct disorder, delinquency, depression, and drug use. To date there are only a few that have evaluated prevention programs focusing on psychosis or schizophrenia. The ease by which a program can be tested usually depends on having a small study with relatively short follow-up. Thus, high-risk preventive interventions often get tested first, even though their successful implementation could mean low or moderate overall effects at the population level. What follows is a relatively short guide to sample sizes needed when putting in place a preventive field trial.

High-risk studies of people with prodromal signs of schizophrenia, such as that now under way at the Melbourne PACE clinic, indicate that about one-third of those who receive a nonspecific behavioral intervention but do not receive low-dose neuroleptics go on to develop a full psychotic episode within 1 year. Also, about 25% of the high-risk group is likely to drop out of the study by 1 year. In order to have 80% power to detect a 50% reduction in 1-year risk, one would need to randomize approx 335 subjects. A smaller sample size would be required

if matching variables could be used in the design or covariates and survival methods used in the analysis.

With a lower risk group, say targeting adolescent first-degree relatives (RR = 10), testing the same 50% reduction in risk from 2% to 1% within a year would require approx 6700 subjects overall. This assumes an anticipated 25% loss to follow-up. When the risk group has only minimally larger risk than the general population (RR = 2), testing again for a 50% reduction in risk from 1% to 0.5% would require about 13,300 subjects. These are rough guides; smaller sample sizes could well be used if more refined analyses are used. In addition, other design factors involving multistage designs (9) or case-cohort designs can produce excellent design efficiencies.

SUMMARY

This chapter presents a number of methodologic concepts guiding the development of prevention programs and suggests ways to apply these methods to the prevention of schizophrenia. To date, a number of important risk factors for schizophrenia have been identified. These present options for developing prevention programs. A few prevention programs that focus exclusively on high-risk groups (especially those showing prodromal symptoms of schizophrenia) are now being tested in randomized trials.

To date, there has yet to be any attempts at evaluation of broader population prevention strategies or strategies that apply screening methods to the population to create high-risk groups. For example, reducing OCs may have some impact on reducing the prevalence of schizophrenia and of other disorders for which such complications are risk factors. Alternatively, it may be feasible to screen births for OCs relevant to the subsequent development of schizophrenia. Within that high-risk sample, one could screen for other risk factors such as family history of schizophrenia, or early signs of inattention, poor motor skills, or poor socialization.

At this juncture, we should work to diminish gaps in our knowledge about the development of schizophrenia in the population. Future work needs to answer several key questions:

1. What are the best early predictors of subsequent schizophrenia?
2. Can these predictors predict illness with sufficient accuracy to justify preventive intervention programs?
3. What are the PAR figures for schizophrenia risk factors?
4. Are these large enough to justify prevention efforts?
5. What types of treatments would prevent schizophrenia in high-risk people?

As we have shown in this chapter, the methodological and statistical technologies needed to answer these questions are available. If these are combined with

the contemporary tools of neuroscience and treatment research, answers to these questions, and the eventual prevention of schizophrenia, should be achievable.

ACKNOWLEDGMENTS

We would like to thank Drs. Jane Pearson, Ming Tsuang, Sheppard Kellam, and George Patton, for many helpful comments and insights on this chapter. Our colleagues in the Prevention Science and Methodology Group (PSMG) reviewed presentations of this work and provided many additional comments. The first author's work on this article was supported by NIMH and NIDA through "Designs and Analyses for Mental Health Preventive Trials" grant MH40859.

REFERENCES

1. Botvin GJ, Baker E, Dusenbury L, Botvin EM, Diaz T. Long-term follow-up results of a randomized drug abuse prevention trial in a white middle-class population. JAMA 1995; 273:1106..1112.
2. Ialongo NS, Werthamer L, Kellam SG, Brown CH, Wang S, Lin Y. Proximal impact of two first-grade preventive interventions on the early risk behaviors for later substance abuse, depression, and antisocial behavior. Am J Community Psychol 1999; 27:599..641.
3. Reid JB, Eddy JM, Fetrow RA, Stoolmiller M. Description and immediate impacts of a preventive intervention for conduct problems. Am J Community Psychol 1999; 27:483..517.
4. Conduct Problems Prevention Research Group. A developmental and clinical model for the prevention of conduct disorder: The FAST Track Program. Dev Psychopathol 1992; 4.
5. Beardslee WR, Versage EM, Wright EJ, et al. Examination of preventive interventions for families with depression: evidence of change. Dev Psychopathol 1997; 9:109..130.
6. Clarke G. Prevention of depression in at-risk samples of adolescents. In: Essau C, Petermann F, eds. Depressive Disorders in Children and Adolescents: Epidemiology, Risk Factors, and Treatment. Northvale, NJ: Jason Aronson, Inc., 1999:341..360.
7. Olds D, Henderson CR Jr, Cole R, et al. Long-term effects of nurse home visitation on children's criminal and antisocial behavior: 15-year follow-up of a randomized controlled trial. J Am Med Association 1998; 280:1238..1244.
8. Mrazek P, Haggerty R. Reducing risks for mental disorders: frontiers for preventive intervention research. Washington, DC: National Academy of Sciences, Institute of Medicine, 1994.
9. Brown C, Indurkhya A, Kellam S. Power calculations for data missing by design with application to a follow-up study of exposure and attention. J Am Statistics Association 2000; 95: 383..395.
10. Brown C. Design principles and their application in preventive field trials. In: Bukoski W, Sloboda Z, eds. Handbook of Drug Abuse Theory, Science, and Practice. New York: Plenum, 2003:523..540.
11. Chow S, Liu J. Design and Analysis of Clinical Trials: Concepts and Methodologies. New York: Wiley, 1998.
12. Coie JD, Watt NF, West SG, et al. The science of prevention. A conceptual framework and some directions for a national research program. Am Psychol 1993; 48:1013..1022.
13. Kraemer HC, Kazdin AE, Offord DR, Kessler RC, Jensen PS, Kupfer DJ. Coming to terms with the terms of risk. Arch Gen Psychiatry 1997; 54:337..343.
14. Lindamer LA, Lohr JB, Harris MJ, Jeste DV. Gender, estrogen, and schizophrenia. Psychopharmacol Bull 1997; 33:221..228.

15. Tsuang MT, Faraone SV. The case for heterogeneity in the etiology of schizophrenia. Schizophr Res 1995; 17:161..175.
16. Faris R, Dunham H. Mental Disorders in Urban Areas: An Ecological Study of Schizophrenia and Other Psychoses. New York: Praeger, 1939.
17. Faraone SV, Tsuang D, Tsuang MT. Genetics of Mental Disorders: A Guide for Students, Clinicians, and Researchers. New York: Guilford, 1999.
18. Goldstein JM, Faraone SV, Chen WJ, Tsuang MT. Genetic heterogeneity may in part explain gender differences in the familial risk for schizophrenia. Biol Psychiatry 1995; 38:808..813.
19. Thomas JC, Clark M, Robinson J, Monnett M, Kilmarx PH, Peterman TA. The social ecology of syphilis. Soc Sci Med 1999; 48:1081..1094.
20. Kalbfleisch J, Prentice R. The Statistical Analysis of Failure Time Data. New York: Wiley, 1980.
21. Eaton W, Day R, Kramer M. The use of epidemiology for risk factor research in schizophrenia: an overview and methodologic critique. In: Tsuang MT, Simpson JC, eds. Handbook of Schizophrenia 3: Nosology, Epidemiology and Genetics. Amsterdam, the Netherlands: Elsevier Science, 1988:151..168.
22. Greenland S. Quantitative methods in the review of epidemiologic literature. Epidemiolog Rev 1987; 9:1..30.
23. Geddes JR, Lawrie SM. Obstetric complications and schizophrenia: a meta-analysis. Br J Psychiatry 1995; 167:786..793.
24. Buka SK, Goldstein JM, Seidman LJ, et al. Prenatal complications, genetic vulnerability, and schizophrenia: the New England longitudinal studies of schizophrenia. Psychiatric Annals 1999; 29:151..156.
25. Holzer C, Shea B, Swanson J, Leaf P. The increased risk for specific psychiatric disorders among persons of low socioeconomic status. Am J Social Psychiatry 1986; 6:259..271.
26. Gottesman II. Schizophrenia Genesis: The Origin of Madness. New York: Freeman, 1991.
27. Tsuang MT, Faraone SV. Epidemiology and behavioral genetics of schizophrenia. In: Watson SJ, ed. Biology of Schizophrenia and Affective Disease. New York: Raven, 1994:163..195.
28. Kendler KS. Overview: a current perspective on twin studies of schizophrenia. Am J Psychiatry 1983; 140:1413..1425.
29. Kety SS, Rosenthal D, Wender PH, Schulsinger F. The types and prevalence of mental illness in the biological and adoptive families of adopted schizophrenics. J Psychiatric Res 1968; 1:345..362.
30. Kety SS, Wender PH, Jacobsen B, et al. Mental illness in the biological and adoptive relatives of schizophrenic adoptees. Replication of the Copenhagen study in the rest of Denmark. Arch Gen Psychiatry 1994; 51:442..455.
31. Tsuang MT, Faraone SV. The frustrating search for schizophrenia genes. Am J Med Genet 2000; 97:1..3.
32. Faraone SV, Tsuang MT. Quantitative models of the genetic transmission of schizophrenia. Psychol Bull 1985; 98:41..66.
33. Risch N. Linkage strategies for genetically complex traits. I. Multilocus models. Am J Human Genet 1990; 46:222..228.
34. Tsuang MT, Stone WS, Faraone SV. Schizophrenia: a review of genetic studies. Harv Rev Psychiatry 1999; 7:185..207.
35. Kinney DK, Holzman PS, Jacobsen B, et al. Thought disorder in schizophrenic and control adoptees and their relatives. Arch Gen Psychiatry 1997; 54:475..479.
36. Tienari P. Interaction between genetic vulnerability and family environment: the Finnish adoptive family study of schizophrenia. Acta Psychiatr Scand 1991; 84:460..465.

37. Tienari P, Wynne LC, Moring J, et al. the Finnish adoptive family study of schizophrenia. Implications for family research. Br J Psychiatry 1994; 163:20..26.
38. Wahlberg K-E, Wynne LC, Oja H, et al. Gene-environment interaction in vulnerability to schizophrenia: findings from the Finnish adoptive family study in schizophrenia. Am J Psychiatry 1997; 154:355..362.
39. Lane EA, Albee GW. Comparative birthweights of schizophrenics and their siblings. J Psychol 1966; 64:227..231.
40. Woerner MG, Pollack M, Klein DF. Birthweight and length in schizophrenics, personality disorders and their siblings. Br J Psychiatry 1971; 118:461.
41. McNeil TF, Kaij L. Obstetric factors in the development of schizophrenia: complications in the births of preschizophrenics and in reproduction by schizophrenic parents. In: Wynne LC, Cromwell RL, Matthysse S, eds. The Nature of Schizophrenia. New Approaches to Research and Treatment. New York: Wiley, 1978:401..429.
42. Jacobsen B, Kinney DK. Perinatal complications in adopted and non-adopted schizophrenics and thier controls: preliminary results. Acta Psychiatr Scand 1980; 285(Suppl):337.
43. McNeil TF. Obstetric factors and perinatal injuries. In: Tsuang MT, Simpson JC, eds. Nosology, Epidemiology and Genetics of Schizophrenia. Vol. 3. New York: Elsevier, 1988: 319..344.
44. Cannon TD, Mednick SA, Parnas J. Genetic and perinatal determinants of structural brain deficits in schizophrenia. Arch Gen Psychiatry 1989; 46:883..889.
45. Zornberg GL, Buka SL, Tsuang MT. Hypoxic-ischemia-related fetal/neonatal complications and risk of schizophrenia and other nonaffective psychoses: a 19-year longitudinal study. Am J Psychiatry 2000; 157:196..202.
46. Buka SL, Tsuang MT, Lipsitt LP. Pregnancy/delivery complications and psychiatric diagnosis. A prospective study. Arch Gen Psychiatry 1993; 50:151..156.
47. O'Callaghan E, Larkin C, Kinsella A, Waddington JL. Obstetric complications, the putative familial-sporadic distinction, and tardive dyskinesia in schizophrenia. Br J Psychiatry 1990; 157:578..584.
48. Kinney DK, Jacobsen S. Environmental factors in schizophrenia: new adoption evidence. In: Wynne LC, Cromwell RL, Matthysse S, eds. The Nature of Schizophenia: New Approaches to Research and Treatment. New York: Wiley, 1978:38..51.
49. Reveley AM, Reveley MA, Murray RM. Cerebral ventricular enlargement in non-genetic schizophrenia: a controlled twin study. Br J Psychiatry 1984; 144:89..93.
50. Schwarzkopf SB, Nasrallah HA, Olson SC, Coffman JA, McLaughlin JA. Preinatal complications and genetic loading in schizophrenia: preliminary findings. Psychiatry Res 1989; 27: 233..239.
51. McNeil TF, Cantor-Graae E, Torrey EF, et al. Obstetric complications in histories of monozygotic twins discordant and concordant for schizophrenia. Acta Psychiatr Scand 1994; 89: 196..204.
52. Onstad S, Skre I, Torgersen S, Kringlen E. Birthweight and obstetric complications in schizophrenic twins. Acta Psychiatr Scand 1992; 85:70..73.
53. Pollin W, Stabenau JR. Biological, psychological and historical differences in a series of monozygotic twins discordant for schizophrenia. In: Rosenthal D, Kety S, eds. The Transmission of Schizophrenia. New York: Pergamon, 1968.
54. Shields J, Gottesman II. Obstetric complications and twin studies of schizophrenia: clarification and affirmation. Schizophr Bull 1977; 3:351..354.
55. DeLisi LE, Dauphinais ID, Gershon ES. Perinatal complications and reduced size of brain limbic structures in familial schizophrenia. Schizophr Bull 1988; 14:185..191.

56. Mednick SA. Breakdown in individuals at high risk for schizophenia: possible predispositional perinatal factors. Ment Hygiene 1970; 54:50.
57. Parnas J, Schulsinger F, Teasdale TW, Feldman PM, Mednick SA. Preinatal complications and clinical outcome within the schizophrenia spectrum. Br J Psychiatry 1982; 140:416..420.
58. Torrey EF, Kaufmann CA. Schizophrenia and neuroviruses. In: Nasrallah HA, Weinberger DR, eds. The Neurology of Schizophrenia. Vol. 1. Amsterdam, New York, Oxford: Elsevier Science, 1986:361..376.
59. Dalen P. Season of Birth   A Study of Schizophrenia and Other Mental Disorders. Amsterdam: Elsevier, 1975.
60. Hare E, Price J, Slater E. Mental disorder and season of birth. Br J Psychiatry 1974; 124:81..86.
61. Hare E. The season of birth of siblings of psychiatric patients. Br J Psychiatry 1976; 129: 49..54.
62. Ganguli R, Rabin BS, Kelly RH, Lyte M, Ragu U. Clinical and laboratory evidence of autoimmunity in acute schizophrenia. Ann NY Acad Sci 1987; 496:676..685.
63. Kaufmann CA, Weinberger DR, Yolken RH, Torrey EF, Potkin SF. Viruses and schizophrenia. Lancet 1983; 2:1136..1137.
64. Kirch DG, Kaurmann CA, Papadopoulous NM, Martin B, Weinberger DR. Abnormal cerebrospinal fluid indices in schizophrenia. Biol Psychiatry 1985; 20:1039..1046.
65. Libikova H, Breir S, Kosikova M, Pagady J, Stunzer D, Ujhazyova D. Assay of interferon and viral antibodies in the cerebrospinal fluid in clinical neurology and psychiatry. Acta Biol Medica Germanica 1979; 38:879..893.
66. Rapaport MH, McAllister CG, Pickar D, Nelson DL, Paul SM. Elevated levels of soluble interleukin 2 receptors in schizophrenia. Arch Gen Psychiatry 1989; 46:291..292.
67. Torrey EF, Yolken RH, Winfrey CJ. Cytomegalovirus antibody in cerebrospinal fluid of schizophrenic patients detected by enzyme immunoassay. Science 1982; 216:892..893.
68. van Kammen DP, Mann L, Scheinin M, van Kammen WB, Linnoila M. Spinal fluid monoamine metabolites and anti-cytomegalovirus antibodies and brain scan evaluation in schizophrenia. Psychopharmacol Bull 1984; 20:519..522.
69. Goldin LR, DeLisi LE, Gershon ES. Genetic aspects to the biology of schizophrenia. In: Henn FA, DeLisi LE, eds. Neurochemistry and Neuropharmacology of Schizophrenia. Vol. 2. Amsterdam, New York, Oxford: Elsevier, 1987:467..487.
70. Wright J, Gill M, Murray RM. Schizophrenia: genetics and the maternal immune response to viral infection. Am J Med Genet (Neuropsychiatric Genetics) 1993; 48:40..46.
71. Mednick SA, Machon RA, Huttunen MO, Bonett D. Adult schizophrenia following prenatal exposure to an influenza epidemic. Arch Gen Psychiatry 1988; 45:189..192.
72. Kendell RE, Kemp JW. Maternal influenza in the etiology of schizophrenia. Arch Gen Psychiatry 1989; 46:878..882.
73. Torrey EF, Rawlings R, Waldman IN. Schizophrenic births and viral diseases in two states. Schizophr Res 1988; 1:73..77.
74. Barr CE, Mednick SA, Munk-Jorgensen P. Exposure to influenza epidemics during gestation and adult schizophrenia. A 40-year study. Arch Gen Psychiatry 1990; 47:869..874.
75. Sham PC, O'Callaghan E, Takei N, Murray GK, Hare EH, Murray RM. Schizophrenia following prenatal exposure to influenza epidemics between 1939 and 1960. Br J Psychiatry 1992; 160:461..466.
76. Crow TJ, Done DJ. Prenatal exposure to influenza does not cause schizophrenia. Br J Psychiatry 1992; 161:390..393.
77. Takei N, Sham P, O'Callaghan E, Murray GK, Glover G, Murray RM. Prenatal influenza and schizophrenia: is the effect confined to females? Am J Psychiatry, in press.

78. Goldstein JM, Santangelo SL, Simpson JC, Tsuang MT. The role of gender in identifying subtypes of schizophrenia: a latent class analytic approach. Schizophr Bull 1990; 16:263..275.
79. Roy M-A, Flaum MA, Gupta S, Jaramillo L, Andreasen NC. Epidemiological and clinical correlates of familial and sporadic schizophrenia. Acta Psychiatr Scand 1994; 89:324..328.
80. O'Callaghan E, Gibson T, Colohan HA, et al. Season of birth in schizophrenia. Evidence for confinement of an excess of winter births to patients without a family history of mental disorder. Br J Psychiatry 1991; 158:764..769.
81. Shur E. Season of birth in high and low genetic risk schizophrenics. Br J Psychiatry 1982; 140:410..415.
82. Pulver AE, Liang K-Y, Brown CH, et al. Risk factors in schizophrenia season of birth, gender, and familial risk. Br J Psychiatry 1992; 160:65..71.
82a. Brown CH. Statistical methods for preventive trials in mental health. Stat in Med 1993; 12: 289..300.
82b. Brown CH. Analyzing preventive trials with generalized additive models. Amer J Comm Psych 1993; 21:635..664.
83. Dolan L, Kellam S, Brown C, et al. The short-term impact of two classroom based preventive intervention trials on aggressive and shy behaviors and poor achievement. J Appl Dev Psychology 1993; 14:317..345.
84. Wolchik SA, West SG, Sandler IN, et al. An experimental evaluation of theory-based mother and mother-child programs for children of divorce. J Consult Clin Psychol 2000; 68:843..856.
85. Sandler IN, Tein JY, West SG. Coping, stress, and the psychological symptoms of children of divorce: a cross-sectional and longitudinal study. Child Dev 1994; 65:1744..1763.
86. Vinokur AD, Schul Y, Vuori J, Price RH. Two years after a job loss: long-term impact of the JOBS program on reemployment and mental health. J Occup Health Psychol 2000; 5:32..47.
87. Gainey RR, Catalano RF, Haggerty KP, Hoppe MJ. Participation in a parent training program for methadone clients. Addict Behav 1995; 20:117..125.
88. McGlashan TH. Early detection and intervention in schizophrenia: research. Schizophr Bull 1996; 22:327..345.
89. McGlashan TH, Johannessen JO. Early detection and intervention with schizophrenia: rationale. Schizophr Bull 1996; 22:201..222.
90. McGorry PD, Edwards J, Mihalopoulos C, Harrigan SM, Jackson HJ. EPPIC: an evolving system of early detection and optimal management. Schizophr Bull 1996; 22:305..326.
91. McGorry PD, McFarlane C, Patton GC. The prevalence of prodromal features of schizophrenia in adolescence: a preliminary survey. Acta Psychiatr Scand 1995; 92:241..249.
92. Falloon IRH, Kydd RR, Coverdale JH, Laidlaw TM. Early detection and intervention for initial episodes of schizophrenia. Schizophr Bull 1996; 22:271..282.
93. Faraone SV, Green AI, Seidman LJ, Tsuang MT. "Schizotaxia": clinical implications and new directions for research. Schizophr Bull 2001; 27:1..18.
94. Tsuang MT, Stone WS, Faraone SV. Towards the prevention of schizophrenia. Biol Psychiatry 2000; 48:349..356.
95. Holzman PS, Kringlen E, Matthysse S, et al. A single dominant gene can account for eye tracking dysfunctions and schizophrenia in offspring of discordant twins. Arch Gen Psychiatry 1988; 45:641..647.
96. Holzman PS, Solomon CM, Levin S, Waternaux CS. Pursuit eye movement dysfunction in schizophrenic patients and their relatives. Arch Gen Psychiatry 1984; 44:1140..1141.
97. Holzman PS, Kringlen E, Levy DL, Proctor LR, Haberman SJ, Yasillo NJ. Abnormal-pursuit eye movements in schizophrenia: evidence for a genetic indicator. Arch Gen Psychiatry 1977; 34:802..805.

98. Erlenmeyer-Kimling L, Cornblatt B, Friedman D, et al. Neurological, electrophysiological, and attentional deviations in children at risk for schizophrenia. In: Henn FA, Nasrallah HA, eds. Schizophrenia as a Brain Disease. New York: Oxford University Press, 1982:61..98.
99. Friedman D, Squires-Wheeler E. Event-related potentials (ERPs) as indicators of risk for schizophrenia. Schizophr Bull 1994; 20:63..74.
100. Seidman LJ, Faraone SV, Goldstein JM, et al. Thalamic and amygdala-hippocampal volume reductions in first degree relatives of schizophrenic patients: an MRI-based morphometric analysis. Biol Psychiatry 1999; 46:941..954.
101. Seidman LJ, Faraone SV, Goldstein JM, et al. Reduced subcortical brain volumes in non-psychotic siblings of schizophrenic patients: a pilot MRI Study. Am J Med Genet (Neuropsychiatric Genetics) 1997; 74:507..514.
102. Faraone SV, Seidman LJ, Kremen WS, Toomey R, Pepple JR, Tsuang MT. Neuropsychological functioning among the nonpsychotic relatives of schizophrenic patients: the effect of genetic loading. Biol Psychiatry 2000; 48:120..126.
103. Faraone SV, Seidman LJ, Kremen WS, Pepple JR, Lyons MJ, Tsuang MT. Neuropsychological functioning among the nonpsychotic relatives of schizophrenic patients: a diagnostic efficiency analysis. J Abnorm Psychol 1995; 104:286..304.
104. Gould MS, Kraemer HC. Youth suicide prevention. Suicide Life Threat Behav 2001; 31:6..31.
105. Brown CH, Liao J. Principles for designing randomized preventive trials in mental health: an emerging developmental epidemiology paradigm. Am J Community Psychol 1999; 27:673..710.
106. Lincoln C, McGorry P. Pathways to care in early psychosis: clinical and consumer perspectives. In: McGorry P, Jackson H, eds. The Recognition and Management of Early Psychosis: A Preventive Approach. New York: Cambridge University Press, 1999:51..79.
107. Costello E, Angold A. Developmental epidemiology: a framework for developmental psychopathology. In: Sameroff A, Lewis M, Miller S, eds. Handbook of Developmental Psychopathology. New York: Kluwer Academic/Plenum, 2000:57..73.
108. Kellam S, Rebok G. Building developmental and etiological theory through epidemiologically based preventive intervention trials. In: McCord J, Tremblay R, eds. Preventing Antisocial Behavior: Interventions from Birth Through Adolescence. New York: Guilford, 1992:162..195.
109. Bronfenbrenner U, Ceci SJ. Nature-nurture reconceptualized in developmental perspective: a bioecological model. Psychol Rev 1994; 101:568..586.
110. Bronfenbrenner U. Developmental ecology through space and time: a future perspective. In: Moen P, Elder G, Luscher K, eds. Examining Lives in Context: Perspectives on the Ecology of Human Development. Washington, DC: American Psychological Association, 1995: 619..647.
111. Muthen B, Curran P. General longitudinal modeling of individual differences in experimental designs: a latent variable framework for analysis and power estimation. Psychol Methods 1997; 2:371..402.
112. Curran PJ, Muthen BO. The application of latent curve analysis to testing developmental theories in intervention research. Am J Community Psychol 1999; 27:567..595.
113. Muthen B, Shedden K. Finite mixture modeling with mixture outcomes using the EM algorithm. Biometrics 1999; 55:463..469.
114. Muthen BO, Brown CH, Masyn K., et al. General growth mixture modeling for randomized preventive interventions. Biostatistics 2002; 3:459..475.
115. Nagin D. Analyzing developmental trajectories: a semiparametric, group-based approach. Psychol Methods 1999; 4:18..34.
116. Nagin D, Tremblay RE. Trajectories of boys' physical aggression, opposition, and hyperactivity on the path to physically violent and nonviolent juvenile delinquency. Child Dev 1999; 70:1181..1196.

117. Jemmott LS, Jemmott JB. Increasing condom-use intentions among sexually active Black adolescent women. Nurs Res 1992; 41:273.279.

118. Kelly JA, St. Lawrence JS, Stevenson LY, Hauth AC. Community AIDS/HIV risk reduction: the effects of endorsements by popular people in three cities. Am J Public Health 1992; 82:1483..1489.

119. O'Leary A, Ambrose TK, Raffaelli M, et al. Effects of an HIV risk reduction project on sexual risk behavior of low-income STD patients. AIDS Educ Prev 1998; 10:483.492.

120. Fishbein M. The role of theory in HIV prevention. AIDS Care 2000; 12:273.278.

121. Pillow DR, Sandler IN, Braver SL, Wolchik SA, Gersten JC. Theory-based screening for prevention: focusing on mediating processes in children of divorce. Am J Community Psychol 1991; 19:809..836.

122. Brown CH. Comparison of mediational selected strategies and sequential designs for preventive trials: comments on a proposal by Pillow et al. Am J Community Psychol 1991; 19:837.846.

123. Kellam SG, Koretz D, Moscicki EK. Core elements of developmental epidemiologically based prevention research. Am J Community Psychol 1999; 27:463.482.

124. Labarthe D. Epidemiology and Prevention of Cardiovascular Diseases: A Global Challenge. Gaithersburg, MD: Aspen, 1998.

125. Kellam S, Branch J, Agrawal A, Ensminger M. Mental health and going to school: the Woodlawn program of assessment, early intervention, and evaluation. Chicago: University of Chicago Press, 1975.

126. Mirsky AF, Yardley SL, Jones BP, Walsh D, Kendler KS. Analysis of the attention deficit in schizophrenia: a study of patients and their relatives in Ireland. J Psychiatr Res 1995; 29:23..42.

127. Kellam SG, Ling X, Merisca R, Brown CH, Ialongo N. The effect of the level of aggression in the first grade classroom on the course and malleability of aggressive behavior into middle school. Dev Psychopathol 1998; 10:165..185.

128. Fish B, Marcus J, Hans SL, Auerbach JG, Perdue S. Infants at risk for schizophrenia: sequelae of a genetic neurointegrative defect. A review and replication analysis of pandysmaturation in the Jerusalem infant development study. Arch Gen Psychiatry 1992; 49:221.235.

129. Olin S-cS, Mednick SA. Risk factors of psychosis: identifying vulnerable populations premorbidly. Schizophr Bull 1996; 22:223.240.

130. Erlenmeyer-Kimling L. Personal Communication, 1997.

131. Walker E, Lewine RJ. Prediction of adult-onset schizophrenia from childhood home movies of the parents. Am J Psychiatry 1990; 147:1052..1056.

132. Muthen B, Muthen LK. Integrating person-centered and variable-centered analyses: growth mixture modeling with latent trajectory classes. Alcohol Clin Exp Res 2000; 24:882.891.

133. Hawkins J, Lishner D, Catalano R. Childhood predictors and the prevention of adolescent substance abuse. National Institute on Drug Abuse: Research Monograph Series. Vol. 56: Washington, DC: U.S. Department of Health & Human Services, 1985.

134. Rebok G, Smith C, Pascualvaca D, Mirsky A, Anthony B, Kellam S. Developmental changes in attentional performance in urban children from eight to thirteen years. Child Neuropsychol 1997; 3:28..46.

135. Lorion R. Basing preventive interventions on theory: stimulating a field's momentum. Prev Human Serv 1989; 7..31.

136. Olfson M, Klerman GL. Depressive symptoms and mental health service utilization in a community sample. Soc Psychiatry Psychiatr Epidemiol 1992; 27:161..167.

137. Chesney MA, Morin M, Sherr L. Adherence to HIV combination therapy. Soc Sci Med 2000; 50:1599..1605.

138. Cornblatt B, Obuchowski M, Schnur D, O'Brien JD. Hillside study of risk and early detection in schizophrenia. Br J Psychiatry Suppl 1998; 172:26..32.

13

The Treatment of Schizotaxia

Ming T. Tsuang, MD, PhD, DSc,
Sarah I. Tarbox, BA, *Levi Taylor,* PhD,
and William S. Stone, PhD

INTRODUCTION

Schizotaxia is characterized by meaningful clinical symptoms that reflect an underlying liability to schizophrenia. Two research paradigms have provided the most data about the basic features of schizotaxia: studies of adult, first-degree relatives of schizophrenic patients, and studies of children of schizophrenic patients. It is useful to distinguish adult and child relatives because adults, unlike children, have lived through at least some of the highest risk period for schizophrenia. Although each age group includes schizotaxic individuals (20.50% of adult, first-degree relatives show symptoms of schizotaxia [1,2]), schizotaxia in most adults (at least over the age of 35) is likely to be a relatively stable condition. In contrast, most children have yet to pass through the period of highest risk, and thus contain a higher percentage of individuals who will express psychosis. Thus, schizotaxia represents both a stable, clinically meaningful condition in its own right (in both adults and children) and, especially in a subset of children, a risk factor for subsequent psychopathology.

The prevalence and clinical significance of schizotaxia in relatives of schizophrenic patients inevitably raises the possibility of intervention. Given the differences in morbid risk between age groups, one strategy for exploring treatments is to discuss adult schizotaxia and child schizotaxia separately. In this chapter, we begin by focusing on the treatment of adult schizotaxia. This is a natural place to start because treatment risks are lower and current intervention efforts are already

From: *Early Clinical Intervention and Prevention in Schizophrenia*
Edited by: W. S. Stone, S. V. Faraone, and M. T. Tsuang © Humana Press Inc., Totowa, NJ

focused there. Clinical implications of treating adult schizotaxia are reviewed, along with options for treatment. The remainder of the chapter focuses on the eventual goal of treating childhood schizotaxia and preventing the development of schizophrenia. This discussion is organized by clinical outcome. Childhood schizotaxia that remains stable through adulthood is contrasted with childhood schizotaxia that progresses into psychosis. Logistical and ethical implications of treating both groups are examined, followed by an exploration of current treatment options and future research directions.

ADULT SCHIZOTAXIA

Why Treat Adult Schizotaxia?: Implications for the Individual, the Family, and the Patient

The risk for schizophrenia declines by the fourth decade of life, even in individuals who were previously at higher risk (3–5). Therefore, most adults with schizotaxia are not as vulnerable for schizophrenia as when they were younger, and proposed treatments of such individuals cannot be predicated on the notion that they will prevent the disorder. Instead, treatments should be aimed primarily at alleviating the negative symptoms, neuropsychological impairment, and social dysfunction of schizotaxia itself. In addition, the psychological vulnerabilities of schizotaxic people may be exacerbated by stress, which may include the emotional burdens and practical complexities of dealing with schizophrenic relatives, along with the usual life events and psychosocial conflict that occur in nonschizophrenic families. It is likely that alleviating the symptoms of schizotaxia would have a positive impact not only on the schizotaxic individual, but on other family members as well, including the schizophrenic patient.

As families are often involved in treatment programs for patients with schizophrenia, it is probable that many schizotaxic persons participate in the treatment of their schizophrenic relative. Psychoeducational family therapies ask family members to learn facts about the disorder and methods of coping with their ill relative (6). Moreover, response acquisition methods are often used to teach communication skills to family members (6). Because family members need to learn, recall, and generalize the use of these skills, therapists engage family members in a variety of tasks requiring intact neuropsychological functioning.

Some aspects of treatment might be difficult for neuropsychologically impaired family members (7). For example, the distractibility of schizotaxic relatives may make it difficult for them to follow lessons and absorb information. Memory deficits will likely compromise their ability to learn skills and use them outside the treatment session. Relatives with abstraction deficits will not be able to integrate

course material and plan for its use in the home environment. Considering that family interventions also tax the capacity of family members to tolerate difficult emotions and face family conflict, the added burden of neuropsychological deficits may make it hard for family members to learn skills or to generalize them from treatment sessions to real-world settings. Thus, full participation in family interventions will likely be compromised by the neuropsychological impairments of schizotaxia. Moreover, it is possible that therapist observations of inattentiveness, slow learning, or poor memory for lessons may be misinterpreted as indicating resistance on the part of the family member. That could lead to counterproductive therapeutic strategies. These factors do not mitigate the value of treatment, but underscore the importance of taking them into account to attain positive treatment outcomes.

How Should Schizotaxia Be Treated?

Currently, there is no specific therapy for schizotaxia. There are, however, several potential approaches, both psychological and pharmacological, which may be beneficial.

PSYCHOLOGICAL INTERVENTIONS

The treatment of schizotaxia may benefit from methods effective in the psychotherapy of other neurodevelopmental conditions (e.g., adult attention deficit hyperactivity disorder) that share some clinical features with schizotaxia. Seidman (7) pointed out several issues to inform the treatment of patients with subtle neuropsychological impairments.

Among these, first, the therapist should have an objective understanding of the patient's neuropsychological strengths and weaknesses. This knowledge helps patients and the significant people in their lives to gain awareness of the behavioral consequences of cognitive dysfunction. For example, schizotaxic people with deficits in attention and verbal memory may view themselves as "stupid" because they cannot learn in the many educational settings that require these skills. Therapy can help them reinterpret these difficulties, better appreciate their strengths, and develop coping strategies. Moreover, teaching patients with schizotaxia about their neuropsychological profile might help them develop realistic expectations and plan their occupational and educational pursuits more efficiently.

Clinicians could also help patients develop cognitive-behavioral strategies to cope with specific deficits. For example, relatives with memory deficits would benefit from learning mnemonic strategies, and those with abstraction deficits could be taught systematic methods of planning and organizing their activities. Thus, standard tools used to aid recall (e.g., appointment books, calendars, "memory notebooks") could be brought into the therapeutic toolbox.

Therapists can also utilize knowledge of neuropsychological weaknesses to facilitate empathic approaches to the issues of shame, inferiority, and performance anxiety that often accompany such disorders *(7)*. Such maladaptive emotions may stem directly from the experiences of failure caused by the schizotaxic, neuropsychological syndrome, they may be reactions to the stress and stigma of having a schizophrenic relative, or they may derive from the relative's fear of developing schizophrenia. Furthermore, deficits in self-regulation may make it difficult to articulate awareness of these feelings. Without therapeutic attention, these emotional consequences might worsen cognitive performance and lead to a downward spiral toward further dysfunction. On the other hand, psychotherapeutic interventions can help schizotaxic patients identify and cope with negative emotions without becoming overwhelmed by them. The promise of psychological interventions for schizotaxia will be realized most efficiently by research to determine which psychotherapeutic approaches are most effective with specific clinical presentations.

PSYCHOPHARMACOLOGICAL INTERVENTIONS

In addition to psychological or psychosocial interventions, schizotaxia or associated emotional problems may also be attenuated by psychopharmacological treatments. When considering potential agents, antipsychotic medications would appear to be a reasonable first step, as the pattern of psychiatric and cognitive difficulties found in schizotaxia share etiological and psychopathological elements with schizophrenia. Unfortunately, although typical antipsychotic drugs (e.g., haloperidol) attenuated some symptoms of schizotypal personality disorder (e.g., refs. *8–10*), many patients discontinued treatment (~50%), at least partly because medication side effects were tolerated poorly *(8,11)*. Moreover, typical antipsychotic medications are limited in their ability to treat the negative symptoms and neuropsychological impairment that are core features of schizotaxia (e.g., refs. *12,13*).

In contrast, the newer "atypical" or novel antipsychotic drugs are more promising for the treatment of schizotaxia. Unlike the typical antipsychotics, atypical antipsychotic agents improve some negative symptoms *(12,14–17)* and cognitive functions (e.g., attention, working memory, and long-term memory) *(18–22)* in patients with schizophrenia. Moreover, atypical antipsychotic medications typically produce fewer extrapyramidal side effects (at least at lower doses) than do typical antipsychotic agents *(23)*.

Clozapine, the first atypical agent, improves negative symptoms *(24,25)* and probably some neurocognitive deficits *(19,22)* in severely ill, treatment-refractory patients with schizophrenia. In addition, a few groups have reported positive outcomes using clozapine to treat schizophrenic patients in their first episode of psychosis *(26)*. The potential toxicity of clozapine, however, proscribes its use

in the absence of clear psychotic symptoms. Even then, it is usually reserved for treatment-resistant cases.

Unfortunately, there is little information in the literature on the use of atypical antipsychotic medications in nonpsychotic populations: even when not prescribed for schizophrenia, most of the disorders treated still include symptoms of psychosis (e.g., affective disorders with psychotic features, and dementia). There is growing evidence, however, that risperidone and olanzapine may be effective treatments for Tourette's syndrome *(27–29)*, and for selective serotonin reuptake inhibitor (SSRI)-refractory patients with obsessive-compulsive disorder *(30,31)*. Risperidone may also show efficacy in the treatment of intrusive thoughts and emotional reactivity in posttraumatic stress disorder *(32)*.

Treatment of Adult Schizotaxia With Risperidone

Given the relative safety of atypical antipsychotics, and their likely value in treating negative symptoms and neurocognitive deficits, we conducted a pilot study to assess the effects of one of them, risperidone, on schizotaxia in adults *(33,34)*. Briefly, Tsuang et al. *(33)* operationalized research criteria for schizotaxia based on a combination of negative symptoms and neuropsychological deficits, two of the most robust findings in first-degree relatives of patients with schizophrenia. The criteria used to determine clinical eligibility involved negative symptoms and neuropsychological deficits, both of at least moderate severity. Negative symptoms were assessed using the Scale for the Assessment of Negative Symptoms (SANS) *(35)*. The criteria required that at least six items be rated 3 or higher. The neuropsychological assessment focused on three cognitive domains, including: (a) vigilance/working memory, using the Auditory Continuous Performance Test (A-CPT), with Interference (A-CPT-INT) *(36)* and the Visual CPT, Identical Pairs version *(37)*; (b) verbal memory, using the Logical Memory subtest from the Wechsler Memory Scale. Revised, and Buschke's Selective Reminding Test; and (c) executive functions, using the Delayed Alternation Test and the Object Alternation Test *(37)*.

Based on these diagnostic criteria, 27 nonpsychotic, first-degree relatives of patients with schizophrenia received full evaluations for schizotaxia, of whom 19 did not meet criteria and 8 did. Six of the eight subjects who met criteria agreed to enter into a brief 6-week trial of low-dose risperidone (up to 2 mg per day) vs placebo. Side effects of treatment were temporary and mainly mild, and all six subjects completed the treatment protocol.

Subjectively, five of the six individuals reported increased cognitive abilities during the risperidone trial. Three of the six individuals reported greater levels of interest in, and enjoyment of, social activities. Objective assessments showed reduced SANS scores in five out of six subjects, particularly in the Anhedonia-

Asociality section. Substantial improvements in attention and working memory were evident in A-CPT scores for all six cases. Five out of six cases also showed improvement in memory as evidenced by gains in Total Recall on the Selective Reminding Test, although this was not a general effect: there was little difference on the Delayed Recall condition of that test, and no apparent effect of treatment on the Logical Memory test. There were no clear improvements on tests of executive function. The improvements were thus selective, although psychometric differences between tasks do not allow for direct comparison of treatment effects *(38)*.

Overall, the results of the pilot treatment trial are encouraging. The attenuation of clinical symptoms and attentional dysfunctions by risperidone in these six cases has at least two important implications. First, it demonstrates that key clinical and neuropsychological problems in nonpsychotic, nonschizotypal relatives of patients with schizophrenia are reversible, at least in part. Second, it shows that the impairments in such people may be ameliorated safely through risperidone treatment. Our experience with these six relatives raises the possibility that eventually, risperidone may be an effective treatment for a population of people whose lives are impaired by similar or related problems. Nevertheless, these results should be considered preliminary. They require replication in larger, controlled studies before they can be considered as a basis for treatment.

The Next Steps

As pharmacologic treatment studies of schizotaxia proceed, larger, double-blind investigations with adequate power will be needed to evaluate the efficacy of available medications systematically, assess the potential occurrence of side effects, and clarify the dose and titration schedules suitable for schizotaxic adults. As more is learned about individuals who meet diagnostic criteria for schizotaxia, methods of diagnosing the syndrome will likely improve. This will facilitate the pairing of appropriate treatments with those who will benefit most from them. If the syndrome continues to receive validation *(39)*, it is also likely that it will evolve to incorporate qualitatively different types of symptoms *(40)*, and will then present a fuller and more precise picture of the disorder. This in turn will more clearly define who has schizotaxia, will provide more targets for treatment trials, and will aid in the development of new treatments designed specifically to alleviate schizotaxic symptoms. Perhaps most important, the validation of schizotaxia in adults will lead to intervention and prevention efforts in adolescents and children.

CHILDHOOD SCHIZOTAXIA

Eventually, if the successful remediation of schizotaxic symptoms is demonstrated in adults, and a homogeneous target population is defined accurately, then

treatments at earlier ages may be considered. As mentioned at the beginning of this chapter, two outcomes of childhood schizotaxia will be considered when discussing potential treatment: one that consists of a stable cluster of symptoms, and one that ultimately progresses to schizophrenia. The first outcome appears to be similar to adult schizotaxia, involving many, if not all, of the same symptoms and deficits. As with other disorders such as depression, however, it is possible that some symptoms will present differently in children. Although the symptoms observed in children with stable childhood schizotaxia may change or worsen slightly through adolescence into adulthood (e.g., fewer than 10% may develop schizotypal personality disorder [1,2]), these individuals will remain essentially stable, and will not develop psychosis. Individuals with the second subtype, however, will likely develop prodromal symptoms (most likely during adolescence) and then psychosis.

Establishing Criteria

Once schizotaxia can be identified in child relatives of schizophrenic individuals, it will be crucial to differentiate the two outcomes discussed above (stable vs progressive childhood schizotaxia). In other words, assuming that similarities exist among all schizotaxic children, it will be necessary to identify the nonoverlapping characteristics of these groups and establish valid criteria for predicting who will go on to develop schizophrenia.

One option is to wait until an individual manifests prodromal symptoms during adolescence, but two problems arise with this strategy. First, these symptoms are often nonspecific. For example, McGorry et al. *(41)* showed that 15.50% of high school students manifest *DSM–III–R* prodromal symptoms for schizophrenia. It does not seem wise to intervene (especially with antipsychotic medication) on the basis of such imprecise indicators. Second, it may not be prudent to postpone intervention until adolescence, especially if prodromal symptoms are already evident. At that point it may be too late to prevent the onset of psychosis in individuals with progressive schizotaxia.

A more effective strategy (at least conceptually) would be to ascertain which schizotaxic individuals are at the highest risk for developing schizophrenia *before* they reach adolescence. Although we do not yet have criteria for differentiating the schizotaxic outcomes in childhood, three current topics of research may provide valuable information in this area: predictive risk factors, protective factors, and genetic liability. Specifically, findings in these areas may help distinguish particular symptoms and characteristics that, when present or occurring in combination with other symptoms (in the case of risk factors), or if absent (in the case of protective factors), would provide criteria for predicting who will and will not develop schizophrenia.

RISK FACTORS

In contrast to current criteria used to diagnose schizophrenia (i.e., psychotic symptoms), many of the features of schizotaxia may be closer to the genetic and other adverse etiological factors that produce the liability for schizophrenia *(42)*. Consequently, measures of schizotaxia may improve risk prediction to the level where it would be useful in determining which schizotaxic children are at very high risk for developing schizophrenia. Moreover, schizotaxic symptoms may come to represent particularly promising treatment targets for prevention protocols. For example, in two independent studies of children of schizophrenic patients, Fish et al. *(43)* described a syndrome of motor abnormalities that predicted subsequent schizophrenia or related disorders. Similarly, in both the Copenhagen and New York High-Risk projects, neuromotor impairment predicted the onset of schizophrenia *(44,45)*. These findings are consistent with Walker and Lewine's *(46)* finding of poorer fine and gross motor coordination in videotapes of children who subsequently became schizophrenic.

In addition to neuromotor impairment, attentional deficits and social impairment also predict subsequent schizophrenia and related disorders (e.g., ref. *45*). In the Israeli High-Risk study, subjects who eventually developed schizophrenia-related disorders had been shy and withdrawn or aggressive and antisocial as children *(47)*. Walker and Lewine's *(46)* videotape study described the children who developed schizophrenia as having had poorer eye contact, more negative affect and diminished social responsiveness. Similarly, in the Copenhagen High-Risk study, teacher-rated social behaviors were predictive of subsequent schizophrenia *(44)*.

As research progresses in this area, additional risk factors in children that predict subsequent schizophrenia may be established (e.g., psychophysiological or neuroanatomical characteristics). For example, Ross et al. *(48)* demonstrated that, in comparison to children without a family history of schizophrenia, children of schizophrenic patients had significantly higher levels of anticipatory saccades on eye-tracking tasks. As measures of anticipatory saccades can also distinguish between schizophrenic patients and normal controls, and are fairly stable in children after 8 years of age *(49)*, such measures could be useful in assessing risk in children *(50–52)*. However, despite these advances, more needs to be known about the diagnostic accuracy of these traits   i.e., their sensitivity and specificity as predictors of psychosis *(53)*   before they can be used to establish divergent criteria for the different outcomes.

PROTECTIVE FACTORS

The term *protective factors* refers to variables that actually reduce risk, as opposed to the absence of variables that confer it. So far, the majority of studies on this topic have compared adult schizophrenic patients either with their non-

schizophrenic parents, or with their nonschizophrenic, adult siblings. Less is known about moderating variables that might serve as protective factors to mitigate the effects of risk factors in schizotaxic children *(54)*. However, findings in adults are very promising and hopefully will generate similar studies in children.

For example, Waldo et al. *(55)* compared three pathophysiological factors in schizophrenic individuals and their siblings. All three factors, including auditory sensory gating, hippocampal size, and catecholamine metabolism, were reported previously as abnormal in schizophrenic individuals (e.g., refs. *56–58*). As expected, the schizophrenic patients demonstrated a deficit in P50 sensory gating, decreased hippocampal volume, and increased plasma levels of homovanillic acid (a measure of dopamine metabolism). In contrast, the unaffected siblings who demonstrated a P50 sensory gating deficit (8 out of 20 siblings) also had a large amplitude N100 wave, large hippocampal volume, and decreased plasma levels of homovanillic acid. Potentially, these findings point to protective factors in relatives who carry the P50 deficit. For instance, increased N100 waves and a larger hippocampus may protect these siblings from the sensory overload produced by the P50 gating deficit *(55,59)*. Thus, schizotaxic children with the P50 deficit, who also have these factors, may be predisposed toward the more stable form of schizotaxia. Children with smaller hippocampi and small amplitude N100 waves may be more disposed toward progressive schizotaxia.

GENETIC LIABILITY

Finally, risk prediction should improve dramatically after molecular genetic studies discover genes for schizophrenia. So far, linkage studies have discovered several regions of the genome that may harbor schizophrenia genes. Promising chromosomal regions include the following: 1q21-22, 6p21-p24, 8p22-21, 10p15-p11, 15q13-q14, and 22q11-q13 *(60–62)*. Although these findings are hopeful, specific schizophrenia genes have yet to be discovered. After geneticists identify the mutations leading to schizophrenia, these results can be used in combination with schizotaxic signs to differentiate children with stable schizotaxia from schizotaxic children who are at very high risk for schizophrenia.

Implications and Ethical Issues of Treatment

Eventually, an understanding of how risks and protective factors combine to produce an overall level of risk, consistent with a diathesis. stress model *(63)*, will be used to predict an individual's level of risk and to tailor individual treatment plans. In addition to establishing criteria for stable and progressive childhood schizotaxia, it will be important to define treatment goals and to weigh the benefits of treatment against the possible hazards. As the projected courses of childhood schizotaxia differ considerably, these issues need to be explored separately for each outcome.

PROGRESSIVE OUTCOME—TREATMENT GOALS

The ultimate objective of treating progressive childhood schizotaxia is the prevention of schizophrenia itself. The idea of prevention through the treatment of childhood schizotaxia is a logical extension of Wyatt's *(64)* notion that early intervention for schizophrenia might modify the course of the illness. His review of 21 controlled studies found that patients who were treated with antipsychotic medicine during their first or second hospitalization showed better outcomes than patients who were not treated early in the course of illness. Others have suggested that early treatment (e.g., of prodromal states, or during the first episode), especially with newer agents, might preserve brain plasticity and reduce the clinical deterioration of chronic schizophrenia *(26,65,66)*. It is also possible that early treatment will mitigate the social consequences of schizophrenic psychopathology and improve the stress tolerance of at-risk persons.

If neuroprotective effects can be shown for pharmacological treatment of schizophrenic patients early in the course of their illness, might pharmacologic treatment show neuroprotective effects for children at risk for developing schizophrenia? If so, would these medications protect them from the first onset of psychosis? A model for successful prevention can be found in the case of several other disorders associated with psychosis, including vascular dementia, syphilis, and epilepsy. If left untreated, each of these disorders can produce psychotic symptoms. However, awareness of early risk factors and treatment of initial symptoms (e.g., hypertension in the case of vascular dementia) can alter the course of the disorder and prevent additional deterioration (including psychosis).

PROGRESSIVE OUTCOME—ETHICAL ISSUES

Although the benefits of preventing psychosis are clear, a case must still be made that they outweigh the risks of treating children and adolescents with progressive schizotaxia. In particular, prevention studies with children and adolescents may have the unintended effect of labeling them as future schizophrenic patients. This raises the very real possibility of stigmatization and emotional harm to the subject and to his or her family. Moreover, the type of medications likely to be used in prevention trials, at least at first, may pose greater risks to children and adolescents than to adults. For example, the use of antipsychotic medications in children has been limited, in part because of concerns about side effects *(67)*. Concerns about stigmatization and medication effects preclude the use of medication without solid evidence of efficacy, but even nonpharmacological interventions could be psychologically harmful if their use is not predicated on a solid rationale. For these reasons, any proposed preventive intervention for schizotaxic adolescents, which would be initiated prior to the onset of prodromal symptoms, would demand a high level of ethical scrutiny and would presuppose a compelling

rationale for any proposed treatment along with the ability to accurately predict who will and will not develop schizophrenia.

STABLE OUTCOME—TREATMENT GOALS

Analogous to adult schizotaxia, children with stable schizotaxia are at less risk for developing schizophrenia. Proposed treatments, therefore, are not aimed primarily at preventing the disorder. Instead, proposed treatments should be focused on improving the social dysfunction, negative symptoms, and neuropsychological impairment of childhood schizotaxia. In addition, as schizotaxic children get older, treatments may also prevent further (nonpsychotic) deterioration including: worsening of negative symptoms and cognitive deficits, and the development of stable, maladaptive ways of dealing with their environments (i.e., personality disorders).

STABLE OUTCOME—ETHICAL ISSUES

Ethical concerns similar to those discussed above also need to be addressed before treating children with stable schizotaxia. For example, although the stable outcome does not presuppose the same level of risk for developing schizophrenia, it is still higher than that of the general public, and may not prevent the child from being stigmatized as preschizophrenic. In addition, medication side effects are also of concern, at least prior to the development of treatments that specifically target schizotaxic symptoms and have improved side effect profiles. Therefore, given that the goals of treating stable childhood schizotaxia are less focused on the prevention of schizophrenia than they are with progressive schizotaxia, the value of treating the stable form potentially demands even more ethical scrutiny.

Treatment Options

Once diagnostic criteria are established for both the stable and progressive outcomes of childhood schizotaxia, treatment goals are defined, and an acceptable risk . benefit ratio is reached, research can move toward finding appropriate treatments. Certainly treatment studies of schizotaxic adults will provide a major source of information for the treatment of schizotaxic children and adolescents. This research strategy assumes that the following: (a) adult schizotaxia is mainly a later stage of stable childhood schizotaxia; (b) treatments that successfully ameliorate symptoms of schizotaxia in adults would also be beneficial in children; (c) in the case of progressive childhood schizotaxia, adult schizotaxia provides a suitable model of the pathophysiology of premorbid schizophrenia; and (d) treatments that ameliorate adult schizotaxia do so through neural mechanisms involved in the onset of psychosis in schizotaxic adolescents. If validation studies can verify this hypothesis, then an effective medication for adult schizotaxia might be the

logical choice as a treatment for stable childhood schizotaxia. In addition to information derived from the study of adult schizotaxia, data from longitudinal and prediction studies, such as those discussed above, may guide the modifications of such treatments for use with children who have progressive schizotaxia in primary-prevention trials of schizophrenia.

WHAT ARE FIRST-LINE MEDICATIONS FOR SCHIZOTAXIA?

We have already suggested antipsychotic medication (e.g., risperidone) as a potential treatment for adult schizotaxia. In fact, there is a small literature documenting the treatment of children and adolescents with antipsychotic medication. In the treatment of child- and adolescent-onset schizophrenia, typical antipsychotic medications (e.g., haloperidol) have been of limited use due to the high risk of side effects (67). The atypical antipsychotics (e.g., clozapine, olanzapine, and risperidone) are considered more effective as they target negative as well as positive schizophrenic symptoms and have a better safety profile (67). For example, Frazier et al. (68) treated 11 adolescents with childhood-onset schizophrenia with a 6-week trial of clozapine and reported improvement in Brief Psychiatric Rating Scale ratings, compared to haloperidol.

Atypical antipsychotic medication is also prescribed to treat children and adolescents with nonpsychotic disorders. Of the atypicals, risperidone has been most widely used in this manner. Positive effects have been reported in risperidone treatment of autism (e.g., ref. 69), chronic tic disorders including Tourette's syndrome (e.g., ref. 70), pediatric autoimmune neuropsychiatric disorders associated with streptococcal infections (PANDAS) (e.g., ref. 71), phenylketonuria (PKU) (e.g., ref. 72), and social functioning in children with behavioral disturbances (e.g., ref. 73).

It is important to note that these medications still produce significant side effects (67,74), which warrant additional concern in the treatment of children and adolescents. For example, clozapine frequently produces hypersalivation and weight gain in adolescents (75), olanzapine elevates prolactin levels in children (76), and risperidone produces significant weight gain in adolescents (77). Besides the negative social consequences of such side effects, the effects of antipsychotic medication on adolescent development are still unknown.

In addition to the use of antipsychotic medication, there is support for treating schizophrenic symptoms with medications other than antipsychotics. For example, Kulkarni et al. (78) showed that estradiol (estrogen), used as a supplement to antipsychotic medication, improved symptoms of psychosis in schizophrenic women. Beta-adrenergic receptor antagonists (β-blockers) also have been used as an adjunct to antipsychotic medication. However, in a recent review, Cheine et al. (79) concluded that there was not sufficient evidence to support the use of β-blockers in the treatment of schizophrenia. There is also evidence that the omega-

3 fatty acid, eicosapentaenoic acid (EPA), improves positive and negative symptoms in schizophrenia *(80,81)*. Other medications that recently have been implicated as potential alternative treatments include diazepam *(82)* and nefazodone *(83)*. Perhaps these treatments, in combination with atypical antipsychotic medication, could provide a strategy for a pilot prevention trial with at-risk, schizotaxic children and adolescents. Once the effective mechanisms of antipsychotic medication and other treatments are identified (and replicated), more specific medications, with fewer side effects and less social stigma, may be utilized or developed.

CONCLUSION

There are several implications of developing interventions for schizotaxia. Treatment of schizotaxia in nonpsychotic relatives could serve to alleviate clinically meaningful symptoms and improve quality of life in these individuals. Effective therapies, be they psychological or psychopharmacologic, might improve the neuropsychological deficits and negative symptoms typically found in both child and adult relatives. Improvements in these domains should lessen the distress of the individuals themselves and allow them to function better in family, occupational, and societal roles *(84)*. Moreover, improving the welfare of schizotaxic family members would indirectly benefit their schizophrenic relatives by decreasing stress in the home and facilitating the progress of family interventions. Even more important, the successful treatment of schizotaxia in adults might serve as a foundation for the eventual development of strategies aimed at the prevention of schizophrenia in vulnerable individuals prior to the onset of prodromal or psychotic symptoms. Although we are not there yet, the accurate identification of one or more schizotaxic syndromes may also allow for the eventual classification of young schizotaxic individuals into lower (i.e., stable) and higher (i.e., progressive) risk categories, which will serve to further focus efforts aimed at the ultimate goal of preventing schizophrenia.

REFERENCES

1. Faraone SV, Kremen WS, Lyons MJ, Pepple JR, Seidman LJ, Tsuang MT. Diagnostic accuracy and linkage analysis: how useful are schizophrenia spectrum phenotypes? Am J Psychiatry 1995; 152:1286..1290.
2. Faraone SV, Seidman LJ, Kremen WS, Pepple JR, Lyons MJ, Tsuang MT. Neuropsychological functioning among the nonpsychotic relatives of schizophrenic patients: a diagnostic efficiency analysis. J Abnorm Psychol 1995; 104:286..304.
3. Faraone SV, Chen WJ, Goldstein JM, Tsuang MT. Gender differences in the age at onset of schizophrenia: fact or artifact. Br J Psychiatry 1994; 164:625..629.
4. Sham PC Jones P, Russell A, et al. Age at onset, sex, and familial psychiatric morbidity in schizophrenia. Camberwell collaborative psychosis study. Br J Psychiatry 1994; 165:466..473.
5. Pulver AE, Brown CH, Wolyniec P, et al. Schizophrenia: age at onset, gender and familial risk. Acta Psychiatr Scandin 1990; 82:344..351.

6. Falloon IRH, Boyd JL, McGill CW, et al. Family management in the prevention of morbidity of schizophrenia. Clinical outcome of a two-year controlled study. Arch Gen Psychiatry 1986; 42:887..896.

7. Seidman LJ. Listening, meaning, and empathy in neuropsychological disorders: Case examples of assessment and treatment. In: Ellison JM, Weinstein CS, Hodel-Malinofsky T, eds. The Psychotherapist's Guide to Neuropsychiatry. American Psychiatric Press, Washington, DC: 1994:1..22.

8. Hymowitz P, Frances A, Jacobsberg LB, Sickles M, Hoyt R. Neuroleptic treatment of schizotypal personality disorders. Compr Psychiatry 1986; 27(4):267.271.

9. Gitlin MJ. Pharmacotherapy of personality disorders: conceptual framework and clinical strategies. J Clin Psychopharmacol 1993; 13(5):343..353.

10. Coccaro EF. Clinical outcome of psychopharmacologic treatment of borderline and schizotypal personality disordered subjects. J Clin Psychiatry 1998; 59(Suppl 1):30..35.

11. Stein G. Drug treatment of the personality disorders. Br J Psychiatry 1992; 161:167..184.

12. Marder S, Meibach R. Risperidone in the treatment of schizophrenia. Am J Psychiatry 1994; 151:825..835.

13. Cassens G, Inglis AK, Appelbaum PS, Gutheil TG. Neuroleptics: effects on neuropsychological function in chronic schizophrenic patients. Schizophr Bull 1990; 16(3):477..499.

14. Rabinowitz J. Risperidone versus haloperidol in long-term hospitalized chronic patients in a double blind randomized trial: a post hoc analysis. Schizophr Res 2001; 50:89..93.

15. Sauriol L, Laporta M, Edwardes M, Deslandes M, Ricard N, Suissa S. Meta-analysis comparing newer antipsychotic drugs for the treatment of schizophrenia: evaluating the indirect approach. Clin Ther 2001; 23:942..956.

16. Beasley CM, Sanger T, Satterlee W, et al. Olanzapine versus placebo: results of a double-blind, fixed-dose olanzapine trial. Psychopharmacology 1996; 124:159..167.

17. Small JG, Hirsch SR, Arvantis LA, Miller BG, Link CC, Group TSS. Quetiapine in patients with schizophrenia: a high and low dose double-blind comparison with placebo. Arch Gen Psychiatry 1997; 54(6):549..557.

18. Umbricht D, Javitt D, Novak G, et al. Effects of risperidone on auditory event-related potentials in schizophrenia. Int J Neuropsychopharmcol 1999; 2:299..304.

19. McGurk SR. The effects of clozapine on cognitive functioning in schizophrenia. J Clin Psychiatry 1999; 60(Suppl 12):24..29.

20. Harvey PD, Keefe RSE. Cognition and the new antipsychotics. J Advances Schizophr Brain Res 1998; 1:2..8.

21. Sharma T, Mockler D. The cognitive efficacy of atypical antipsychotics in schizophrenia. J Clin Psychopharmacol 1998; 18(Suppl):12s..19s.

22. Green MF, Braff DL. Translating the basic and clinical cognitive neuroscience of schizophrenia to drug development and clinical trials of antipsychotic medications. Biol Psychiatry 2001; 49:374..384.

23. Tamminga CA. The promise of new drugs for schizophrenia treatment. Can J Psychiatry 1997; 42:265..273.

24. Carpenter WT, Conley RR, Buchanan RW, Breier A, Tamminga CA. Patient response and resource management: another view of clozapine treatment with schizophrenia. Am J Psychiatry 1995; 152:827..832.

25. Meltzer HY. Editorial: clozapine: is another view valid? Am J Psychiatry 1995; 152:821..826.

26. Green AI, Schildkraut JJ. Should clozapine be a first-line treatment for schizophrenia? The rationale for a double-blind clinical trial in first-episode patients. Harv Rev Psychiatry 1995; 3:1..9.

27. Bruggeman R, van der Linden C, Buitelaar JK, et al. Risperidone versus pimozide in Tourette's disorder: a comparative double-blind parallel-group study. J Clin Psychiatry 2001; 62(1):50..56.
28. Bruun RD, Budman CL. Risperidone as a treatment for Tourette's syndrome. J Clin Psychiatry 1996; 57(1):29..31.
29. Budman CL, Gayer A, Lesser M, Shi Q, Bruun RD. An open-label study of the treatment efficacy of olanzapine for Tourette's disorder. J Clin Psychiatry 2001; 62(4):290..294.
30. McDougle CJ, Epperson CN, Pelton GH, Wasylink S, Price LH. A double-blind, placebo-controlled study of resperidone addition in serotonin reuptake inhibitor-refractory obsessibe-compulsive disorder. Arch Gen Psychiatry 2000; 57(8):794..801.
31. Bogetto F, Bellino S, Vaschetto P, Ziero S. Olanzapine augmentation of fluvoxamine-refractory obsessive-compulsive disorder (OCD): a 12-week open trial. Psychiatry Res 2000; 96(2): 91..98.
32. Krashin D, Oates EW. Risperidone as an adjunct therapy for post-traumatic stress disorder. Mil Med 1999; 164(8):605..606.
33. Tsuang MT, Stone WS, Seidman LJ, et al. Treatment of nonpsychotic relatives of patients with schizophrenia: four case studies. Biol Psychiatry 1999; 41:1412..1418.
34. Tsuang MT, Stone WS, Tarbox SI, Faraone SV. Treatment of nonpsychotic relatives of patients with schizophrenia: a pilot study. Neuropsychiatric Genet 2002; 114:943..948.
35. Andreasen NC. The Scale for the Assessment of Negative Symptoms (SANS). Iowa City: University of Iowa Press,1983.
36. Seidman LJ, Biederman J, Weber W, Hatch M, Faraone SV. Neuropsychological functioning in adults with ADHD. Biol Psychiatry 1998; 44:260..268.
37. Cornblatt B, Winters L, Erlenmeyer-Kimling L. Attentional markers of schizophrenia: evidence from the New York high-risk study. In: Schulz SC, Tamminga CA, eds. Schizophrenia: Scientific Progress. New York: Oxford University Press, 1989:83..92.
38. Chapman LJ, Chapman JP. The measurement of differential deficit. J Psychiatric Res 1978; 14:303..311.
39. Stone WS, Faraone SV, Seidman LJ, Green AI, Wojcik JD, Tsuang MT. Concurrent validation of schizotaxia: a pilot study. Biol Psychiatry 2001; 50(6):434..440.
40. Tsuang MT, Stone WS, Faraone SV. Understanding predisposition to schizophrenia: toward intervention and prevention. Can J Psychiatry 2002; 47:518..526.
41. McGorry PD, McFarlane C, Patton GC. The prevalence of prodromal features of schizophrenia in adolescence: a preliminary survey. Acta Psychiatr Scandin 1995; 92:241..249.
42. Tsuang MT, Stone WS, Faraone SV. Towards reformulating the diagnosis of schizophrenia. Am J Psychiatry 2000; 147:1041..1050.
43. Fish B, Marcus J, Hans SL, Auerbach JG, Perdue S. Infants at risk for schizophrenia: sequelae of a genetic neurointegrative defect. A review and replication analysis of pandysmaturation in the Jerusalem infant development study. Arch Gen Psychiatry 1992; 49:221..235.
44. Olin SCS, Mednick SA. Risk factors of psychosis: identifying vulnerable populations premorbidly. Schizophr Bull 1996; 22:223..240.
45. Erlenmeyer-Kimling L, Personal Communication, 1997.
46. Walker E, Lewine RJ. Prediction of adult-onset schizophrenia from childhood home movies of the parents. Am J Psychiatry 1990; 147(8):1052..1056.
47. Hans SL, Marcus J, Henson L, Auerbach JG, Mirsky AF. Interpersonal behavior of children at risk for schizophrenia. Psychiatry 1992; 55:314..335.
48. Ross RG, Hommer DW, Radant AD, Roath M, Freedman R. Early expression of smooth pursuit eye movement abnormalities in children of schizophrenic parents. J Am Acad Child Adolesc Psychiatry 1996; 35:941..949.

49. Ross RG, Radant AD, Hommer DW. A developmental study of smooth pursuit eye movements in normal children from 7 to 15 years of age. J Child Adolesc Psychiatry 1993; 32:783..791.
50. Ross RG, Harris JG, Olincy A, Radant A, Adler LE, Freedman R. Familial transmission of two independent saccadic abnormalities in schizophrenia. Schizophr Res 1998; 30:59..70.
51. Ross RG, Olincy A, Harris JG, Radant A, Adler LE, Freedman R. Anticipatory saccades during smooth pursuit eye movements and familial transmission af schizophrenia. Biol Psychiatry 1998; 44:690..697.
52. Radant AD, Hommer DW. A quantitative analysis of saccades and smooth pursuit during visual pursuit tracking: a comparison of schizophrenics with normals and substance abusing controls. Schizophr Res 1992; 6:225..235.
53. Faraone SV, Tsuang MT. Measuring diagnostic accuracy in the absence of a gold standard. Am J Psychiatry 1994; 151:650..657.
54. Tsuang MT. Genes, environment, and mental health wellness. Am J Psychiatry 2000; 157: 489..491.
55. Waldo MC, Cawthra E, Adler LE, et al. Auditory sensory gating, hippocampal volume, and catecholamine metabolism in schizophrenics and their siblings. Schizophr Res 1994; 12:93..106.
56. Adler LE, Pachtman E, Franks R, Pecevich M, Waldo MC, Freedman R. Neurophysiological evidence for a defect in neuronal mechanisms involved in sensory gating in schizophrenia. Biol Psychiatry 1982; 17:639..654.
57. Adler LE, Gerhardt GA, Franks R, et al. Sensory physiology catecholamines in schizophrenia and mania. Psychiatry Res 1990; 31:297..309.
58. Nelson M, Saykin A, Flashman L, Riordan H. Hippocampal volume reduction in schizophrenia as assessed by magnetic resonance imaging: a meta-analytic study. Arch Gen Psychiatry 1998; 55:433..440.
59. Waldo MC, Adler LE, Leonard S, et al. Familial transmission of risk factors in the first-degree relatives of schizophrenic people. Biol Psychiatry 2000; 47:231..239.
60. Tsuang MT, Stone WS, Faraone SV. Schizophrenia: a review of genetic studies. Harv Rev Psychiatry 1999; 7:185..207.
61. Levinson DF, Holmans P, Straub RE, et al. Multicenter linkage study of schizophrenia candidate regions on chromosomes 5q, 6q, 10p, and 13q: schizophrenia linkage collaborative group III. Am J Hum Genet 2000; 67(3):652..663.
62. Gurling HM, Kalsi G, Brynjolfson J, et al. Genomewide genetic linkage analysis confirms the presence of susceptibility loci for schizophrenia, on chromosomes 1q32.2, 5q33.2, and 8p21-22 and provides support for linkage to schizophrenia, on chromosomes 11q23.3-24 and 20q12.1-11.23. Am J Hum Genet 2001; 68(3):661..673.
63. Gottesman II. Schizophrenia Genesis: The Origin of Madness. New York: Freeman, 1991,
64. Wyatt RJ. Early intervention for schizophrenia: can the course of the illness be altered? Biol Psychiatry 1995; 38:1..3.
65. McGlashan TH, Johannessen JO. Early detection and intervention with schizophrenia: rationale. Schizophr Bull 1996; 22:201..222.
66. Lieberman JA. Atypical antipsychotic drugs as a first-line treatment of schizophrenia: a rationale and hypothesis. J Clin Psychiatry 1996; 57(Suppl 11):68..71.
67. Findling RL, Schulz SC, Reed MD, Blumer JL. The antipsychotics. A pediatric perspective. Pediatr Clin North Am 1998; 45(5):1205..1232.
68. Frazier JA, Gordon CT, McKenna K, Lenane MC, Jih D, Rapoport JL. An open trial of clozapine in 11 adolescents with childhood-onset schizophrenia. J Am Acad Child Adolesc Psychiatry 1994; 33:658..663.

69. Findling RL, Maxwell K, Wiznitzer M. An open clinical trial of risperidone monotherapy in young children with autistic disorder. Psychopharmacol Bull 1997; 33(1):155..159.
70. Lombroso PJ, Scahill L, King RA, et al. Risperidone treatment of children and adolescents with chronic tic disorders: a preliminary report. J Am Acad Child Adolesc Psychiatry 1995; 34(9):1147..1152.
71. Kleinsasser BJ, Misra LK, Bhatara VS, Sanchez JD. Risperidone in the treatment of choreiform movements and aggressiveness in a child with "PANDAS." South Dakota J Med 1999; 52(9):345..347.
72. Shiwach RS, Sheikha S. Delusional disorder in a boy with phenylketonuria and amine metabolites in the cerebrospinal fluid after treatment with neuroleptics. J Adolesc Health 1998; 22(3): 244..246.
73. Van Bellinghen M, De Troch C. Risperidone in the treatment of behavioral disturbances in children and adolescents with borderline intellectual functioning: a double-blind, placebo-controlled pilot trial. J Child Adolesc Psychopharmacol 2001; 11:5..13.
74. Whitaker A, Rao U. Neuroleptics in pediatric psychiatry. Pediatr Clin North Am 1992; 15(1): 243..276.
75. Remschmidt H, Fleischhaker C, Hennighausen K, Schulz E. Management of schizophrenia in children and adolescents. The role of clozapine. Paediatr Drugs 2000; 2(4):253..262.
76. Wudarsky M, Nicolson R, Hamburger SD, et al. Elevated prolactin in pediatric patients on typical and atypical antipsychotics. J Child Adolesc Psychopharmacol 1999; 9(4):239..245.
77. Kelly DL, Conley RR, Love RC, Horn DS, Ushchak CM. Weight gain in adolescents treated with risperidone and conventional antipsychotics over six months. J Child Adolesc Psychopharmacol 1998; 8(3):151..159.
78. Kulkarni J, Riedel A, de Castella AR, et al. Estrogen   a potential treatment for schizophrenia. Schizophr Res 2001; 48(1):137..144.
79. Cheine M, Ahonen J, Wahlbeck K. Beta-blocker supplementation of standard drug treatment for schizophrenia. Cochrane Database of Systematic Reviews [computer file], 2000; (2):CD000234.
80. Puri BK, Richardson AJ, Horrobin DF, et al. Eicosapentaenoic acid treatment in schizophrenia associated with symptom remission, normalization of blood fatty acids, reduced neuronal membrane phospholipid turnover and structural brain changes. Intl J Clin Pract 2000; 54(1): 57..63.
81. Richardson AJ, Easton T, Puri BK. Red cell and plasma fatty acid changes accompanying symptom remission in a patient with schizophrenia treated with eicosapentaenoic acid. Eur Neuropsychopharmacol 2000; 10(3):189..193.
82. Carpenter WRJ, Buchanan RW, Kirkpatrick B, Breier AF. Diazepam treatment of early signs of exacerbation in schizophrenia. Am J Psychiatry 1999; 156(2):299..303.
83. Rosenberg PB, Rosse RB, Schwartz BL, Deutsch SI. Nefazodone in the adjunctive therapy of schizophrenia: an open-label exploratory study. Clin Neuropharmacol 2000; 23(4):222..225.
84. Cornblatt BA, Keilp JG. Impaired attention, genetics, and the pathophysiology of schizophrenia. Schizophr Bull 1994; 20:31..46.

14 Treatment of the Schizophrenia Prodrome

Barbara Cornblatt, PhD,
Todd Lencz, PhD,
Christopher Smith, MA,
and Andrea Auther, PhD

INTRODUCTION

A series of rapidly emerging research events has generated both optimism and concern about the administration of antipsychotic medication prior to the onset of psychosis: hope that early intervention will lead to the prevention of full-blown schizophrenia, but concern that this belief may be premature. Although the supporting research is encouraging, it is still in its infancy. The handful of early findings *(1–3)* are encouraging, but are in no way conclusive, and the possibility of prevention remains open. In this chapter, we discuss both the promise and the problems characterizing this area of research. We begin by addressing two very preliminary questions: (1) Why is schizophrenia, arguably the most severe and difficult to treat of the mental illnesses, considered preventable? and (2) Why does pharmacological intervention during the prodromal phase of schizophrenia appear justified or even acceptable as a starting point in prevention programs? We discuss the evidence that supports the use of early pharmacotherapy as well as some of the controversies that have emerged in response to the early clinical interventions. We conclude by reporting the early treatment findings emerging from the Hillside Recognition and Prevention (RAP) program, which has attempted to integrate a high-risk research methodology within a treatment framework and has, as a result, adopted a somewhat different strategy than most of the other prodromal studies now under way.

From: *Early Clinical Intervention and Prevention in Schizophrenia*
Edited by: W. S. Stone, S. V. Faraone, and M. T. Tsuang © Humana Press Inc., Totowa, NJ

WHY DO WE THINK
THAT SCHIZOPHRENIA IS PREVENTABLE?

Prevention is suggested by the neurodevelopmental nature of schizophrenia. Over the past two decades or so, schizophrenia has become widely viewed as a brain disease with its roots in very early, probably prenatal, development. Yet florid psychosis, the end point of the illness, typically does not emerge until late teens or early 20s, suggesting that an extensive period of time exists during which preventive intervention can take place. One major challenge is accurate identification of vulnerable individuals sufficiently early to enable the initiation of effective interventions; this has traditionally been the task of genetic high-risk (GHR) studies. A second critical challenge is establishing the nature of the most effective type of treatment. In the sections to follow, we argue that intervention has, to date, been approached from the perspective of previous treatment trials, but that in the case of prodromal intervention (which involves treatment of an "at-risk" population), elements of traditional high-risk studies should also be incorporated.

Neurodevelopmental Hypothesis

The neurodevelopmental hypothesis was originally proposed as a theoretical alternative to the traditional view of schizophrenia as a neurodegenerative illness. The notion that schizophrenia follows a degenerative course dates back to E. Kraepelin *(4)*, who believed that schizophrenia was an early form of dementia (i.e., dementia praecox). Recent studies provide evidence countering the degenerative hypothesis. Several studies have indicated that structural anomalies such as enlarged ventricles are found in schizophrenic patients at their initial episode of illness and do not appear to increase as the illness progresses (e.g., refs. *5, 6–8,* but *see* DeLisi et al. *[9]*). Moreover, clinically, it appears that few patients show the progressive deterioration characteristic of the dementias and, in fact, some patients improve over time. The alternative viewpoint   that at least some aspects of schizophrenia are neurodevelopmental   has evolved far more recently and is supported by indirect but consistent data. Developmental abnormalities on the cellular level, including abnormal synaptic pruning, defects in embryonic cell migration, and abnormal myelination of axons, have been reported that support the neurodevelopmental model *(10–14)*.

A neurodevelopmental perspective suggests that preventive intervention should be quite possible, since the unfolding of the clinical illness is a long-term process. As illustrated in Fig. 1, according to most views, this process most likely begins with an early (prenatal) series of biological insults or errors that include the presence of a disease genotype and may also involve other factors (e.g., infection, environmental trauma, etc.). As a result, the brain develops abnormalities, which might be structural, functional, or biochemical, or some combination of the

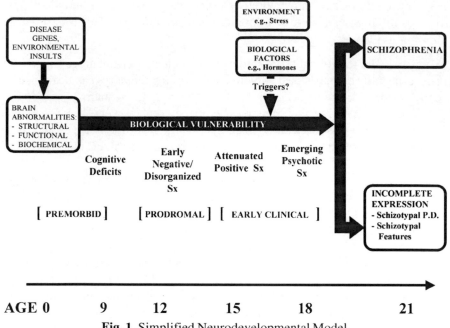

Fig. 1. Simplified Neurodevelopmental Model.

three. Whatever the exact nature of the brain disturbance, it is currently believed to be the source of the susceptibility or vulnerability to later schizophrenia.

Although frequently described as being "clinically silent" throughout much of adolescence, it has been increasingly recognized that the biological substrate of illness is reflected in subtle premorbid neurocognitive deficits and nonspecific prodromal behavioral/clinical disturbances. This underlying susceptibility is likely to be essential for future illness, although it may not be sufficient. For example, full disease expression may require some sort of "trigger," such as an independent environmental or biological stressor (not as yet identified). It therefore follows that if the underlying susceptibility is successfully treated, it may be possible to eliminate or reduce the impact of the trigger(s). The resulting questions are: which of the markers or risk factors should be targeted; which are most amenable to treatment; when should treatment be initiated; and what types of medication should be used?

Causal Risk Factors

Neurocognitive Deficits

Kraemer et al. *(15)* suggest that only causal risk factors are reasonable targets for intervention. We propose that neurocognitive deficits are strong candidates

since they are among the most widely studied early risk factors and also appear to be causally involved in the development of schizophrenia. This is based on the following evidence:

1. Findings from traditional GHR studies have indicated that neurocognitive deficits (especially compromised attention and working memory) can be detected in early childhood, and precede other types of symptoms by many years *(16–20)*. These deficits have been referred to as "biobehavioral markers" because they are intermediate between basic biological functions and more complex clinical behaviors and are thought to be direct reflections (or markers) of the underlying brain abnormalities.
2. Data collected over 20 years in the New York High-Risk Project (NYHRP) has indicated that the attentional deficits detected in childhood (typically by age 9) are stable across development and appear to be causally related to subsequent social difficulties in adolescence and to increasing social isolation in adulthood (e.g., refs. *20–26*).
3. Impaired attention, in particular, and neurocognitive dysfunctions, in general, do not appear to be related to positive symptoms *(23,27,28)*. This indicates that neurocognition is a separate domain, most likely involved in the underlying vulnerability that precedes the emergence of positive (psychotic) symptoms.
4. Cognitive disturbances have been reported to relate more directly to functional outcome in affected patients than do either positive or negative symptoms *(28,29)*.

These findings suggest that treating preillness cognitive markers may substantially impact the extent to which subsequent "triggers" will result in the expression of the full psychotic illness. Moreover, it can be speculated that treating long-standing cognitive deficits may reduce the social difficulties and functional disability associated with the range of schizophrenia spectrum disorders.

ATTENUATED NEGATIVE AND DISORGANIZED FEATURES

Although neurocognitive deficits have traditionally been the most widely studied preillness risk factors, a number of other clinical and functional abnormalities have also been identified. There is considerable evidence, especially from prospective and follow-back high-risk studies, to suggest that attenuated negative symptoms, such as deficits in social functioning, are important characteristics of the prodromal phase of illness (e.g., refs. *30–34*). Incorporating these research findings as well as early data from the RAP program, we have proposed *(35)* a specific profile in adolescence that appears to reflect risk for schizophrenia-related disorders. This is referred to as the CASID cluster and consists of Cognitive, Academic, and Social Impairments as well as Disorganization/odd behaviors. Academic in this context primarily reflects withdrawal from school (and often increasing refusal to attend school) rather than "acting-out" difficulties, and is typically accompanied by a decline in academic performance. This view is similar

but not identical to the concept of schizotaxia proposed by Tsuang and colleagues *(34,36,37)*. Consistent with Tsuang's view of schizotaxia, it is assumed that the CASID cluster does not inevitably lead to full-blown schizophrenia, but appears to be a risk factor for it. Therefore, treatment targeting these difficulties would be assumed to decrease that risk.

Although each of the features entering into this cluster is quite nonspecific and can signal any number of emerging difficulties, it is possible that it is the particular combination of features that is predictive of later schizophrenia. Thus, it is proposed that this cluster of preillness features may serve two roles: First, as a combined profile, it may function as a way to accurately predict later illness. (Future research will determine whether predictive validity will be improved by the addition of attenuated positive symptoms.) Second, it may inform prevention efforts by providing risk factors that represent optimal targets for early treatment.

This view has substantial implications for intervention. As discussed in detail here, the prodromal intervention programs now in progress focus on positive symptoms consistent with clinical trials involving already psychotic patients. This, in turn, leads to the assumption that antipsychotic medication is the optimal starting point for psychopharmacology. However, an increased emphasis on treatment of cognitive deficits and attenuated negative symptoms prior to the emergence of positive symptoms suggests a broader choice of medication. This is further supported by the widely accepted understanding that in affected patients, antipsychotics are more effective in treating positive symptoms than in improving either negative symptoms or cognitive deficits.

PRODROMAL INDICATORS

Because interest in the schizophrenia prodrome is very new, the signs and symptoms defining this phase of the illness are just beginning to be established *(38–44)*. Developmentally, the prodrome can be viewed as the transition between the premorbid and psychotic stages of illness. Prodromal indicators therefore emerge at a later time point than the premorbid neurocognitive risk factors just discussed. Because they are closer to the onset of illness, it is assumed that prodromal indicators will have considerably greater predictive accuracy than either the neurocognitive or other CASID cluster markers discussed here. However, the extent to which this is actually the case remains to be determined.

The schizophrenia prodrome is currently identified almost entirely by the presence of mild (i.e., attenuated) positive symptoms, which are psychotic-like but have not reached the intensity of true psychosis. Such attenuated symptoms are considered the forerunners of psychosis. These signs and symptoms are therefore not causal risk factors for psychosis, but, instead, are its first manifestations   i.e., are part of the disease process itself. As a result, interventions based on the identification of positive symptom indicators are, at best, early secondary

prevention, since the illness has already begun. This is in contrast to primary or preillness intervention that can result from treatment of the CASID predictors, once these are firmly established.

However, even if prodromal intervention is started after the illness has actually begun, it can be seen as having considerable value in preventing further deterioration and disability. It is also possible to conduct such programs now, whereas preillness interventions are still many years away. However, there are a number of problems still to be resolved. Despite assumptions that prodromal indicators accurately signal impending schizophrenia, it has become clear that considerably more research is needed. To date, prediction is in the 40.50% range *(40,45,46)*. This means that using the current criteria consisting primarily of attenuated positive symptoms, around 50% of the individuals targeted for treatment in prodromal programs will be false positives. This is problematic, especially for the design of clinical intervention trials.

Selection criteria focusing on positive symptoms have been inherited from the treatment tradition. It is quite possible that predictive accuracy will be considerably improved by adding some of the risk factors identified by high-risk studies, especially those making up the CASID cluster of risk factors as discussed earlier. To do so, however, may change the way treatment is approached in the next generation of prodromal intervention programs.

PHARMACO-INTERVENTION:
JUSTIFICATION AND CONTROVERSIES

BENEFITS OF EARLY TREATMENT

A number of studies have now suggested that the earlier medication begins after the onset of psychosis, the better the outcome *(47–53)*. The notion that the longer psychosis remains untreated, the poorer the prognosis, is typically referred to as the duration of untreated psychosis (DUP) effect, and is tied to the belief (as yet not well supported) that psychosis, in and of itself, may be toxic to the brain *(52–54)*. This has led McGlashan *(51)* to suggest that the DUP effect justifies prodromal intervention in spite of the possibility of false-positive identifications. However, the importance of the DUP has been increasingly challenged by several recent studies *(56–58)* that report no association between the DUP and outcome. Furthermore, several researchers have raised questions about the direction of causality, maintaining that even if there is a correlation between the DUP and prognosis, this may simply reflect other factors, such as severity of illness or level of premorbid functioning *(59,60)*. Nevertheless, whether or not the DUP does directly impact prognosis, as pointed out by McGorry and Edwards *(61)*, intervention during the prodromal stage can still result in many psychosocial, psychological, educational, and other advantages.

INTRODUCTION OF SECOND-GENERATION ANTIPSYCHOTIC MEDICATIONS

Until recently, intervention could not be attempted, regardless of whether stable risk factors could be identified. This was because standard neuroleptics, the most effective pharmacological treatment previously available, were associated with quite severe side effects (e.g., tardive dyskinesia and other types of movement disorders). Given the likelihood of involving a relatively high rate of false-positive identifications, prodromal intervention was not considered either feasible or ethical. However, the emergence of second-generation antipsychotics (SGAPs) has changed this situation and has provided the tools for preventive intervention. Given the reduced side effects of the antipsychotic medications currently available *(62–64)*, intervening early in the illness process, before psychosis sets in, has been increasingly regarded as ethically acceptable *(65)*. Nevertheless, a major question can be raised about whether antipsychotics should be the first-line treatment of prodromal symptoms.

TYPE OF MEDICATION

It is assumed by most treatment-oriented prodromal researchers that SGAPs are the most effective tools for achieving the prevention of psychosis. This is because administration of antipsychotic medication to prodromal individuals appears to be a logical extension of treatment for the fully expressed disorder. However, this strategy is justified only if attenuated positive symptoms are accepted as the first-line targets for intervention, which, from a high-risk research perspective, can be challenged.

By definition, individuals considered to be prodromal do not display florid psychotic symptoms, the symptoms most improved by antipsychotic medication. They do, however, typically display the range of features included in the CASID cluster discussed above. Nevertheless, little attention has been directed toward designing treatments for these other risk features.

The need for an alternate treatment strategy is illustrated by Fig. 2. Rather than viewing the unfolding of the illness as a single linear process (as shown earlier in Fig. 1), here there are two defined pathways, with the implication that many additional pathways to psychosis may, in reality, be involved. However, even from the simplified viewpoint in Fig. 2, it is clear that the two pathways are likely to involve different types of intervention. To begin with, the vulnerability pathway (bottom arrow) consists of enduring traits that begin at a developmentally earlier time point. The top arrow, representing emerging positive symptoms, begins considerably later, most likely has its origins in a different part of the brain, and may benefit from early treatment with antipsychotics. It may be that only by treating both pathways can the illness be fully eliminated.

Of particular interest here is what effect treating one pathway will have on the other. Treating the clinical (top) pathway with antipsychotics may reduce the

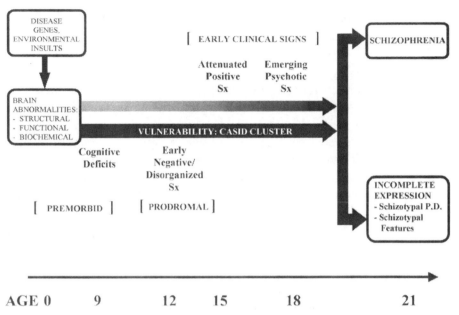

Fig. 2. Expanded Neurodevelopmental Model, with at least two independent pathways required for schizophrenia to be fully expressed.

likelihood of psychosis, but still result in an individual characterized by schizotypal personality disorder or other schizophrenia-spectrum features or personality disorders. If the vulnerability (bottom) process is reduced by early intervention, it may be possible to reduce or eliminate not only the later-emerging psychotic symptoms, but to also reduce the disability associated with the vulnerability deficits.

HETEROGENEITY OF THE PRODROME

Schizophrenia is considered to be a heterogeneous disorder by most researchers heterogeneous in terms of clinical characteristics and in terms of etiology (e.g., ref. 66). It is therefore logical that the prodromal stage that precedes the fully expressed illness is equally heterogeneous. This will pose still further complications when attempting to evaluate treatment effectiveness, because different prodromal patterns may respond differently to a common intervention.

An illustration of this is the highly influential diagnostic system developed by McGorry, McGlashan, and their colleagues (38,43,44,46,66), which consists of three separate categories of selection criteria. Category 1 requires at least one of the following attenuated positive symptoms: ideas of reference, odd beliefs or magical thinking; perceptual disturbance; odd thinking and speech; paranoid

ideation; and odd behavior or appearance. Category 2 consists of individuals who have experienced transient psychotic symptoms that have spontaneously resolved within 1 week. Category 3 combines genetic risk (i.e., being the first-degree relative of an individual with a diagnosis of schizophrenia) with state change in functioning (must have undergone a substantial decline in the previous year). An individual meeting any one of these three categories is considered to be prodromal for schizophrenia, with the prodrome itself viewed as a single clinical entity.

This type of approach incorporates several potential difficulties. First, there is no evidence to indicate that the three categories involve a common etiology. Second, if etiologically different, it is likely that each category involves a different conversion rate. Third (and related to points 1 and 2), different treatment approaches may be optimal for each of the three categories. When combined into a single broad group, treatment successes or failures may well be masked. However, separation into individual cells increases the problems associated with small sample sizes and further complicates clinical trials by requiring much broader recruitment.

DEVELOPMENTAL CONCERNS

An additional concern involves the lack of solid information describing the developmental course of the prodromal phase. As now conceptualized, this period can last from weeks to years *(44,67)* and involves a complex developmental picture. The extent to which there are common stages of the prodrome (e.g., initial emergence of attenuated negative symptoms followed by attenuated positive symptoms; *see* discussion of RAP program) is unknown. Such information would contribute to an understanding of when treatment should be most profitably initiated, what type of treatment is most appropriate for each prodromal phase, and the criteria most helpful in evaluating short-term treatment effects (i.e., in delaying or preventing the progression of illness). We propose that naturalistic research can help to clarify such unresolved descriptive issues. This approach provides the framework for the Hillside RAP program, which is the focus of the balance of this chapter.

THE HILLSIDE RAP PROGRAM

In contrast with most of the other prodromal studies now in progress, the Hillside RAP program integrates components of both genetic high-risk research and traditional clinical trials. This results from our notion that treatment programs developed for patients who already have schizophrenia may not be appropriate for prodromal adolescents who are "at risk" for developing psychosis. In particular, the way to measure outcome (i.e., the successfulness of the intervention) is unclear in a high-risk as opposed to an affected patient population. To a

considerable extent, this difficulty results from the absence of well-established conversion rates. If the rate of conversion from the prodrome to schizophrenia without treatment has not yet been established, how can it be determined that an intervention is effective in reducing the number of new cases (incidence) of the disorder? Although some researchers have suggested conversion rates in placebo controls will provide this information, this solution has been judged highly flawed, at least at this stage of prodromal research (65).

To address the lack of base-rate information, the RAP program was designed to collect fundamental clinical data before moving on to clinical trials. We have incorporated a prospective research methodology borrowed from traditional genetic high-risk studies (18,25), many of which involve long-term naturalistic follow-up of at-risk adolescents with no attempt to intervene (e.g., for over 30 years in the NYHRP). The RAP program is following this strategy by obtaining baseline data and then naturalistically following all research participants. However, unlike the earlier GHR adolescents who were typically symptom-free, all RAP adolescents are symptomatic. Ethically, they require treatment. We have therefore incorporated the clinic component into our naturalistic framework. There is no attempt to do any sort of systematic treatment intervention or to conduct prevention trials in the current RAP program. Instead, we are tracking the course the prodrome follows when treated as it would be in the community. We expect this approach both the naturalistic follow-up and the naturalistic treatment program   to provide much of the basic information now missing from the field: for example, to establish the validity of the diagnostic criteria now in use, the heterogeneity of the prodrome, its developmental course, and the best type of medication that should be used at particular stages of the prodrome.

DESCRIPTION OF PROGRAM

The RAP Program is jointly sponsored by the Zucker Hillside Hospital and Schneider Children's Hospital of the North Shore. Long Island Jewish Health System in New York. The program consists of a clinic treating prodromal adolescents and a number of related high-risk and naturalistic treatment research projects. The RAP clinic provides treatment to all adolescents between the ages of 12 and 18 (in some cases, however, participants may be as old as 22 when admitted) who meet the entry criteria, whether or not they participate in any of the research protocols. Following admission into the clinic, patients and their families are asked if they are interested in enrolling in the research program. Approximately 80% of the patients undergoing treatment in the RAP clinic participate in research (with full consent obtained from parents and assent from minors).

The primary research project involves baseline neurocognitive, biobehavioral, and clinical assessments and then at least 3 years of prospective follow-up of all

participants (whether or not they continue to receive treatment in the RAP clinic). For research purposes, we refer to this as the clinical high-risk (CHR) project because the label "prodrome," widely used clinically, implies a greater likelihood of developing subsequent illness than can currently be definitively established. In fact, as discussed previously, establishing the validity of prodromal indicators has not yet been solidly established and is one of the major goals of the RAP research program. It is therefore not inevitable, or even highly likely, that youngsters displaying these symptoms will develop schizophrenia. At present, they are assumed, at most, to be at elevated risk for illness, but the extent of that elevation is another major issue to be resolved by the RAP program. We therefore label all adolescents displaying signs and symptoms considered prodromal to be at CHR (to differentiate them from individuals at genetic high risk [GHR]) in the balance of this chapter.

The RAP program has recently completed a 3-year pilot phase, which was conducted from 1998 to 2001. In addition to establishing the baseline characteristics of prodromal adolescents, the pilot study included a treatment component that followed the naturalistic strategy mentioned earlier. As a result, RAP clinic psychiatrists treated presenting symptoms as they would in their routine practice. It should be noted here that the RAP clinic is independent of the research program. Treating psychiatrists in the clinic do not attend research meetings and are not familiar with the hypotheses.

INITIAL SELECTION STRATEGY

In the absence of well-defined selection criteria matching our theoretical orientation, the initial recruitment strategy during the pilot phase was to circulate two lists of putative prodromal indicators to the intake staff at Schneider Children's Hospital. These lists were derived to a great extent from the early work of McGorry and collaborators (e.g., refs. *44,68*). The first list consisted of nonspecific, attenuated negative characteristics of schizophrenia considered to be early features of the prodrome and included depressed mood, social withdrawal, deterioration in functioning, impairment in personal hygiene, reduced concentration reduced motivation, sleep disturbance, and anxiety. The second list, directed at the more positive schizophrenia-like symptoms assumed to appear later in the prodrome, included suspiciousness, peculiar behavior, inappropriate affect, vague or overelaborate speech, circumstantial speech, odd beliefs, magical thinking, and unusual perceptual experiences. Intake staff were asked to refer any adolescents displaying these symptoms   no specific combination or minimum number were required. Each referral was considered by the RAP intake team on an individual basis. As mentioned, on acceptance into the clinic, each individual and his or her family was fully informed about the research protocol and invited to participate.

RAP Diagnostic Model

Treatment Sample Phase I (n=54)

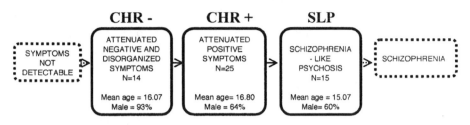

Fig. 3. RAP program developmental clinical model.

CLINICAL SUBGROUPS

A total of 81 patients (mean 15.7 years; age range, 11. 22 years; 70% male) completed baseline testing at the close of the Phase I pilot study. Based on analyses of the structured and semistructured Axis I K-SADS (Schedule for Affective Disorders and Schizophrenia for School-Age Children. Epidemiologic Version, 5th Revision; ref. *69*), Axis II SIDP-IV (Structured Interview for *DSM–IV* Personality; ref. *70*), and prodromal symptoms (SIPS: Structured Interview for Prodromal Symptoms, and SOPS: Schedule of Prodromal Symptoms; ref. *38*) interviews, a rigorous algorithm was developed to divide the sample into three clinical subgroups. (*See* ref. *70a* for more details.) We consider these subgroups to reflect prodromal symptoms as they naturally occur in the types of clinical populations commonly treated by health care professionals (especially psychiatrists and pediatricians).

As shown in the Fig. 3, going from left to right, subgroup 1 represents the least severe RAP patients who are characterized by either attenuated negative symptoms (in particular, social withdrawal/isolation and school withdrawal/difficulties) or attenuated disorganized symptoms (such as odd behaviors or poor grooming and hygiene). We refer to this group as the CHR– (characterized by attenuated negative/disorganized symptoms) subgroup. We hypothesize that these subjects may represent the earliest stage at which true prodromal subjects can be identified.

The middle subgroup consists of patients considered to be prodromal according to criteria similar to those developed by McGlashan *(38)* and by McGorry and colleagues *(68)*. We refer to this group as the CHR+ (attenuated positive symptoms). We consider these patients to be in the later stages of the prodrome because they display attenuated positive symptoms in addition to the attenuated negative features they share with the CHR– subgroup.

Somewhat to our surprise, when assessed in depth, just over one-third of the patients accepted into the RAP clinic displayed symptoms that had already reached psychotic intensity. These individuals, represented by the third box, do not meet criteria for schizophrenia because they lack the number or chronicity of psychotic symptoms or the level of functional deterioration required. This group is labeled as having a Schizophrenia-Like Psychosis (SLP). It should be noted that although the SLPs are no longer within the strictly defined prodromal phase of illness, they are nevertheless of considerable interest within the RAP program. From a clinical perspective, the primary goal for both the CHR– and CHR+ subgroups is to prevent the onset of psychosis. Although it is too late to prevent psychosis in the SLPs, it is still possible to prevent chronic schizophrenia, which is the major goal for SLPs in the RAP intervention program.

From a research perspective, all three of these subgroups seem to formulate a coherent developmental model that is fully compatible with the neurodevelopmental hypothesis of schizophrenia. Based on this model, we hypothesize that schizophrenia typically involves a premorbid period (not included in the model), during which only subtle neurocognitive deficits are evident, followed by a phase of relatively mild, nonspecific, and attenuated negative symptoms. The early prodromal stage then flows into the mid- to late prodromal phases, when positive symptoms begin to emerge in attenuated form. Untreated, these attenuated symptoms will gradually increase in intensity until they reach the level of psychosis, and, eventually, full-blown schizophrenia will take hold.

Of the 81 youngsters who completed the pilot study, 54 had complete medication data and at least 6 months of clinical follow-up. We refer to these 54 adolescents as the Phase I Treatment Sample (TS-I). As shown in Fig. 3, of the 54 youths, 14 were in the CHR– group, 25 in the CHR+ group, and 15 were SLPs. Across the three subgroups, the mean age ranged from 15 to 16 years. There were also more males than females in all three groups, but the difference is particular marked in the CHR– group, where 93% of that group was male. Given the small sample size, continued recruitment into this subgroup will be necessary before it can be determined whether the sex disparity reflects an ascertainment bias or is legitimate, and, if so, what the implications are for diagnosis and outcome.

PRELIMINARY CLINICAL OUTCOME

Deterioration in the RAP program refers to a symptom exacerbation of sufficient magnitude to require a shift in clinical subgroup (i.e., from CHR– to CHR+ or from CHR+ to SLP, etc.; *see* ref. *70a* for more details). Conversion indicates that criteria for *DSM–IV* schizophrenia or schizoaffective disorder were met. By the end of Phase I, 12 of the 54 youngsters had deteriorated (22%), with 9 (17%) converting to schizophrenia. Broken down by subgroup, in the CHR– group, two subjects (14%) deteriorated, with one converting to schizophrenia (7%). Among

CHR+ subjects, there was a similar pattern, with four subjects deteriorating (16%) and two of these four converting (8%). For the SLP subgroup, however, as might be expected, the risk was far higher, with 6 of the 15 adolescents deteriorating (40%) and all 6 converting to schizophrenia.

These early findings are of interest from a number of perspectives. To begin with, the initial pattern of deterioration/conversion displayed by RAP adolescents is not fully consistent with our expectations or with the literature. We had predicted that the CHR– group, characterized by nonspecific symptoms and therefore likely to have the highest false-positive rate, would show the lowest number of deterioration/conversions. We further expected that the CHR+ group would have conversion in the 40% range, consistent with the literature, and that the rate would be higher still for subjects in the SLP group.

Contrary to expectation, rates of both conversion and deterioration were equivalent for the two prodromal groups (i.e., CHR– and CHR+) and, for both, were considerably lower than those reported in the literature. About 15% of each of the two prodromal subgroups deteriorated during follow-up, which was, on average, just under a year. Approximately 7.5% of each group converted to schizophrenia. As expected, conversions within the SLP subgroup were much higher than the other two, but, to our surprise, were very similar to the 40% rate reported by other prodromal research groups.

Several factors must be considered when evaluating these data. First, our subjects are considerably younger than the prodromal samples studied by both McGorry and McGlashan, who tend to focus on young adults *(2,40)*. As a result, it may be that interventions begun in adolescence are particularly effective in delaying/eliminating symptoms. Alternatively, it may require several more years before the full symptom picture emerges, with symptom stability during adolescence not fully indicative of later outcome. These competing possibilities can only be resolved with long-term follow-up, which is currently under way.

Differences in diagnostic procedures must also be taken into account, in that in some cases it is possible that subjects considered prodromal by other diagnostic systems are classified within the SLP group according to our algorithm (*see* ref. *70a* for more details). This possibility is supported by the similarity in conversion rates between the SLP subgroup and the more general prodromal populations reported by McGlashan, McGorry, and their colleagues *(2,40)*. In the end, though, the possibility must also be recognized that our sample simply has a considerably lower conversion rate to schizophrenia than was initially expected.

This early outcome data also provides some very preliminary support for the developmental model. The 12 adolescents who deteriorated tended to follow a lawful progression, moving from box to box in the model. This suggests that for at least some schizophrenia patients, the developmental sequences proposed in the model may hold.

EARLY TREATMENT FINDINGS

As noted earlier, throughout the RAP pilot study, treatment was provided within a naturalistic framework. Treating clinicians were asked to provide medication as they would in standard practice and were given no guidelines or special instructions. The primary goals of our naturalistic treatment study were to: (a) determine the way prodromal symptoms are typically treated, and (b) evaluate the extent to which standard care is effective in reducing or eliminating prodromal signs and symptoms.

How Are Prodromal Symptoms Typically Treated?

The primary initial observation resulting from the pilot data addressing this question is that there is a very high level of polypharmacy. About 75% of the prodromal adolescents participating in the CHR study received some type of pharmacotherapy, with a considerable majority of these subjects treated with more than one class of medication. The categories most commonly used included SGAPs, antidepressants (ADs mainly selective serotonin reuptake inhibitors [SSRIs]), mood stabilizers, anxiolytics, and, in some cases, stimulants. A number of factors undoubtedly lead to this high level of polypharmacy in standard care: for example, pressure from the parents and the schools for immediate symptom reduction, lack of criteria for clear physician choice of medication, and, probably most important, the high rate of comorbidity.

COMORBIDITY

Many of the prodromal adolescents participating in the CHR project meet criteria for other AXIS I disorders, in many cases more than one. The five most common comorbid illnesses are: attention deficit/hyperactivity disorder (ADHD), oppositional defiant disorder, major depression, social phobia, and obsessive-compulsive disorder (OCD). Aside from leading to considerable polypharmacy, this pattern raises a number of diagnostic issues. Of primary interest is the extent to which the additional diagnoses represent independent illnesses with distinct etiologies or, in fact, are actually risk factors for schizophrenia that, on the surface, appear to be other childhood disorders. For example, the attention deficits that are major determinants of the ADHD diagnosis are also well-established childhood precursors of schizophrenia. As a result, ADHD diagnoses in CHR subjects are always somewhat suspect. The high rate of comorbidity should also be evaluated in regard to the population rates of both illnesses. If the two are etiologically independent, ADHD would not be expected in prodromal subjects to any greater extent than in the general population. Yet the rate is considerably higher (>25%).

Similar concerns can be raised about the other disorders. For example, depression has been reported by Hafner and colleagues (e.g., refs. *31,71*) to be the earliest of the prodromal symptoms. Thus, are the depressive symptoms that are ever-

present among prodromal adolescents risk factors or is depression a frequent co-morbid disorder? Similarly, obsessions during adolescence either can signal the presence of OCD or can be the forerunners of delusions. Whether these and other symptoms indicate comorbid disorders or are risk factors for later schizophrenia (or early symptom presentations) is important from a treatment perspective. True comorbidity suggests polypharmacy might be the preferred strategy.

How Effective Is Standard Care in Treating Prodromal Symptoms?

Again, some preliminary answers to this question were provided by the pilot data obtained from the Phase I treatment sample. Outcome for each of the three groups was assessed as a function of type of medication. Medication was divided into ADs (with or without mood stabilizers and/or anxiolytics), SGAPs (with or without any of the other medications), or no medication.

It should first be emphasized that across all three subgroups, the majority of patients treated in the RAP program (77%) have either stabilized or improved clinically, suggesting that early intervention may indeed be beneficial. It should also be noted that all individuals treated within the RAP clinic receive some form of psychosocial treatment: group, family, or individual therapy and in most cases, some combination of these three.

Outcome as a function of medication (or no medication) was quite different for each of the three groups, as follows:

CHR– Subgroup

As would be expected, the highest proportion of subjects not treated pharma-cologically were in the CHR– group (close to 40%). In nearly all cases, this was because psychosocial treatment, frequently group therapy focusing on social skills, was considered the preferred treatment. Only in a handful of cases was medication prescribed but not taken. Approximately 40% of the remaining CHR– subjects were treated with ADs (primarily SSRIs). This finding was in no way surprising, given the nonspecific nature of the attenuated negative and disorganized symp-toms characterizing this group. The balance of the CHR– group (around 20%) received SGAP treatment.

With respect to outcome after 1 year of treatment, most of the adolescents in the CHR– group remained clinically stable over the follow-up period. Neither psychosocial therapy or pharmacological treatment with either ADs or SGAPs resulted in major improvement in any notable number of CHR– subjects. There was also a minimum of deterioration, but in the few cases where this occurred, it was related to nonadherence with prescribed medication.

CHR+ Subgroup

Because this subgroup most closely corresponds with the "prodromal" diag-nosis as it is typically described in the literature, our expectation was that SGAPs

would be the optimal treatment. In fact, about one-half of the subjects in the CHR+ subgroup were treated with SGAPs (mainly olanzapine or risperidone). What was surprising in light of the presence of mild positive symptoms, however, was the high rate of AD treatment: about 30% of CHR+ adolescents received ADs, often in combination with anxiolytics or mood stabilizers, but not SGAPs. Moreover, there was considerable clinical improvement among CHR+ subjects over the follow-up period, but the rate of improvement was comparable whether they were treated with ADs or with SGAPs. The other result of special note was that the balance of the CHR+ group (about one-quarter) were off medication throughout the follow-up period. However, in contrast with CHR– subjects, in most cases this reflected nonadherence to prescribed treatment. Nearly all of the CHR+ individuals who deteriorated/converted were considered nonadherent.

SLP Subgroup

All individuals within the SLP subgroup were prescribed an SGAP to treat the psychotic symptoms already in evidence. However, nearly one-third of the SLP subjects were largely nonadherent. This, as it turns out, had considerable implications for outcome. Of those individuals who were relatively adherent, 100% improved clinically. Of those adolescents in the SLP group who deteriorated i.e., converted to schizophrenia   all were nonadherent to medication.

Treatment Conclusions

The preliminary data collected over the pilot phase of the RAP study suggest that early pharmacological intervention is very helpful in controlling prodromal symptoms. However, these findings challenge the assumption that antipsychotics are necessarily best for first-line treatment, since ADs had a comparably beneficial effect in adolescents free of psychotic symptoms (i.e., CHR– and CHR+ subjects). However, it must be kept in mind that these findings were generated by an open-label, naturalistic study without random assignment. Controlled research is necessary to conclusively establish the comparability of antipsychotics and antidepressants in prepsychosis intervention. Possibly the strongest finding, however, is the effect of adherence with medication. Refusal to take prescribed medication   regardless of whether antidepressant or antipsychotic   appears to be the strongest risk factor for subsequent conversion to schizophrenia. The reasons for this effect will be a subject of intense scrutiny throughout the newly initiated 5-year RAP research program.

SUMMARY

Interest in pharmacological intervention prior to the onset of psychosis has undergone a dramatic increase over the past 5 years. This has largely resulted from three research developments: (a) widespread acceptance of the neurodevelopmental view of schizophrenia; (b) emerging evidence that the earlier treatment is initiated

after onset of psychosis, the better the outcome   leading to the assumption that treatment initiated before onset will be better still; and (c) by the introduction of the SGAPs, with reduced side effects. The convergence of these three events has generated considerable enthusiasm for the possibility that schizophrenia can be prevented. However, a great deal of preliminary groundwork is necessary to support full-scale prevention trials. Information about the predictive validity of the prodromal indicators currently in use is essential. In addition, considerable research is needed to address such questions as the developmental course and heterogeneity of the prodrome, the identity of the causal risk factors that should be targeted for early treatment, and what the treatment should consist of. The Hillside RAP program is a naturalistic, prospective clinical high-risk study that has been designed to answer many of these preliminary questions.

Preliminary findings from Phase I, the initial 3-year pilot phase of the RAP program, have highlighted three major areas of particular interest. First, a cluster of early features   including cognitive, academic, and social impairments, along with disorganized/odd behaviors (referred to as the CASID cluster)   appear to precede positive symptoms and may constitute a core risk profile for schizophrenia and related spectrum disorders. Second, medications other than antipsychotics may be effective for treating early prodromal symptoms, challenging the widely held hypothesis that antipsychotics should always be the first-line preventive treatment. Third, the single most important risk factor for clinical deterioration identified during the early treatment phase is noncompliance with medication, whether antipsychotics or antidepressants. Based on these and other findings, it can be concluded that the prodrome is a developmentally complex phase of schizophrenia, and that considerably more research is essential for optimizing intervention programs.

REFERENCES

1. McGlashan TH, Miller TJ, Woods SW. Pre-onset detection and intervention research in schizophrenia psychoses: current estimates of benefit and risk. Schizophr Bull 2001; 27:563..570.
2. McGorry PD, Yung A, Phillips L. Ethics and early intervention in psychosis: keeping up the pace and staying in step. Schizophr Res 2001; 51:17..29.
3. Heinssen RK, Perkins DO, Appelbaum PS, Fenton WS. Informed consent in early psychosis research: National Institute of Mental Health Workshop, November 15, 2000. Schizophr Bull 2001; 27:571..583.
4. Kraepelin E. Dementia Praecox and Paraphrenia. Huntington, NY: Robert Krieger, 1919/1971.
5. Degreef G, Ashtari M, Bogerts B, et al. Volumes of ventricular system subdivisions measured from magnetic resonance images in first-episode schizophrenic patients. Arch Gen Psychiatry 1992; 49:531..537.
6. DeLisi LE, Strikzke P, Riordan H, et al. The timing of brain morphological changes in schizophrenia and their relationship to clinical outcome. Biol Psychiatry 1992; 31:241..254.
7. Hoffman WF, Ballard L, Turner EH, Casey DE. Three-year follow-up of older schizophrenics: extrapyramidal syndromes, psychiatric symptoms, and ventricular brain ratio. Biol Psychiatry 1991; 30:913..926.

8. Cannon TD. Abnormalities of brain structure and function in schizophrenia: implications for etiology and pathophysiology. Ann Med 1996; 28:533.539.
9. DeLisi LE. A prospective follow-up study of brain morphology and cognition in first-episode schizophrenic patients: preliminary findings. Biol Psychiatry 1995; 38:349.360.
10. Kovelman JA, Scheibel AB. A neurohistological correlate of schizophrenia. Biol Psychiatry 1984; 19:1601..1621.
11. Jakob H, Beckmann H. Prenatal developmental disturbances in the limbic allocortex in schizophrenics. J Neural Transm 1986; 65:303..326.
12. Falkai P, Bogerts B, Rozumek M. Limbic pathology in schizophrenia: the entorhinal region a morphometric study. Biol Psychiatry 1988; 24:515.521.
13. Cannon TD. Genetic and perinatal influences in the etiology of schizophrenia: a neurodevelopmental model. In: Lenzenweger M, Dworkin RH, eds. Origins and Development of Schizophrenia: Advances in Experimental Psychopathology. Washington, DC: APA, 1998, pp. 67.92.
14. Berman I, Merson A, Viegner B, Losonczy MF, Pappas D, Green AI. Obsessions and compulsions as a distinct cluster if symptoms in schizophrenia: a neurological study. J Nerv Ment Dis 1998; 186:150..156.
15. Kraemer HC, Stice E, Kazdin A, Offord D, Kupfer DJ. How do risk factors work together? Mediators, moderators, and independent, overlapping and proxy risk factors. Am J Psychiatry 2001; 158:848.856.
16. Cornblatt B, Obuchowski M, Roberts S, Pollack S, Erlenmeyer-Kimling L. Cognitive and behavioral precursors of schizophrenia. Dev Psychopathol 1999; 11:487.508.
17. Cornblatt BA, Keilp JG. Impaired attention, genetics, and the pathophysiology of schizophrenia. Schizophr Bull 1994; 20:31.46.
18. Cornblatt B, Obuchowski M. Update of high-risk research: 1987..1997. Int Rev Psychiatry 1997; 9:437.447.
19. Cannon TD, Mednick SA. The schizophrenia high-risk project in Copenhagen: three decades of progress. Acta Psychiatr Scand Suppl 1993; 370:33.47.
20. Erlenmeyer-Kimling L, Rock D, Roberts SA, et al. Attention, memory, and motor skills as childhood predictors of schizophrenia-related psychoses: the New York High-Risk Project. Am J Psychiatry 2000; 157:1416..1422.
21. Cornblatt B, Erlenmeyer-Kimling L. Global attentional deviance as a marker of risk for schizophrenia: specificity and predictive validity. J Abnorm Psychol 1985; 94:470.486.
22. Cornblatt BA, Lenzenweger MF, Dworkin RH, Erlenmeyer-Kimling L. Childhood attentional dysfunctions predict social deficits in unaffected adults at risk for schizophrenia. Br J Psychiatry 1992; 161:59..64.
23. Cornblatt B, Obuchowski M, Schnur D, O'Brien JD. Hillside study of risk and early detection in schizophrenia. Br J Psychiatry Suppl 1998; 172:26..32.
24. Erlenmeyer-Kimling L, Cornblatt B. Attentional measures in a study of children at high-risk for schizophrenia. J Psychiatric Res 1978; 14:93..98.
25. Erlenmeyer-Kimling L, Cornblatt B. High-risk research in schizophrenia: a summary of what has been learned. J Psychiatric Res 1987; 21:401.411.
26. Erlenmeyer-Kimling L, Cornblatt BA. Summary of attentional findings in the New York high-risk project. J Psychiatric Res 1992; 26:405.426.
27. Cornblatt B, Obuchowski M, Schnur DB, O'Brien JD. Attentional and clinical symptoms in schizophrenia. Psychiatr Q 1997; 68:343.359.
28. Green MF, Kern RS, Braff DL, Mintz J. Neurocognitive deficits and functional outcome in schizophrenia: are we measuring the "right stuff"? Schizophr Bull 2000; 26:119..136.
29. Green MF. What are the functional consequences of neurocognitive deficits in schizophrenia. Am J Psychiatry 1996; 153:321.330.

30. Davidson M, Reichenberg A, Rabinowitz J, Weiser M, Kaplan Z, Mark M. Behavioral and intellectual markers for schizophrenia in apparently healthy male adolescents. Am J Psychiatry 1999; 156:1328..1335.
31. Hafner H, Loffler W, Maurer K, Hambrecht M, Heiden W. Depression, negative symptoms, social stagnation and social decline in the early course of schizophrenia. Acta Psychiatr Scand 1999; 100:105..118.
32. Jones PB, Done DJ. From birth to onset: a developmental perspective of schizophrenia in two national birth cohorts. In: Keshavan MS, Murray RM, eds. Neurodevelopment and Adult Psychopathology. Cambridge, England: Cambridge University Press, 1997, pp. 119..136.
33. Cannon TD, Rosso IM, Bearden CE, Sanchez LE, Hadley T. A prospective cohort study of neurodevelopmental processes in the genesis and schizophrenia. Dev Psychopathol 1999; 11: 467..485.
34. Tsuang MT, Stone WS, Faraone SV. Towards the prevention of schizophrenia. Biol Psychiatry 2000; 48:349..356.
35. Cornblatt BA. From the prediction of schizophrenia to prevention: New York High Risk Project to the Hillside Recognition and Prevention (RAP) Program. Am J Med Genet 2002; 114:956..966.
36. Tsuang MT, Stone WS, Faraone SV. Towards reformulating the diagnosis of schizophrenia. Am J Psychiatry 2000; 147:1041..1050.
37. Tsuang MT. Genes, environment, and mental health wellness. Am J Psychiatry 2000; 157: 489..491.
38. Miller TJ, McGlashan TH, Woods SW, et al. Symptom assessment in schizophrenic prodromal states. Psychiatr Q 1999; 70:273..287.
39. McGlashan TH, Johannessen JO. Early detection and intervention with schizophrenia: rationale. Schizophr Bull 1996; 22:201..222.
40. McGlashan TH, Miller TJ, Woods SW, Hoffman RE, Davidson L. Instrument for the assessment of prodromal symptoms and states. In: Miller TJ, ed. Early Intervention in Psychotic Disorders. Dordrecht, Netherlands: Kluwer Academic, 2001, pp. 135..149.
41. McGorry PD, McKenzie D, Jackson HJ, Waddell F, Curry C. Can we improve the diagnostic efficiency and predictive power of prodromal symptoms for schizophrenia? Schizophr Res 2000; 42:91..100.
42. McGorry PD, McKenzie D, Jackson HJ, Waddell F, Curry C. Can we improve the diagnostic efficiency and predictive power of prodromal symptoms for schizophrenia? Schizophr Res 2000; 42:91..100.
43. Yung AR, McGorry PD, McFaarlane CA, Jackson HJ, Patton GC, Rakkar A. Monitoring and care of young people at incipient risk of psychosis. Schizophr Bull 1996; 22:283..304.
44. Yung AR, McGorry PD. The prodromal phase of first-episode psychosis: past and current conceptualizations. Schizophr Bull 1996; 22:363..370.
45. Phillips L, Yung A, Hearn N, McFarlane C, Hallgren M, McGorry PD. Preventative mental health care: accessing the target population. Aust N Z J Psychiatry 1999; 33:241..247.
46. Yung AR, Phillips LJ, McGorry PD, et al. Prediction of psychosis. A step towards indicated prevention of schizophrenia. Br J Psychiatry Suppl 1998; 172:14..20.
47. Haas GL, Garratt LS, Sweeney JA. Delay to first antipsychotic medication in schizophrenia: impact on symptomatology and clinical course of illness. J Psychiatric Res 1998; 32:151..159.
48. Larsen TK, Johannessen JO, Opjordsmoen S. First-episode schizophrenia with long duration of untreated psychosis. Br J Psychiatry Suppl 1998; 172:45..52.
49. Loebel AD, Lieberman JA, Alvir JMJ, Mayerhoff DI, Geisler SH, Szymanski DO. Duration of psychosis and outcome in first-episode schizophrenia. Am J Psychiatry 1992; 149:1183..1188.
50. Lieberman JA, Koreen AR. Neurochemistry and neuroendocrinology of schizophrenia: a selective review. Schizophr Bull 1993; 19:371..429.

51. McGlashan TH. Early detection and intervention in schizophrenia: research. Schizophr Bull 1996; 22:327..345.
52. Wyatt RJ. Neuroleptics and the natural course of schizophrenia. Schizophr Bull 1991; 17:325..351.
53. Wyatt RJ, Green MF, Tuma AH. Long-term morbidity associated with delayed treatment of first admission schizophrenic patients: a re-analysis of the Camarillo State Hospital data. Psychol Med 1997; 27:261..268.
54. Lieberman JA. Is schizophrenia a neurodegenerative disorder? A clinical and neurobiological perspective. Biol Psychiatry 1999; 46:729..739.
55. McGlashan TH. Duration of untreated psychosis in first-episode schizophrenia: marker or determinant of course. Biol Psychiatry 1999; 46:899..907.
56. Craig TJ, Bromet EJ, Fennig S, Tanenberg-Karant M, Lavelle J, Galambos N. Is there an association between duration of untreated psychosis and 24-month clinical outcome in a first-admission series. Am J Psychiatry 2000; 157:60..66.
57. Ho BC, Andreasen NC, Flaum M, Nopoulos P, Miller D. Untreated initial psychosis: its relation to quality of life and symptom remission in first-episode schizophrenia. Am J Psychiatry 2000; 157:808..815.
58. Robinson D, Woerner MG, Alvir JM, et al. Predictors of relapse following response from a first episode of schizophrenia or schizoaffective disorder. Arch Gen Psychiatry 1999; 56:241..247.
59. Harvey PD, Davidson M. Schizophrenia: course over the lifetime. In: Davis KL, Charney DS, Coyle JT, Nemeroff CB, eds. Neuropsychopharmacology: The Fifth Generation of Progress. Nashville, TN: American College of Neuropsychopharmacology, 2002, pp. 641..656.
60. Verdoux H, Liraud F, Bergey C, Assens F, Abalan F, van Os J. Is the association between duration of untreated psychosis and outcome confounded? A two year follow-up study of first-admitted patients. Schizophr Res 2001; 49:2331..2241.
61. McGorry PD, Edwards. Response to: "the prevention of schizophrenia: what interventions are safe and effective?" (letter). Schizophr Bull 2002; 28:177..180.
62. DeQuardo JR, Tandon R. Do atypical antipsychotic medications favorably alter the long-term course of schizophrenia? J Psychiatric Res 1998; 32:229..242.
63. Brown CS, Markowitz JS, Moore TR, Parker NG. Atypical antipsychotics: Part II: adverse effects, drug interactions, and costs. Ann Pharmacother 1999; 33:210..217.
64. Lewis R. Typical and atypical antipsychotics in adolescent schizophrenia: efficacy, tolerability, and differential sensitivity to extrapyramidal symptoms. Can J Psychiatry 1998; 43:596..604.
65. Cornblatt B, Lencz T, Kane JM. Treatment of the schizophrenia prodrome: is it presently ethical? Schizophr Res 2001; 51:31..38.
66. Venables PH. Schizotypal status as a developmental stage in studies of risk for schizophrenia. In: Raine A, Lencz T, Mednick SA, eds. Schizotypal Personality. Cambridge: Cambridge University Press, 1995:107..131.
67. Beiser M, Erickson D, Fleming J, Iacono W. Establishing the onset of psychotic illness. Am J Psychiatry 1993; 150:1349..1354.
68. McGorry PD, McFarlane C, Patton GC, et al. The prevalence of prodromal features of schizophrenia in adolescence: a preliminary survey. Acta Psychiatr Scand 1995; 92:241..249.
69. Orvaschel H, Puig-Antich J. Schedule for Affective Disorders and Schizophrenia for School-Age Children. Epidemiologic Version. Pittsburgh, PA: Western Psychiatric, 1994.
70. Pfohl B, Blum N, Zimmerman M. Structured Interview for DSM-IV Personality (SIDP-IV). Arlington VA: American Psychiatric Press, 1995.
70a. Lencz T, Smith CW, Auther A, Correll CU, Cornblatt BA. The assessment of "prodromal schizophrenia": unresolved issues and future directions. Schizophr Bull, in press.
71. Hafner H, Nowotny B. Epidemiology of early-onset schizophrenia. Eur Arch Psychiatry Clin Neurosci 1995; 245:80..92.

15 The Role of Genetic Counseling

Debby W. Tsuang, MD, MSc,
Stephen V. Faraone, PhD,
and Ming T. Tsuang, MD, PhD, DSc

INTRODUCTION

There are many misunderstandings about the heritability of psychiatric disorders. Like other medical conditions, some are inherited, whereas others are not. The primary purpose of genetic counseling is to educate those seeking counseling (the *consultands*) and to provide them with relevant information concerning the disorder of interest. The recent explosive growth in the number of genes identified through the efforts of the National Institutes of Health has been exciting. Currently, more than 9000 diseases are known to be genetic *(1)*, and diagnostic tests are available for more than 800 genetic disorders (GeneTest www.genetests.org). However, new knowledge can and often does create new confusion. As more genetic tests become available, the use and interpretation of those tests will become critical.

PURPOSES OF PSYCHIATRIC GENETIC COUNSELING

Many misconceptions concerning human genetics and psychiatric illness exist. Genetic counseling can alleviate some of the following common but mistaken beliefs:

1. *If a disorder is genetic, it inevitably occurs in those who carry the harmful gene(s).* The influence of genetic factors in psychiatric disorders is highly variable. Because most psychiatric disorders are believed to be *multifactorial* disorders, there are important environmental and genetic interactions in their expression *(2)*. Even in single-gene disorders such as Huntington's disease (HD), there is considerable variability in age of onset *(3)*, suggesting that other environmental or genetic modifiers exist. Therefore, even if susceptible gene(s) are present, individuals may not necessarily develop the disorder.

From: *Early Clinical Intervention and Prevention in Schizophrenia*
Edited by: W. S. Stone, S. V. Faraone, and M. T. Tsuang © Humana Press Inc., Totowa, NJ

2. *If a disorder is genetic, it is untreatable.* Although many heritable conditions are currently untreatable, most psychiatric disorders are treatable and may be preventable. For example, individuals with a positive family history of schizophrenia may not develop the disorder if they avoid substance abuse and/or dependence (in particular stimulant use). As susceptibility genes for psychiatric conditions are discovered, there may be many diagnostic and treatment implications. One hypothetical scenario includes close monitoring of individuals at high genetic risk for developing bipolar affective disorder. If and when symptoms occur in these individuals, early interventions may include treatment with mood stabilizers, which may improve the prognosis. Other alternatives yet to be explored include the benefits and burdens of presymptomatic treatment.

3. *Genetic counseling is associated with eugenics and genocide.* This belief, based on memories of Nazi Germany, is unjustifiable. Contemporary genetic counseling is nondirective, with emphasis on individual autonomy and decision-making abilities. The goal of genetic counseling is to disseminate current scientific knowledge concerning the disorder at hand and to help the consultand(s) in making the best possible decision. The overall purpose of genetic counseling is to reduce the burden of human suffering.

CLINICAL APPLICATIONS

As the advances in molecular genetic technology and bioinformatics have rapidly made genetic information much more accessible, mental health practitioners in turn need to provide this type of information to their patients. In order to do this, we need to understand the principles of genetic counseling, potential future use of genetic testing, and some of the associated social and ethical implications of providing these genetic tests.

Stages of Genetic Counseling

Genetic counseling is a time-consuming process, but it can be extremely valuable in educating those at risk for specific disorders. In the following, we outline the guidelines that ensure the best outcome *(4,5)*.

STAGE 1: CONFIRM THE DIAGNOSIS

The first step in genetic counseling is to verify the diagnosis of the disorder in the consultand or his or her family members. This implies obtaining a cross-sectional clinical picture as well as a longitudinal history of the consultand's lifetime psychiatric history. A thorough review of medical and psychiatric records is necessary. Counseling under a mistaken diagnosis is far more dangerous than counseling without the knowledge of the underlying mode of transmission. Certain disorders that appear the same may, in fact, be genetically heterogeneous. On

the other hand, patients with the same genetic liability may have variable clinical pictures (*variable expressivity*). The importance of obtaining accurate medical and/or psychiatric diagnoses before proceeding with counseling is critical.

STAGE 2: OBTAIN FAMILY HISTORY

The second stage of genetic counseling involves diagramming a complete and accurate pedigree. Standard symbols used in pedigree construction can be found in Bennett et al. *(6)*. A pedigree should include first-degree relatives (parents and siblings), second-degree relatives (aunts and uncles), and third-degree relatives (grandparents and cousins). The family history should include such information as parental age, ethnic background, childhood behavioral or learning problems, abortions, stillbirths, other deaths, and the ages, sexes, and health of living siblings and children. Sensitive information such as *nonpaternity* (when the designated father is not the biological father) as well as pregnancy termination may arise during this time. Confidentiality, even from other family members, should be assured.

Structured diagnostic instruments for establishing psychiatric diagnoses in relatives are also available (e.g., the Family Interview for Genetic Studies [FIGS]; *[7]*). The clinician may need to obtain additional information from other relatives who are more knowledgeable about the affected individuals. In addition, it is important to obtain consent to conduct a thorough review of medical and/or psychiatric records to best establish psychiatric diagnoses. Underreporting of relatives' psychiatric diagnosis is more common than overreporting *(8)*. Collecting such information is time consuming but this step is crucial prior to proceeding with subsequent steps.

STAGE 3: ASSESS THE RECURRENCE RISK

The inheritance pattern of a disorder is often established by careful examination of the pedigree. For a review of the various modes of inheritance, interested readers should refer to Chapter 4 in *The Genetics of Mental Disorders (2)*. Each family should be categorized into one of three basic groups: (a) an isolated case within a family, (b) a complex family with psychiatric disorders in several family members (either the same or different disorders), or (c) a specific subtype of the psychiatric disorder that may have an underlying genetic mechanism already identified (e.g., psychosis in HD *[9]* or learning disability in velocardiofacial syndrome *[10]*).

Most patients with psychiatric disorders are *sporadic* cases (with no other affected relatives). On the other hand, patients may have relatives with other psychiatric diagnoses, which may have some (or no) shared genetic liability. In either case, the counselor should refer to established risk estimates for discussion regarding recurrence risks for specific disorders. For example, the population base rate for alcoholism is estimated to be 14% for men and 3% for women. However, the

risk increases if there are other affected relatives. The risk to a female sibling of an individual with alcoholism is 5%, but the risk increases to 17% if a parent is also alcoholic. A table reviewing risk estimates for major psychiatric disorders can be found in Chapter 6 of *The Genetics of Mental Disorders (2)*.

STAGE 4: EVALUATION OF THE CONSULTAND

Before conveying genetic risks and burdens to the consultand, the clinician must assess the intellectual and emotional capacity of the individual. Does the consultand seek information only, or does she or he also seek advice? Do they want advice for themselves or for their relatives? Consultands may be anxious, stressed, or depressed because of their underlying concerns about their genetic risks. Additional psychiatric assessment and treatment may be necessary following the initial appointment. Humane and effective genetic counseling must account for the emotional and intellectual capacity of the consultand(s).

STAGE 5: EVALUATING BURDENS AND BENEFITS

After communicating the recurrence risks, clinicians must help consultands integrate the information with the perceived burdens and benefits. This can be a complex process. Disorders that have a high recurrence risk but that can be stabilized by treatment and do not significantly affect quality of life may be viewed as more acceptable than disorders that have a low recurrence risk but dramatically reduce quality of life. For example, a 5% risk of a chronically debilitating psychiatric disorder may be perceived as more of a burden than a 50% risk of a relatively mild episodic and treatable disorder. Because there are many combinations of risks, benefits, and burdens, genetic counseling must include an in-depth evaluation of the consultands' values, expectations, and future plans. Genetic counseling must provide a means of quantifying the tolerability of the risk for a disorder in the context of its risks and benefits.

STAGE 6: FORMING A PLAN OF ACTION

Once the risk.benefit ratio is understood, the clinician is responsible for assisting the consultand in forming a reasonable plan of action for deciding among his or her options. For conditions that have known genetic etiology (e.g., velocardiofacial syndrome), cytogenetic tests may be indicated *(11)*. Because susceptibility genes for most psychiatric disorders remain unknown, presymptomatic and prenatal testing are not currently options. In the future, once molecular genetic studies identify susceptibility genes for a condition, genetic testing may become an option in risk assessments. The responsibility of the counselor is to help consultands make informed decisions that are the most consistent with their cultural, religious, and ethnic background.

As genetic tests for psychiatric disorders become available, experience from other genetic disorders for which presymptomatic testing is available will be appli-

cable. For example, genetic testing in HD suggests that testing in children should only be done in symptomatic individuals *(12)*. For childhood-onset disorder, presymptomatic testing may be indicated only if clinical benefits (disease prevention) clearly outweigh the individual's autonomy and the risk of any intervention. Current guidelines in genetic testing of HD will be discussed in the following section.

STAGE 7: FOLLOW-UP

The final stage of genetic counseling is follow-up. Typically, this involves writing a follow-up letter that summarizes the discussion. This letter serves as a written summary for the consultand and it provides him or her information to share with interested relatives. A follow-up appointment allows continued assessment of the consultand's understanding of the previous discussions. In addition, it gives the clinician an opportunity to obtain more information, such as subsequent births or news of other family members becoming affected. If the mode of inheritance becomes apparent with the additional information, then recurrence risks can be revised for greater accuracy.

GENETIC TESTING

We briefly review the types of genetic testing currently available. Understanding the uses of genetic tests will help to provide the knowledge base for future psychiatric genetic testing.

Use of Direct DNA Testing

DNA-based tests provide the latest technology to test for the presence or absence of genetic disorders *(13)*. These techniques involve direct examination of the DNA molecule itself (e.g., determination of the number of trinucleotide CAG repeats in the HD gene). Other currently available genetic tests include those that detect gene products (e.g., for phenylketonuria) and those that detect chromosomal changes by microscopic examination of fluorescent chromosomes (e.g., fluorescent *in situ* hybridization techniques to determine if the genetic condition associated with velocardiofacial syndrome exists). Genetic tests are used for several reasons, including the following:

Presymptomatic testing for prediction of adult-onset disorders.
Diagnostic testing for symptomatic individuals.
Prenatal diagnostic testing.
Newborn screening.
Carrier screening.
Forensic testing.

We elaborate on presymptomatic and diagnostic testing in the following section. Readers interested in the clinical application of the other types of testing should

refer to Robinson and Linden *(14)* for additional information. For many asymptomatic individuals with family members with a heritable disorder (*at risk*), the availability of direct DNA-based genetic tests provides the opportunity to relieve uncertainty and to better plan for the future. This is called *presymptomatic* testing. For treatable disorders such as some genetic forms of cancer, a positive test can also lead to a higher level of surveillance as well as intervention to reduce risk *(15)*.

Diagnostic testing in *symptomatic* individuals exists for other adult-onset disorders. For example, genetic testing is available for a small subset of individuals with early-onset Alzheimer's disease (AD). At present, there are three known genes that have been identified in rare autosomal-dominant, early-onset families *(16)*, one gene on chromosome 1 [presenilin-2 (PS-2)], 14 [presenilin-1 (PS-1)], and 21 [amyloid precursor protein (APP)]. Although these three genes account for less than 5% of all cases with AD, the discovery of these mutations has been important in AD research. Testing for PS-1 is available on a commercial basis; whereas PS-2 and APP mutation screening are available only on a research basis and are applicable only to individuals in these high-risk families.

The genetics of "garden-variety" or late-onset (>65 years old) AD appear to be more complicated. It is likely that the majority of these AD cases are attributable to multifactorial inheritance *(17)*. One important genetic risk factor that has been identified is the apolipoprotein E gene on chromosome 19 *(18)*. It is apparent that carriers of ε4 homozygotes are at high risk for developing AD. However, these individuals constitute only 2.3% of the general population and 15.20% of AD patients. Since about 35.50% of all AD patients do not have an inherited ε4 allele, other etiologic factors must play a role *(19)*. Some have advocated APOE testing as an adjunct in the diagnostic evaluation of demented persons *(20)*. However, a community-based study suggests that such testing only adds a small amount of additional certainty to diagnostic accuracy *(21)*. The American Society of Human Genetics *(22)* and the American Academy of Neurology *(23)* do not recommend APOE testing in routine clinical diagnosis or in predictive testing because of its limited sensitivity and specificity *(22)*.

The discovery of new disease genes occurs weekly. However, it may take months or years (a) to confirm the initial results, (b) to determine the frequency of these mutations in clinical samples, and (c) to determine the *penetrance* (probability of developing the disease given the presence of a mutation) of these genes. This delay in genetic test availability can be very frustrating for at-risk families. In addition, different mutations (in the same or different gene) can result in disease. Conversely, the same mutation may manifest differently in some families. Commercially available tests for some disorders do not screen for all know mutations. Therefore, "negative" results from commercial tests that screen for the most common mutations may be misleading. In addition, most psychiatric disorders are presumed to be *complex* genetic disorders. Therefore, future susceptibility gene-

tic testing is likely to be much more difficult to interpret and may lead to more uncertainty. Clinicians need to understand the genetics of the disorder and competently interpret the specific laboratory tests in order to avoid false reassurances.

GUIDELINES IN PRESYMPTOMATIC TESTING

The major guidelines in presymptomatic testing of adult-onset disorders arose from the experience in genetic testing of HD *(24)*, which include:

1. *Individuals must consent to predictive testing and undergo pretest counseling to learn about predictive testing.* Members from the same family may be very strongly for or against testing. Unlike other laboratory test results, genetic testing results not only affect the individual being tested but may have an impact on other family members as well. Unintentional risk alteration may occur when disclosing test results concerning one family member because those results could also reveal the risk status of another family member. For example, the presence of the HD mutation in a symptomatic child would indicate that one of his or her parents also has the mutation. Thus, testing in *asymptomatic* children is considered inappropriate, even if requested by parents or other authorities, such as adoption agencies *(12)*.
2. *Decisions to test and test results must be strictly confidential.* The question of who has the right to know has become problematic in the era of presymptomatic testing. Employers and insurance companies could consider it a right to know test results and in the foreseeable future, health, life, and disability insurance companies may require genetic screening results prior to insurance approval. The ethical dilemmas associated with future predictive testing for psychiatric disorders are complicated and problematic *(25)*.
3. *Pretesting follow-up must be conducted.* Serious concerns have been raised as to whether it was ethical to offer predictive testing for a disease for which no treatments are available. When the HD gene test first became available, genetic counselors conducted primarily pre- and immediate posttesting follow-ups. There has been increasing concern that individuals who undergo HD presymptomatic testing may be at higher risk for catastrophic outcomes such as suicide attempts or completions compared to the general population. These adverse outcomes also occurred in individuals who received the news of their *decreased* risk *(26,27)*. In general, persons undergoing presymptomatic testing should be followed long-term. Additional ongoing psychological and/or psychiatric support may be necessary, even in individuals who are informed of their decreased risk.

Guidelines that pertain to HD may not be applicable to future genetic testing in psychiatric disorders because HD most likely represents the simplest model of human genetic conditions. In addition, very few DNA tests are as highly accurate and specific as the HD gene test (99% accurate) *(28)*. These differences may have a bearing on genetic counseling:

1. *HD is inherited in an autosomal dominant fashion.* Therefore, an offspring is at 50% risk for inheriting the gene. This is in contrast to most psychiatric conditions, which are believed to be multifactorial.
2. *Almost all individuals who carry the HD gene develop the disease by age 80.* In other words, it is completely penetrant. In contrast, most psychiatric disorders are thought to be incompletely penetrant, and the presence of clinical symptoms may be modified by many genetic and environmental factors.
3. *The mutation in HD is the same in all affected individuals.* The mutation in HD has been identified as an elongation of a genetic sequence. Individuals with an elongation greater than 38 CAG repeats in the HD gene are considered to have inherited the mutated gene. There is only one mutation in HD. In contrast, there are currently more than 50 different known mutations in the presenilin-1 gene on chromosome 14 that may result in one type of familial AD. Unless a specific mutation is known in an affected family member, "negative" results (or absence of a known mutation) could provide a false sense of security and in fact be misleading.
4. *There are very few sporadic cases of HD.* In the majority of HD families, there are other affected family members. In most psychiatric conditions, the absence of other affected family members is the rule rather than the exception. Many uncertainties involving genetic testing in common medical disorders exists *(29)*. Guidelines will evolve as susceptibility genes for psychiatric disorders are identified.

On a positive note, presymptomatic genetic testing of psychiatric conditions has many advantages over testing of neurodegenerative conditions like HD. HD is an incurable disease with midlife onset, whereas schizophrenia and bipolar affective disorder have onset in early adulthood, and effective treatments are available for both disorders. In this light, presymptomatic identification of genetically susceptible individuals may allow early intervention in high-risk individuals.

ETHICAL ISSUES IN GENETIC TESTING

The guiding principle assuring the ethics of clinical practice and genetics research (including genetic testing) is the idea of informed consent *(30)*. Consultands choosing genetic testing for clinical reasons should be thoroughly informed about the risks and benefits of the procedure and should always have the option to terminate at any time. The counselor should inform them of the potential social consequences related to genetic testing *(31)*. Unlike other laboratory tests, genetic tests may reveal information about other family members, who may or may not want access to this information. Part of the consent process should routinely describe the confidentiality of the data, although clinicians must inform the consultand that the genetic information is part of his or her medical records. Stigmatization may occur as a consequence of test results. Therefore, consultands should review their life and disability insurance prior to proceeding with testing as insurance companies have argued that they should have access to presymptomatic genetic testing results.

To compute the costs of health and life insurance, actuaries take into account many factors known to predict disease and death. Few people can argue with the rationale that smokers should pay higher health insurance premiums than non-smokers. However, does a parallel argument justify the use of genetic information? Theoretically, insurance companies should have access to genetic profiles of individuals who apply for insurance. Should those who are at genetic risk for untreatable or chronically debilitating disorders pay higher insurance premiums? Should insurance companies have the right to deny coverage to those individuals? There are no clear or easy answers.

In the same vein, employers may want access to employee records regarding medical information including risk factors for genetic disorders. Because potential at-risk employees could eventually both become less productive and incur higher health care costs, there is justifiable concern that discrimination based on genetic testing results could occur. Although this might seem unjustifiable, proponents have argued that employers should have access to genetic test results for disorders that may impair judgement and job performance in occupations involving the safety of the general public (e.g., commercial airline pilots, physicians).

The implications of the Human Genome Project *(32)* have not escaped the attention of legislators. In the United States, several states have already enacted genetic privacy laws *(31)*. In general, these laws limit the use of genetic data by insurance companies. However, the idea that genetic data should be treated differently from other clinical data has been hotly debated *(33)*. Society can anticipate the ethical and legal debates concerning genetic testing to continue. Indeed, those debates are likely to intensify as the capability to predict behavioral and personality traits become a reality. Society will then have to decide the ethical, legal, and social implications of this new knowledge. Much work is ongoing as part of the Ethical, Legal, and Social Initiative (ELSI) of the Human Genome Project. For additional information, see the ELSI web site (http:/www.ornl.gov/hgmis/elsi/elsi.html). The Human Genome Project will undoubtedly provide an abundance of data for researchers to identify genes that contribute to human behavioral disorders. With a "working draft" of the human genome in hand, identification of genes relevant to human behavior continues. The implications of genetic data for diagnosing and treating psychiatric disorders remain speculative.

As psychiatric genetics enter into the gene identification era, more clinical applications will be discovered. Identification of susceptibility genes for psychiatric disorders will facilitate the eventual discovery of disease pathways, which in turn will both impact risk assessment as well as increase our understanding of underlying pathogenesis (Fig. 1). Genetic analysis of at-risk individuals will provide more precise risk estimates in genetic counseling *(34,35)*. However, guidelines for genetic testing for complex disorders such as psychiatric conditions have not yet been established. In addition, determination of genetic polymorphisms

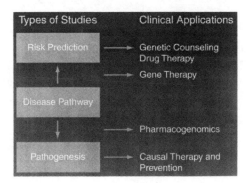

Fig. 1

could provide a basis for individualized pharmacotherapy in the treatment of psychiatric disorders *(36,37)*. Furthermore, as Fig. 1 indicates, identification of disease-causing genes will likely lead to new treatment strategies, including gene therapy *(38)*. Although many obstacles currently exist in the successful clinical application of this strategy, future advances are likely. Other advances include the design of new pharmaceutical agents to target specific molecules and/or proteins associated with the disease process. Pharmacogenomics is the study of drug response at the human genome level and is applicable to new-drug development *(39)*. Finally, our understanding of the underlying pathogenesis will eventually lead to treatments that will not only reverse the disease process, but will also ultimately prevent the development of disease.

Indeed, the future of psychiatric genetics will answer many scientific and clinical questions. However, it will also raise many new questions about the legal, ethical, and social implications of these answers. Although medical and scientific advances may bring many gifts to society in the form of new knowledge, as clinicians and scientists, we should approach this new knowledge with caution as one of these gifts could be a Pandora's box.

INTERNET RESOURCES

Multiple on-line resources are available on the Internet. New discoveries take place at a rapid pace and are updated on a regular basis on-line. Updated information about genetic disorders can be obtained at the following web sites: GeneTests (http://www.genetests.org), GeneClinics (http://www.geneclinics.org), and OMIM (On-line Mendelian Inheritance in Man, Johns Hopkins University (www.ncbi. nlm.nih.gov/omim). The first site provides information about currently available DNA diagnostic tests; the second provides up-to-date clinical information about a variety of disorders; OMIM provides updated clinical descriptions and molecular advances for most known heritable conditions.

CONCLUSION

As the Human Genome Project facilitates the rapid sequencing of the human genome, genes contributing to common psychiatric disorders will soon be discovered. It is uncertain how rapidly these findings will take place. However, the identification of susceptibility genes for psychiatric conditions will change the practice of clinical psychiatry *(40)*. Knowledge of an individual's genetic risks raises many ethical, moral, social, and legal issues. Clinicians must be equipped to face these new and exciting changes with great optimism as well as caution.

REFERENCES

1. McKusick V. Online Mendelian Inheritance in Man (OMIM). Baltimore, MD: Johns Hopkins University, 2001.
2. Faraone S, Tsuang M, Tsuang M. Genetics of Mental Disorders: A Guide for Students, Clinicians and Researchers. New York: Guilford, 1999.
3. Harper P. Huntington's Disease. San Diego: Harcourt, 1996.
4. Tsuang MT. Genetic counseling for psychiatric patients and their families. Am J Psychiatry 1978; 135:1465..1475.
5. Harper P. Practical Genetic Counseling. London: Reed Educational and Professional, 1998.
6. Bennett RL, Steinhaus KA, Uhrich SB, et al. Recommendations for standardized human pedigree nomenclature. Pedigree Standardization Task Force of the National Society of Genetic Counselors. Am J Hum Genet 1995; 56:745..752.
7. Initiative NG. Family Interview for Genetic Studies. Rockville: National Institute of Mental Health, 1992.
8. Andreasen NC, Rice J, Endicott J, Reich T, Coryell W. The family history approach to diagnosis. How useful is it? Arch Gen Psychiatry 1986; 43:421..429.
9. Tsuang D, Almqvist EW, Lipe H, et al. Familial aggregation of psychotic symptoms in Huntington's disease. Am J Psychiatry 2000; 157:1955..1959.
10. Bassett AS, Hodgkinson K, Chow EW, Correia S, Scutt LE, Weksberg R. 22q11 deletion syndrome in adults with schizophrenia. Am J Med Genet 1998; 81:328..337.
11. Hodgkinson KA, Murphy J, O'Neill S, Brzustowicz L, Bassett AS. Genetic counselling for schizophrenia in the era of molecular genetics. Can J Psychiatry 2001; 46:123..130.
12. Points to consider: ethical, legal, and psychosocial implications of genetic testing in children and adolescents. American Society of Human Genetics Board of Directors, American College of Medical Genetics Board of Directors. Am J Hum Genet 1995; 57:1233..1241.
13. Bird TD, Bennett RL. Why do DNA testing? Practical and ethical implications of new neurogenetic tests. Ann Neurol 1995; 38:141..146.
14. Robinson A, Linden M. Applied Genetics. Clinical Genetics Handbook. Boston: Blackwell Scientific, 1993:3..68.
15. Devilee P. BRCA1 and BRCA2 testing: weighing the demand against the benefits. Am J Hum Genet 1999; 64:943..948.
16. Levy-Lahad E, Tsuang D, Bird T. Recent advances in the genetics of Alzheimer's disease. J Geriatr Psychiatry Neurol 1998; 11:42..54.
17. Schellenberg GD, D'Souza I, Poorkaj P. The genetics of Alzheimer's disease. Curr Psychiatry Rep 2000; 2:158..164.
18. Corder EH, Lannfelt L, Bogdanovic N, Fratiglioni L, Mori H. The role of APOE polymorphisms in late-onset dementias. Cell Mol Life Sci 1998; 54:928..934.
19. Farrer LA, Cupples LA, Haines JL, et al. Effects of age, sex, and ethnicity on the association between apolipoprotein E genotype and Alzheimer disease. A meta-analysis. APOE and Alzheimer Disease Meta Analysis Consortium. JAMA 1997; 278:1349..1356.

20. Roses AD, Saunders AM. Apolipoprotein E genotyping as a diagnostic adjunct for Alzheimer's disease. Int Psychogeriatr 1997; 9:277..288; discussion 317..321.
21. Tsuang D, Larson EB, Bowen J, et al. The utility of apolipoprotein E genotyping in the diagnosis of Alzheimer disease in a community-based case series. Arch Neurol 1999; 56:1489..1495.
22. Statement on use of apolipoprotein E testing for Alzheimer disease. American College of Medical Genetics/American Society of Human Genetics Working Group on ApoE and Alzheimer disease. JAMA 1995; 274:1627..1629.
23. Knopman D, DeKosky S, Cummings J, et al. Practice parameter: diagnosis of dementia (an evidence-based review). Report of the Quality Standards Subcommittee of the American Academy of Neurology. Neurology 2001; 56:1143..1153.
24. Guidelines for the molecular genetics predictive test in Huntington's disease. International Huntington Association (IHA) and the World Federation of Neurology (WFN) Research Group on Huntington's Chorea. Neurology 1994; 44:1533..1536.
25. Farmer AE, Owen MJ, McGuffin P. Bioethics and genetic research in psychiatry. Br J Psychiatry 2000; 176:105..108.
26. Almqvist EW, Bloch M, Brinkman R, Craufurd D, Hayden MR. A worldwide assessment of the frequency of suicide, suicide attempts, or psychiatric hospitalization after predictive testing for Huntington disease. Am J Hum Genet 1999; 64:1293..1304.
27. Bird TD. Outrageous fortune: the risk of suicide in genetic testing for Huntington disease. Am J Hum Genet 1999; 64:1289..1292.
28. Welch HG, Burke W. Uncertainties in genetic testing for chronic disease. JAMA 1998; 280:1525..1527.
29. Kremer B, Goldberg P, Andrew SE, et al. A worldwide study of the Huntington's disease mutation. The sensitivity and specificity of measuring CAG repeats. N Engl J Med 1994; 330:1401…1406.
30. Sharpe NF. Informed consent and Huntington disease: a model for communication. Am J Med Genet 1994; 50:239..246.
31. Hall M, Rich S. Genetic privacy laws and patients' fear of discrimination by health insurers: the view from genetic counselors. J Law Med Ethics 2000; 28:245..257.
32. Collins FS. Shattuck lecture   medical and societal consequences of the Human Genome Project. N Engl J Med 1999; 341:28..37.
33. Kapp M. Physicians' legal duties regarding the use of genetic tests to predict and diagnose Alzheimer disease. J Leg Med 2000; 21:445..475.
34. McConnell L, Goldstein M. The application of medical decision analysis to genetic testing: an introduction. Genet Test 1999; 3:65..70.
35. McConnell L, Koenig B, Greely H, Raffin T, Members of the Alzheimer Disease Working Group of the Stanford Program in Genomics E, and Society. Genetic testing and Alzheimer Disease: Recommendations of the Stanford Program in Genomics, Ethics, and Society. Genet Test 1999; 3:3..12.
36. Masellis M, Basile VS, Ozdemir V, Meltzer HY, Macciardi FM, Kennedy JL. Pharmacogenetics of antipsychotic treatment: lessons learned from clozapine. Biol Psychiatry 2000; 47:252..266.
37. Cichon S, Nothen MM, Rietschel M, Propping P. Pharmacogenetics of schizophrenia. Am J Med Genet 2000; 97:98..106.
38. Lesch KP. Gene transfer to the brain: emerging therapeutic strategy in psychiatry? Biol Psychiatry 1999; 45:247..253.
39. Kawanishi Y, Tachikawa H, Suzuki T. Pharmacogenomics and schizophrenia. Eur J Pharmacol 2000; 410:227..241.
40. Rutter M, Plomin R. Opportunities for psychiatry from genetic findings. Br J Psychiatry 1997; 171:209..219.

IV CHALLENGES FOR THE NEAR FUTURE

16 The Biology of Schizotaxia

William S. Stone, PhD,
Stephen J. Glatt, PhD,
and Stephen V. Faraone, PhD

Like schizophrenia, the biology of schizotaxia is multidimensional and complex. This point is underscored by other chapters in this volume that focus on abnormalities in brain imaging and sensory gating in nonpsychotic relatives of patients with schizophrenia. The goal of this chapter is to look forward by considering representative neurochemical areas in schizophrenia that are promising but largely unexplored in schizotaxia. In each case, a brief overview of a neurochemical disturbance in schizophrenia is outlined, followed by the relevance of that area for schizotaxia research. Four representative examples are reviewed, starting with abnormalities in dopamine (DA) neurotransmission. As a point of reference, each of the other areas discussed includes a discussion of how it relates to DA function. Moreover, each succeeding area of discussion focuses on a system that has a broader effect on brain function than does DA alone, to highlight the importance of multiple levels of analysis for an understanding of schizotaxia. After the discussion of DA, glutamate (GLU) function in schizophrenia is reviewed, followed by consideration of abnormalities in membrane phospholipids, and then a discussion of glucose regulation. We begin with a brief introduction to the neurochemistry of schizophrenia.

OVERVIEW
OF THE NEUROCHEMISTRY OF SCHIZOPHRENIA

One strategy for exploring the biology of schizotaxia is to determine whether biological deficits in schizophrenia occur to some degree in patients with schizotaxia. Although this approach is logical, the challenge is daunting. Decades of research show a plethora of neurochemical abnormalities, many of which are

From: *Early Clinical Intervention and Prevention in Schizophrenia*
Edited by: W. S. Stone, S. V. Faraone, and M. T. Tsuang © Humana Press Inc., Totowa, NJ

related to each other, are relatively distal to their underlying etiology, and/or are consequences rather than causes of dysfunction. Moreover, as most cases of schizophrenia likely reflect the influence of multiple genetic and adverse environmental factors (1), it is also likely that etiological factors are at least somewhat heterogeneous across families, populations, and geographical locales.

Nevertheless, decades of research on neurochemical features of schizophrenia show consistencies as well as differences. In this section, some of the major candidate systems are identified, and discussed briefly. In the following sections, selected candidate mechanisms for a neurochemical biology of schizotaxia are considered. The most extensively investigated abnormalities in schizophrenia include demonstrations of dysfunctional neurotransmission in the central nervous system. Neurotransmitters frequently implicated include monoamines such as norepinephrine (NE), serotonin (5-HT), and DA; the excitatory amino acid, GLU; γ-aminobutyric acid (GABA) and acetylcholine (ACh); along with various neuropeptides, phospholipids, prostaglandins, hormones, and measures of neuronal integrity (2–6). The three monoamines are structurally similar and are related metabolically; for example, DA is converted to NE by DA-β-hydroxylase (DBH), and all three neurotransmitters are metabolized, in part, by a common enzyme, monoamine-oxidase-A (MAO-A). Regardless of which neurotransmitter is considered for an etiological role in schizophrenia, most neurotransmitter-based theories of the disorder attempt to explain schizophrenic symptoms as a consequence of abnormalities in transmitter distribution, metabolism, release, receptor interaction, or genetic control. The discussion of relatively specific abnormalities in schizophrenia begins with DA neurotransmission.

DOPAMINE

The most widely tested neurotransmitter hypotheses of schizophrenia involve abnormalities in DA transmission. The "DA hypothesis" was derived partly from observations that typical antipsychotic medications blocked DA D_2 receptors, whereas indirect DA agonists like amphetamine produced psychotic symptoms that in some ways resembled schizophrenia (7). Based on these and subsequent observations, the most basic form of the DA hypothesis is that schizophrenia results from dopaminergic hyperactivity (8). Later formulations focused on relationships between hyperactivity in mesolimbic DA neurons and dopaminergic hypoactivity in the prefrontal cortex (9–11). Activity in the different pathways is related. For example, changes in one pathway may result from abnormal transmission in the other (11,12). Although the status of the DA hypothesis remains inconclusive, owing partly to a paucity of direct evidence for DA hyperactivity in unmedicated patients with schizophrenia (8,13), there is considerable evidence

(the details of which are beyond the scope of this chapter) for both cortical dopaminergic hypoactivity and subcortical dopaminergic hyperactivity.

Much of the recent evidence in favor of the DA hypothesis actually extends beyond the role of DA alone. For example, the relationship between mesolimbic and mesocortical DA projections is modulated by other neurotransmitters, such as GLU *(14)*. In fact, the proposed balance between the activities of these two DA systems is at least modulated, if not regulated, by multiple neurochemical systems. Examples of these systems are described in more detail later.

In theory, any aspect of DA synthesis, release, metabolism, or receptor function that is impaired in schizophrenia is a potential target for study in schizotaxia. One area of interest involves DA metabolism. For example, DBH levels are often lower in patients with schizophrenia than they are in control subjects *(15–17)*. Some data also demonstrate lower plasma levels of homovanillic acid (HVA), a DA metabolite, in patients with schizophrenia *(18)*, although elevated levels were also reported among the most severely psychotic patients *(19)*. These findings are difficult to reconcile, but may be indicative of relative imbalances between distributed DA systems rather than a global hyperactivity of all DA neurons. Moreover, chronic treatments may cause regionally specific tolerance to HVA increases *(20)*, and different methods of sampling (e.g., plasma vs cerebrospinal fluid [CSF]) may produce different results.

A clearer picture does emerge from studies of HVA levels in CSF among schizophrenic patients. Initially, these levels were found to correlate with levels of anxiety and agitation among schizophrenic patients *(21)*; later, the severity of psychosis (and more generally, positive symptoms) in schizophrenia was correlated with HVA levels in CSF *(22)*. The ability of antipsychotic medications to reduce CSF levels of HVA in schizophrenic patients is consistent with the dopamine hypothesis *(23)*. Interestingly, Sedvall and Wode-Helgodt *(24)* observed elevated levels of HVA in the CSF of schizophrenic patients, but only in those individuals with a positive family history of the disorder.

Whereas elevated levels of HVA in schizophrenia are associated primarily with positive symptoms, relatively few studies reported the inverse relationship with negative symptoms (i.e., higher levels of negative symptoms associated with lower levels of HVA *[25]*). It is relevant for the study of schizotaxia, however, that decreased plasma and CSF concentrations of HVA are found not only in chronic schizophrenic patients *(23)*, but also in drug-free and first-episode patients *(26)*. In this context, it is of interest that Waldo et al. *(27)* found lower levels of HVA in relatives of patients with schizophrenia. Amin et al. *(28)* also found lower circulating levels of HVA in the first-degree relatives of schizophrenic patients compared to a normal control group. Since the major peripheral factors that could affect plasma HVA were well controlled in this study, the observed changes can

be attributed to decreased brain DA activity with some confidence. Of further note, plasma HVA was inversely correlated with negative symptom scores and positively correlated with attenuated positive symptom scores on the Positive and Negative Syndrome Scale (PANSS). The inverse correlation with negative symptom scores (i.e., higher levels of negative symptoms associated with lower levels of HVA) is particularly consistent with the diagnostic criterion of elevated negative symptoms in schizotaxia. It is still to be determined whether individuals who meet diagnostic criteria for schizotaxia also show reductions or other abnormalities in HVA.

GLUTAMATE

The diversity of clinical symptoms in schizophrenia, the likely multifactorial polygenic mode of inheritance in most cases (1), the multiple neurochemical actions of atypical antipsychotic medications such as clozapine (4,6), and the demonstration of numerous neurochemical and morphological abnormalities all underlie the view that multiple biochemical deficits contribute to the etiology of schizophrenia. As noted previously, many candidates may contribute to abnormalities in neurotransmission. This section focuses on GLU as a representative example, for three reasons. First, its role in schizophrenia has attracted considerable attention in recent years (29–33). Second, the ubiquity of GLU as an excitatory neurotransmitter in the central nervous system (13) makes it a suitable candidate to interact with and modulate numerous other transmitter systems, including DA. Third, some manipulations of glutamatergic function in schizophrenia reduce negative symptoms and improve cognition (34,35), which is particularly relevant to the diagnostic criteria for schizotaxia.

Several lines of evidence relate GLU dysfunction to schizophrenia. One of these involves the neuroanatomical and functional relationships between GLU and DA. N-methyl-D-aspartate (NMDA) and α-amino-3-hydroxy-5-methyl-4-isoxasolepropionate (AMPA) GLU receptors in the nucleus accumbens modulate dopaminergic neurons in the nucleus accumbens and in the frontal cortex (36–40). The effect of GLU input differs, however, at the two sites. The presence of presynaptic GLU receptors on DA neurons in the frontal cortex facilitates DA function, whereas it inhibits reuptake and facilitates release in the nucleus accumbens (40). This means that agents that interfere with GLU transmission would facilitate cortical dopaminergic hypoactivity and subcortical hyperactivity, which is consistent with the DA hypothesis of schizophrenia.

In fact, NMDA GLU antagonists, such as phencyclidine (PCP), produce symptoms of psychosis that resemble schizophrenia in nonschizophrenic individuals, and exacerbate symptoms in patients with schizophrenia (5,33). PCP acts by binding to a site on the NMDA receptor that blocks the influx of calcium and other cations through the ion channel, which then blocks receptor function. The effects

of NMDA antagonists are not limited to positive symptoms. PCP and ketamine (another drug in this class), for example, produce negative symptoms and cognitive deficits in verbal declarative memory and executive functions in normal subjects *(33,41–44)*. Administration of ketamine to patients with schizophrenia worsens psychotic symptoms and neuropsychological deficits *(44–46)*.

It follows that if GLU antagonists exacerbate symptoms of schizophrenia, then GLU agonists might produce clinical improvements. Although the administration of GLU itself is not feasible *(6,33)*, other types of agonist approaches are available. The NMDA receptor is unique in that it involves multiple recognition sites to function. In addition to a site for GLU and other agonists, a strychnine-insensitive glycine modulatory site must also be filled *(13)*. This latter site may be filled by either glycine, D-serine, or, exogenously, by D-cycloserine. Several studies showed reductions in negative symptoms and/or cognitive impairments when either glycine or D-cycloserine was added to antipsychotic medications *(33,35)*. Other approaches are based on the possibility that NMDA receptor blockade results in enhanced transmission at other sites, such as AMPA receptors, or altered transmission in other transmitter systems, such as GABA. These effects might themselves contribute to the production of schizophrenia-like symptoms *(47,48)*. Consistent with this possibility, lamotrigine, which reduces GLU release, also reduced positive and negative symptoms and cognitive deficits, in normal subjects who received ketamine *(47)*. Lamotrigine alone produced no clinical and few cognitive effects.

The data linking GLU abnormalities to schizophrenia are particularly relevant to the study of schizotaxia for at least two reasons. First, they show that GLU may be associated with the production of negative symptoms and neuropsychological deficits, which comprise the core clinical symptoms of schizotaxia. Second, they show that negative symptoms and neuropsychological deficits may be attenuated with treatments that facilitate transmission at NMDA receptors. This type of treatment response in individuals with schizotaxia would thus provide evidence for the validity of the syndrome.

NIACIN SKIN FLUSH
AND THE MEMBRANE PHOSPHOLIPID HYPOTHESIS

This section focuses on a broader level of hypothesized deficit in schizophrenia than is represented by either the DA or GLU hypotheses. Although DA and GLU, along with their receptors, are present in neurons that are organized both neuroanatomically and neurophysiologically to exert broad influence on neural activity, the deficit reflected by the niacin skin flush response (abnormalities in the constituents of neuronal membranes) is one that potentially affects all nerve cells. This possibility, along with the likelihood that alterations in cell membranes

affect DA and GLU neurotransmission, among other transmitter systems, accounts for its inclusion here.

When healthy individuals ingest nicotinic acid in adequate doses, a global vaso-dilatory response results. Since 1980, however, a growing number of reports have shown since 1980, that some patients with schizophrenia show an attenuated skin flush in response to niacin administration *(49–51)*. Unlike the DA and GLU hypotheses, the phenomenon and its proposed underlying mechanism of action received less attention. In part this reflected controversy about methods of admin-istration and the specificity of the finding. In general, topical administration to the skin is tolerated better and is more sensitive than oral administration *(51,52)*. Using topical administration, for example, Ward et al. *(52)* showed that 83% of a schizophrenic sample, but only 23% of a normal sample, showed a zero or min-imal response to niacin. These figures translated into a sensitivity of 83% and a specificity of 77% for distinguishing patients with schizophrenia from normal controls. Puri et al. *(53)* demonstrated 78% sensitivity and 65% specificity for dif-ferentiating schizophrenic from normal subjects. Messamore et al. *(54)* used a discriminant function analysis to classify 74% of patients and 81% of controls correctly. A comparison of schizophrenic, bipolar, and normal controls (using oral administration of niacin) showed that 43% of schizophrenic patients did not show vasodilation, compared to 6% of bipolar patients and 0% of control subjects.

Thus, the attenuated response occurs somewhat reliably in some, but not all, patients with schizophrenia. Although the response is interesting, its inclusion in this chapter is more a result of its putative underlying mechanisms of action, which involve altered phospholipids. Phospholipids are important because they are major components of neuronal membranes, and are involved in the growth of neurons, in synaptogenesis, and in pruning *(55)*. As part of the subcellular envi-ronment, they contribute to the structure and function of receptors, ion channels, and enzymes, and their metabolism provides substrates that serve as second mes-sengers that regulate or modulate signal transduction and intraneuronal processes *(50)*. Consequently, membrane lipids and fatty acids modulate binding affinities for multiple neurotransmitters, including DA, NMDA, and ACh. Deficits in par-ticular fatty acids result in increased 5-HT2 and decreased DA D2 receptors in the frontal cortex of rats (reviewed in Fenton et al., ref. *50*). Omega-3 deficits also impair learning and behavioral performance in a manner consistent with impaired prefrontal DA transmission *(56)*. Moreover, elevated levels of DA activity may indirectly inhibit the synthesis of essential fatty acids such as arachidonic acid (*see* later discussion), and the subsequent synthesis of several prostaglandins *(57)*.

The phospholipid membrane hypothesis is related to the structure of phospho-lipids (see reviews in refs. *3,50*). Briefly, they consist of a three-carbon backbone, with acyl groups derived from fatty acids in the 1- and 2-positions, and a phos-

phate-containing head group in the 3-position. Phospholipids vary according to the specific acyl groups attached to the 1- and the 2-positions, and according to which molecule is attached to the phosphate group (e.g., choline, ethanolamine, serine, or inositol). Brain phospholipids are rich in unsaturated fatty acids, which are "essential fatty acids" (EFAs), meaning they cannot be manufactured by the body. Two main EFAs are the "n-3" (or omega-3, derived from linolenic acid) and the "n-6" (or omega-6, derived from linoleic acid) chains, which refer to an unsaturated bond at the third or sixth carbon atom (from the methyl end). Multiple enzymes are involved in phospholipid synthesis *(3,50)*; phospholipases A_2 and C are particularly involved in both synthesis and degradation in the brain *(3)*.

Common EFAs in the brain include docosahexaenoic acid (DHA) and eicosapentaenoic acid (EPA) in the n-3 series, and arachidonic acid (AA) and dihomo-gamma-linolenic acid (DGLA) in the n-6 series *(3,50,55,58)*. EFAs also serve as precursor molecules for other significant neurochemicals in the brain, including prostaglandins and eicosanoids. A basic form of the phospholipid membrane hypothesis is that schizophrenia occurs secondary to an abnormal loss of DHA, EPA, AA, and DGLA, possibly because of overactivity of phospholipase or other functionally similar enzymes. Although a detailed review of the membrane phospholipid hypothesis, and the evidence that supports or disconfirms it, is beyond the scope of this discussion, a few points particularly relevant to schizotaxia should be stressed. First, and consistent with the membrane hypothesis, AA and DHA levels are lower in patients with schizophrenia who do not show the niacin skin flush reaction *(52,59)*. Because vasodilatory prostaglandins are important mediators of the skin flush response, and are derived from AA *(54)*, the niacin response may reflect a specific instance of the more general view that lowered inflammatory reactivity is associated with schizophrenia. In fact, observations between fever and clinical remission in schizophrenic patients, and a relative resistance to pain, arthritis, and other inflammatory conditions in schizophrenia, comprise several of the early clinical observations that underlie the membrane hypothesis *(3,50)*.

Second, reduced levels of AA and DHA occur in red blood cell phospholipid membranes of patients with schizophrenia (which may be exacerbated by elevated levels of oxidants) *(3,50)*. Several studies have also reported elevated circulating levels of phospholipase A_2 *(60,61)*. Although neither of these findings, nor the niacin skin flush findings, has yet translated into diagnostic tests for schizophrenia, the relative ease with which they may be measured add to their potential utility in assessing schizotaxia. Third, there are several positive treatment studies of omega-3 EFA treatment in schizophrenia *(50)*, which raises the question of whether such treatment would also attenuate symptoms of schizotaxia.

These three points raise the possibility that physical functions outside the usual purview of the central nervous system might be useful in the assessment and vali-

dation of schizotaxia. These issues are emphasized further in the next section, which focuses on glucose dysregulation.

GLUCOSE REGULATION

Glucose regulation is considered here as an example of a system that has broad modulatory effects on multiple neurochemical systems that are affected in schizophrenia, but also specific neurochemical actions that may be relevant to the disorder. The issue of glucose dysregulation in schizophrenia has several elements in common with the membrane phospholipid hypothesis discussed above. First, as phospholipids are necessary for the normal function of nerve (and other) cells, so is glucose, in its role as the main source of metabolic fuel for neurons *(62)*. Second, if glucose metabolism is impaired, multiple transmitter and other neurochemical systems may be compromised, including those involved in schizophrenia. Moreover, the metabolism of glucose is associated with the synthesis of several neurotransmitters, including ACh and GLU, among others *(63)*, that are likely involved in schizophrenia.

In addition, DA transmission is among the likely neurochemical systems that are altered by glucose dysregulation *(64)*. Studies with rats show, for example, that glucose suppresses DA firing in the striatum *(65)*, whereas DA receptor binding increases in diabetic rats *(66)*. The pattern of decreased firing and increased number or sensitivity of receptors describes a state of receptor supersensitivity, which contributes to a poorly regulated and at least intermittently excessive DA activity. Insulin, however, prevents increases in haloperidol-induced DA receptors *(67)*, and to some extent normalizes DA transmission. Levin confirmed recently that glucose modulates DA release from the substantia nigra, through an adenosine triphosphate-sensitive K^+ channel *(68)*. His data also suggested that low glucose availability (as may occur in chronic hyperglycemia or diabetes) was associated with decreased DA release, whereas high availability was associated with decreased DA release.

Unlike abnormalities in DA or GLU neurotransmission, glucose dysregulation in schizophrenia is only beginning to attract concerted research attention, although reports of impaired regulation appeared over much of the last century. Some of the earlier observations were made before neuroleptic treatments were introduced *(69)*, or later, in unmedicated patients *(70)* and in patients treated with typical neuroleptics *(71)*. Although these observations are consistent with the possibility that impaired glucose regulation is in some way related to schizophrenia, other factors such as poor diet, substance abuse, stress, and/or lack of exercise are common in schizophrenia and could also contribute to impaired glucose regulation *(72)*. Consistent with the notion that glucose dysregulation occurs secondary to environmental causes, the single largest source of interest in the

topic derives from hyperglycemic effects associated with some of the newer, atypical antipsychotic medications *(73–76)*.

Interestingly, however, impaired glucose regulation in schizophrenia is not limited to an association with the newer pharmacological treatments. Although there are methodological problems with many of the early studies (e.g., most do not report relationships between body wt/adiposity and glycemic control), recent studies with appropriate methodological controls confirm relationships between antipsychotic medications and impaired glucose regulation *(76)*. These findings raise the possibility, however, that impaired glucose regulation in schizophrenia is related to the underlying disorder, as well as to the medication used to treat it. Consistent with this view, Mukherjee et al. *(71)* reported elevated rates of non-insulin-dependent diabetes in the relatives of patients with schizophrenia, and Wright et al. *(77)* demonstrated elevated levels of insulin-dependent diabetes in relatives of patients as well.

We recently explored this issue from a different perspective, by performing genetic linkage analyses on a set of genes that code for enzymes that are involved in the regulation of glucose metabolism *(78)*. This approach minimizes the effects of environmental variables, such as medications and diet, and explores the issue of whether impaired glucose regulation might be an intrinsic feature of schizophrenia. Data were utilized from the National Institute of Mental Health (NIMH) Genetics Initiative for Schizophrenia data set, which was described earlier *(79)*. A genome scan with 459 markers spaced at an average interval of 10 cM was conducted using a linkage analysis program. Data from European- and African-American groups were analyzed separately, with the genome-wide significance of linkage between these genes and putative schizophrenia-risk genes assessed using permutation testing.

When results were adjusted for multiple testing within and across ethnic groups, 6-phosphofructo-2-kinase/fructose-2,6-bisphosphatase 2 (PFKFB2; chromosome 1q32.2) achieved genome-wide significance ($p = 0.04$), and hexokinase 3 (HK3; chromosome 5q35.3) showed evidence suggestive of linkage ($p = 0.09$). In the European-American sample, PFKFB2, HK3, and pyruvate kinase 3 (PK3; chromosome 15q23) achieved significance at the 0.05 level. None of the genes showed significance in the African-American sample. These results, though preliminary, provide converging support for the view that genes that regulate glucose metabolism may also influence susceptibility to schizophrenia. The question of whether glucose dysregulation occurs at elevated rates in relatives of patients with schizophrenia, and in particular, in relatives who meet criteria for schizotaxia, remains to be explored.

If glucose dysregulation does contribute to the susceptibility to schizophrenia (along with multiple other genetic and environmental factors), a number of implications might follow. One is that glucose availability in specific brain regions is

not optimal in times of high demand (e.g., when performing cognitive tasks). Several studies have shown, for example, that impaired glucose regulation is associated with poor memory in rodents and people *(80–82)*. Moreover, McNay et al. *(83,84)* showed in rats that learning tasks involving the hippocampus depleted extracellular glucose levels in the hippocampus, but not in other brain regions. On the other hand, glucose administration, which improves memory in schizophrenia and in other conditions *(85,86)* through actions that may include activation of the hippocampal region *(87)*, reverses the deficit *(83)*. These findings, although speculative, raise the question of whether glucose dysregulation/availability contributes to verbal memory deficits in relatives of patients with schizophrenia, or even to hippocampal dysfunction.

SUMMARY

As is clear from the foregoing representative examples, our knowledge about the neurochemistry and pharmacology of schizotaxia is at an early stage. Even at this point, however, a few generalizations may be stressed. First, an understanding of the biology of schizotaxia is likely to extend across several levels of neurobiological function and analysis. For example, abnormalities in schizophrenia that are relevant to schizotaxia ranged from the relative specificity of altered HVA levels to the broader modulatory effects of altered membrane phospholipid levels and the availability of glucose. Second, aspects of the neurobiology of schizophrenia that are likely to be of the greatest value, at least initially, will involve negative symptoms and neuropsychological deficits, which are the core clinical features of schizotaxia. Third, the study of schizotaxia is not limited to the central nervous system. The linkage study relating regulatory enzymes in glycolysis described previously *(78)* is but one example of a genetic approach that is likely to identify numerous candidate genes for schizophrenia whose locations and physiological functions will be determined empirically.

The next steps in the process will be to continue to validate the syndrome of schizotaxia, and to refine it. In the short run, some of the biological measures discussed in this chapter may serve to provide concurrent validation of the syndrome. Eventually, however, some of them, whether they describe an abnormality or a treatment response to a drug, may become incorporated into the definition of the syndrome. The extent to which this occurs will depend on the ability of the measures to discriminate between control and schizotaxic subjects, which is a more exacting standard than simply demonstrating between-group differences *(88)*. In the longer term, as our concept or another concept of schizotaxia is validated, the incorporation of biological measures will hopefully provide specific treatment targets to facilitate the development of early-intervention and prevention strategies.

REFERENCES

1. Gottesman II. Psychopathology through a life-span genetic prism. Am Psychol 2001; 56:864.878.
2. Callicott JH, Egan MF, Bertolino A, et al. Hippocampal N-acetyl aspartate in unaffected siblings of patients with schizophrenia: a possible intermediate neurobiological phenotype. Biol Psychiatry 1998; 44:941.950.
3. Horrobin DF. The membrane phospholipid hypothesis as a biochemical basis for the neurodevelopmental concept of schizophrenia. Schizophr Res 1998; 30:193.208.
4. Meltzer HY. Treatment of schizophrenia and spectrum disorders: pharmacotherapy, psychosocial treatments, and neurotransmitter interactions. Biol Psychiatry 1999; 46:1321..1327.
5. Carlsson A, Waters N, Holm-Waters S, Tedroff J, Nilsson M, Carlsson ML. Interactions between monoamines, glutamate, and GABA in schizophrenia: new evidence. Annu Rev Pharmacol Toxicol 2001; 41:237.260.
6. Sawa A, Snyder S. Schizophrenia: diverse approaches to a complex disease. Science 2002; 296:692..695.
7. Carlsson A, Lindqvist M. Effect of chlorpromazine and haloperidol on formation of 3-methoxytyramine and normetanephrine in mouse brain. Acta Pharmacol Toxicol 1963; 20:140..144.
8. Meltzer H, McGurk S. The effect of clozapine, risperidone, and olanzapine on cognitive function in schizophrenia. Schizophr Bull 1999; 25:233.255.
9. Weinberger DR. Implications of normal brain development for the pathogenesis of schizophrenia. Arch Gen Psychiatry 1987; 44:660..669.
10. Weinberger DR, Berman KF, Illowsky BP. Physiological dysfunction of dorsolateral prefrontal cortex in schizophrenia. III. A new cohort and evidence for a monaminergic mechanism. Arch Gen Psychiatry 1988; 45:609..615.
11. Meyer-Lindenberg A, Miletich RS, Kohn PD, et al. Reduced prefrontal activity predicts exaggerated striatal dopaminergic function in schizophrenia. Nat Neurosci 2002; 5:267.271.
12. Lipska BK, Weinberger DR. Prefrontal cortical and hippocampal modulation of dopamine-mediated effects. Adv Pharmacol 1998; 42:806..809.
13. Cooper JR, Bloom FE, Roth RH. The Biochemical Basis of Neuropharmacology. New York: Oxford University Press, 2003.
14. Finlay JM, Zigmond MJ. The effects of stress on central dopaminergic neurons: possible clinical implications. Neurochem Res 1997; 22:1387..1394.
15. Sternberg DE, VanKammen DP, Lerner P, Bunney WE. Schizophrenia: dopamine beta-hydroxylase activity and treatment response. Science 1982; 216:1423..1425.
16. Wise CD, Stein L. Dopamine-beta-hydroxylase deficits in the brains of schizophrenic patients. Science 1973; 181:344.347.
17. Wyatt RJ, Erdelyi E, Schwartz M, Herman M, Barchas JD. Difficulties in comparing catecholamine-related enzymes from the brains of schizophrenics and controls. Biol Psychiatry 1978; 13:317.334.
18. Davidson M, Davis KL. A comparison of plasma homovanillic acid concentrations in schizophrenic patients and normal controls. Arch Gen Psychiatry 1988; 45:561..563.
19. Green A, Alam M, Sobieraj J, et al. Clozapine response and plasma catecholamines and their metabolites. Psychiatry Res 1993; 46:139..149.
20. Jentsch JD, Redmond DE, Elsworth JD, Taylor JR, Youngren KD, Roth RH. Enduring cognitive deficits and cortical dopamine dysfunction in monkeys after long-term administration of phencyclidine. Science 1997; 277:953..955.
21. Bridges PK, Bartlett JR, Sepping P, Kantamaneni BD, Curzon G. Precursors and metabolites of 5-hydroxytryptamine and dopamine in the ventricular cerebrospinal fluid of psychiatric patients. Psychol Med 1976; 6:399..405.

22. Maas JW, Bowden CL, Miller AL, et al. Schizophrenia, psychosis, and cerebral spinal fluid homovanillic acid concentrations. Schizophr Bull 1997; 23:147..154.

23. Pickar D, Litman RE, Konicki PE, Wolkowitz OM, Breier A. Neurochemical and neural mechanisms of positive and negative symptoms in schizophrenia. Mod Probl Pharmacopsychiatry 1990; 24:124..151.

24. Sedvall GC, Wode-Helgodt B. Aberrant monoamine metabolite levels in CSF and family history of schizophrenia. Their relationships in schizophrenic patients. Arch Gen Psychiatry 1980; 37:1113..1116.

25. Steinberg JL, Garver DL, Moeller FG, Raese JD, Orsulak PJ. Serum homovanillic acid levels in schizophrenic patients and normal control subjects. Psychiatry Res 1993; 48:93..106.

26. Lindstrom LH. Low HVA and normal 5HIAA CSF levels in drug-free schizophrenic patients compared to healthy volunteers: correlations to symptomatology and family history. Psychiatry Res 1985; 14:265..273.

27. Waldo MC, Cawthra E, Adler LE, et al. Auditory sensory gating, hippocampal volume, and catecholamine metabolism in schizophrenics and their siblings. Schizophr Res 1994; 12:93..106.

28. Amin F, Silverman JM, Siever LJ, Smith CJ, Knott PJ, Davis KL. Genetic antecedents of dopamine dysfunction in schizophrenia. Biol Psychiatry 1999; 45:1143..1150.

29. Kim J, Kornhuber H, Shcmid-Burgk W, Hollander B. Low cerebrospinal fluid glutamate in schizophrenic patients and a new hypothesis on schizophrenia. Neurosci Lett 1980; 20:379..383.

30. Olney J, Farber N. Glutamate receptor dysfunction and schizophrenia. Arch Gen Psychiatry 1995; 52:998..1007.

31. Garland Bunney B, Bunney WE, Carlsson A. Schizophrenia and glutamate. In: Bloom FE, Kupfer DJ, eds. Psychopharmacology: The Fourth Generation of Progress. New York: Raven, 1995:1203..1214.

32. Coyle J. The glutamatergic dysfunction hypothesis for schizophrenia. Harv Rev Psychiatry 1996; 3:241..253.

33. Goff DC, Coyle JT. The emerging role of glutamate in the pathophysiology and treatment of schizophrenia. Am J Psychiatry 2001; 158:1367..1377.

34. Goff DC, Tsai G, Manoach DS, Coyle JT. D-Cycloserine added to neuroleptics for negative symptoms in schizophrenia. Am J Psychiatry 1995; 152:1213..1215.

35. Eden Evins A, Amico E, Posever TA, Toker R, Goff DC. D-Cycloserine added to risperidone in patients with primary negative symptoms of schizophrenia. Schizophr Res 2002; 56:19..23.

36. Floresco SB, Blaha CD, Yang CR, Phillips AG. Modulation of hippocampal and amygdalar-evoked activity of nucleus accumbens neurons by dopamine: cellular mechanisms of input selection. J Neurosci 2001; 21:2851..2860.

37. Floresco SB, Todd CL, Grace AA. Glutamatergic afferents from the hippocampus to the nucleus accumbens regulate activity of ventral tegmental area dopamine neurons. J Neurosci 2001; 21: 4915..4922.

38. Floresco SB, Yang CR, Phillips AG, Blaha CD. Basolateral amygdala stimulation evokes glutamate receptor-dependent dopamine efflux in the nucleus accumbens of the anaesthatized rat. Eur J Neurosci 1998; 10:1241..1251.

39. Pralong E, Magistretti P, Stoop R. Cellular perspectives on the glutamate-monoamine interactions in limbic lobe structures and their relevance for some psychiatric disorders. Prog Neurobiol 2002; 67:173..202.

40. Kandel ER. Disorders of thought and volition: schizophrenia. In: Kandel ER, Schwartz JH, Jessell TM, eds. Principles of Neural Science. New York: McGraw-Hill, 2000:1188..1208.

41. Cohen B, Rosenbaum G, Luby E, Gottlieb J. Comparison of phencyclidine hydrochloride (sernyl) with other drugs: simulation of schizophrenic performance with phencyclidine hydro-

chloride (sernyl), lysergic acid diethylamide (LSD-25), and amobarbital (Amytal) sodium, II: symbolic and sequential thinking. Arch Gen Psychiatry 1962; 6:79..85.

42. Malhotra A, Pinals D, Weingartner H, et al. NMDA receptor function and human cognition: the effects of ketamine in healthy volunteers. Neuropsychopharmacology 1996; 14:301..307.

43. Newcomer JW, Farber NB, Jevtovic-Todorovic V, et al. Ketamine-induced NMDA receptor hypofunction as a model of memory impairment and psychosis. Neuropsychopharmacology 1999; 20:106..118.

44. Lahti AC, Weiler MA, Tamara Michaelidis BA, Parwani A, Tamminga CA. Effects of ketamine in normal and schizophrenic volunteers. Neuropsychopharmacology 2001; 25:455..467.

45. Lahti AC, Koffel B, LaPorte D, Tamminga CA. Subanesthetic doses of ketamine stimulate psychosis in schizophrenia. Neuropsychopharmacology 1995; 13:9..19.

46. Malhotra A, Pinals D, Adler C, et al. Ketamine-induced exacerbation of psychotic symptoms and cognitive impairment in neuroleptic-free schizophrenics. Neuropsychopharmacology 1997; 17:141..150.

47. Anand A, Charney DS, Oren DA, et al. Attenuation of the neuropsychiatric effects of ketamine with lamotrigine: support for hyperglutamatergic effects of N-methyl-D-aspartate receptor antagonists. Arch Gen Psychiatry 2000; 57:270..276.

48. Krystal JH, Anand A, Moghaddam B. Effects of NMDA receptor antagonists: implications for the pathophysiology of schizophrenia. Arch Gen Psychiatry 2002; 59:663..664.

49. Horrobin DF. Schizophrenia: a biochemical disorder? Biomedicine 1980; 32:54..55.

50. Fenton WS, Hibbeln J, Knable M. Essential fatty acids, lipid membrane abnormalities, and the diagnosis and treatment of schizophrenia. Biol Psychiatry 2000; 47:8..21.

51. Puri BK, Easton T, Das I, Kidane L, Richardson AJ. The niacin skin flush test in schizophrenia: a replication study. Int J Clin Pract 2001; 55:368..370.

52. Ward PE, Sutherland J, Glen EMT, Glen AIM. Niacin skin flush in schizophrenia: a preliminary report. Schizophr Res 1998; 29:269..274.

53. Puri BK, Hirsch SR, Easton T, Richardson AJ. A volumetric biochemical niacin flush-based index that noninvasely detects fatty acid deficiency in schizophrenia. Prog Neuropsychopharm Biol Psychiatry 2002; 26:49..52.

54. Messamore E, Hoffman WF, Janowsky A. The niacin skin flush abnormality in schizophrenia: a quantitative dose-response study. Schizophr Res 2003; 62:251..258.

55. Horrobin DF, Glen AIM, Vaddadi K. The membrane hypothesis of schizophrenia. Schizophr Res 1994; 13:195..207.

56. Reisbick S, Neuringer M. Omega-3 fatty acid deficiency and behavior: a critical review and directions for future research. In: Yehuda S, Mostafsky D, eds. Handbook of Essential Fatty Acid Biology; Biochemsitry, Physiology, and Behavioral Neurobiology. Totowa, NJ: Humana, 1997:397..426.

57. Holden RJ, Mooney PA. Schizophrenia is a babetic brain state: an elucidation of impaired metabolism. Med Hypotheses 1994; 43:420..435.

58. Horrobin DF. Schizophrenia: the illness that made us human. Med Hypotheses 1998; 50: 269..288.

59. Glen AIM, Cooper JR, Rybaskowski J, Vaddadi K, Brayshaw N, Horrobin DF. Membrane fatty acids, niacin flushing and clinical parameters. Prostaglandins Leukot Essent Fatty Acids 1996; 55:9..15.

60. Gattaz WF, Brunner J. Phospholipase A2 and the hypofrontality hypothesis of schizophrenia. Prostaglandins Leukot Essent Fatty Acids 1996; 55:109..113.

61. Ross BM. Brain and blood phospholipases in schizophrenia. Prostaglandins Leukot Essent Fatty Acids 1997; 57:211.

62. Dienel GA, Hertz L. Glucose and lactate metabolism during brain activation. J Neurosci Res 2001; 66:824..838.
63. Wenk G. An hypothesis on the role of glucose in the mechanism of action of cognitive enhancers. Psychopharmacology 1989; 99:431..438.
64. Dwyer DS, Bradley RJ, Kablinger AS, Freeman AM, 3rd. Glucose metabolism in relation to schizophrenia and antipsychotic drug treatment. Ann Clin Psychiatry 2001; 13:103..113.
65. Saller CF, Chiodo LA. Glucose suppreses basal firing and haloperidol-induced increases in the firing rate of central dopaminergic neurons. Science 1980; 210:1269..1271.
66. Lozovsky DB, Saller CF, Kopin IJ. Dopamine receptor binding is increased in diabetic rats. Science 1981; 214:1031..1033.
67. Lozovsky DB, Kopin IJ, Saller CF. Modulation of dopamine receptor supersensitivity by chronic insulin: implication in schizophrenia. Brain Res 1985; 343:190..193.
68. Levin BE. Glucose-regulated dopamine release from substantia nigra neurons. Brain Res 2000; 874:158..164.
69. Braceland FJ, Meduna LJ, Vaichulis JA. Delayed action of insulin in schizophrenia. Am J Psychiatry 1945; 102:108..110.
70. Schimmelbusch W, Mueller P, Sheps J. The positive correlation between insulin resistance and duration of hospitalization in schizophrenia. Br J Psychiatry 1971; 118:429..436.
71. Mukherjee S, Schnur DB, Reddy R. Family history of type 2 diabetes in schizophrenic patients. Lancet 1989; 1:495.
72. Ryan MCM, Thakore JH. Physical consequences of schizophrenia and its treatment: the metabolic syndrome. Life Sci 2002; 71:239..257.
73. Popli AP, Konicki PE, Jurjus GJ, Fuller MA, Jaskiw GE. Clozapine and associated diabetes mellitus. J Clin Psychiat 1997; 58:108..111.
74. Hagg S, Joelsson L, Mjorndal T, Spigset O, Oja G, Dahlqvist R. Prevalence of diabetes and impaired glucose tolerance in patients treated with clozapine compared with patients treated with conventional depot neuroleptic medications. J Clin Psychiat 1998; 59:294..299.
75. Lindenmayer J-P, Patel R. Olanzapine-induced ketoacidosis with diabetes mellitus. Am J Psychiatry 1999; 156:1471.
76. Newcomer JW, Haupt DW, Fucetola R, et al. Abnormalities in glucose regulation during antipsychotic treatment of schizophrenia. Arch Gen Psychiatry 2002; 59:337..345.
77. Wright P, Sham PC, Gilvarry CM, et al. Autoimmune diseases in the pedigrees of schizophrenic and control subjects. Schizophr Res 1996; 20:261..7.
78. Stone WS, Faraone SV, Su J, Tarbox SI, Van Eerdewegh P, Tsuang MT. Evidence for linkage between regulatory enzymes in glycolysis and schizophrenia in a multiplex sample. Neuropsychiat Genet, in press.
79. Cloninger CR, Kaufmann CA, Faraone SV, et al. Genome-wide search for schizophrenia susceptibility loci: the NIMH Genetics Initiative and Millennium Consortium. Am J Med Genet (Neuropsychiat Genet) 1998; 81:275..281.
80. Hall JL, Gonder-Frederick LA, Chewning WW, Silveira J, Gold PE. Glucose enhancement of performance on memory tests in young and aged humans. Neuropsychologia 1989; 27: 1129..1138.
81. Stone WS, Wenk GL, Olton DS, Gold PE. Poor blood glucose regulation predicts sleep and memory deficits in normal aged rats. J Gerontol: Biol Sci Med Sci 1990; 45:B169..B173.
82. Messier C, Desrochers A, Gagnon M. Effect of glucose, glucose regulation and word imagery value on human memory. Behav Neurosci 1999; 113:431..438.
83. McNay EC, Fries TM, Gold PE. Decreases in rat extracellular hippocampal glucose concentration associated with cognitive demand in a spatial task. Proc Natl Acad Sci USA 2000; 97: 2881..2885.

84. McNay EC, McCarty RC, Gold PE. Fluctuations in brain glucose concentration during behavioral testing: dissociations between brain areas and between brain and blood. Neurobiol Learn Mem 2001; 75:325..337.
85. Newcomer JW, Craft S, Fucetola R, et al. Glucose-induced increase in memory performance in patients with schizophrenia. Schizophr Bull 1999; 25:321..335.
86. Stone WS, Seidman LJ, Wojcik JD, Green AI. Glucose effects on cognition in schizophrenia. Schizophr Res 2003; 62:93..103.
87. Stone WS, Tarbox SI, Wencel H, Seidman LJ. Medial temporal lobe activation following glucose administration in schizophrenia: an fMRI study. Vol. 28. Orlando, FL: Society for Neuroscience Abstracts, 2002.
88. Faraone SV, Kremen WS, Lyons MJ, Pepple JR, Seidman LJ, Tsuang MT. Diagnostic accuracy and linkage analysis: How useful are schizophrenia spectrum phenotypes? Am J Psychiatry 1995; 152:1286..1290.

17 Molecular Medicine and the Prospects for Prevention and Early Intervention in Schizophrenia

William T. Carpenter, Jr., MD
and James I. Koenig, PhD

CONCEPTS OF EARLY INTERVENTION

Early intervention in schizophrenia has three aspects. First, patients with a diagnosis of schizophrenia who have achieved a degree of clinical improvement and course stability are likely to have a future exacerbation of psychotic symptoms. Certain psychosocial therapeutic techniques and antipsychotic medications reduce the relapse rate. A clinical care program that provides close clinical monitoring can detect early warning signs of relapse, and interventions aimed at preventing progression from exacerbation to relapse can be initiated *(1)*. Available intervention techniques include assuring adherence with antipsychotic drugs, administration of antianxiety drugs to target prodromal symptoms *(2)*, and the use of psychosocial techniques to reduce stress, provide personal support, and assure outreach if the patient withdraws. Early intervention in this situation is plausible, effective *(3,4)*, and should be the standard of care. That the majority of patients with chronic forms of schizophrenia do not receive care meeting this standard is a shame in a resource-rich country such as the United States *(5)*.

The second aspect of early intervention involves case detection close to the initial onset of psychosis. There is substantial evidence that behavior changes including subtle manifestations of psychosis appear months to years prior to diagnosis and treatment in most cases *(6)*. Falloon *(7)* first showed that detection was feasible, and psychosocial and pharmacologic interventions had a favorable effect on the course of the first episode. Some authors speculate that psychosis

From: *Early Clinical Intervention and Prevention in Schizophrenia*
Edited by: W. S. Stone, S. V. Faraone, and M. T. Tsuang © Humana Press Inc., Totowa, NJ

is neurotoxic, and that early intervention may have long-lasting benefits *(4,8,9)*. However, no evidence has yet documented the neurotoxicity hypothesis *(10–12)*, and substantial evidence suggests that the duration of untreated psychosis is less important in determining course than are traditional prognostic variables *(13–19)*. For example, insidious-onset schizophrenia develops more slowly and quietly than the better prognostic acute onset subtype. Delay in treatment initiation will be greater in the former, but the poorer outcome is predicted by the prognostic status. Despite the interesting hypotheses and unverified speculations that surround early detection and intervention, a solid foundation for this endeavor is based on two facts. First is clinical prudence. It is a virtual truism that illnesses are best managed if detected early. Second is the availability of effective treatment. In this aspect patients are manifesting early psychosis, and psychosocial and pharmacologic treatments documented as efficacious for the psychotic component of schizophrenia are available. If an adolescent is having school problems caused by beginning hallucinations, delusions, and subtle disorganization of thought, much good may accrue from case identification and therapy. This aspect of early intervention is receiving much attention *(4)*.

It is the third aspect of early intervention for which molecular biology holds greatest promise. Case identification and clinical therapeutic methods are available for early intervention in the first and in subsequent psychotic episodes. New knowledge of molecular targets for therapeutics will, no doubt, lead to more efficacious and safer drugs. But it is in the third aspect of early intervention that both case identification and efficacious therapy are wanting. Here we turn to prepsychotic and phenotypic case assessment methods, and require sufficient sensitivity and specificity to permit intervention. Methods have not yet been defined for either effective intervention or prevention at this very early stage. We outline the problem followed by a consideration of the role of molecular biology

Detection of persons in this third category involves recognition of the disease before even subtle psychotic symptoms are manifest. There are two general approaches: phenotype markers and behavior. Putative phenotypic indicators of vulnerability for schizophrenia include sensory gating impairments (i.e., P50 electrophysiology), oculomotor neurointegrative dysfunction, and late components of evoked potential *(20)*. Behavior includes a range of cognitive impairments and schizophrenia-spectrum psychopathology typical of schizoid and schizotypal personality disorders. Molecular genetics is expected to contribute decisively as gene markers and genes associated with schizophrenia are discovered.

The behavioral manifestations can be viewed as either prepsychotic vulnerability markers or the prepsychotic morbid features of schizophrenia. Pathologic manifestations in a person who later becomes schizophrenic, pathologic manifestations in biologic relatives of a person with schizophrenia, and pathologic mani-

festations in young people at risk for schizophrenia are documented. The concept of schizophrenia-spectrum psychopathology includes subtle impairments in attention and cognition. The identification of children and adolescents with asocial development, magical thinking and perceptual aberrations, anhedonia, and lower than expected performance on tasks of attention and cognition is feasible. However, one encounters several formidable problems that have not yet been adequately addressed:

1. *Sensitivity and specificity.* The cognitive and pathologic features known to be associated with the prepsychotic state are also common in the population. Sensitivity to detect cases, the more young people will be included who are not, in fact, fated for a schizophrenia outcome. There is not yet sufficient positive predictive power to justify case identification and potential stigma. From a scientific and ethics perspective, this obstacle may be overcome by highly selective inclusion criteria for research protocols. For example, manifestation of spectrum pathology and cognitive impairments plus the presence of a phenotype marker in a subject who has a first-degree relative with schizophrenia (*see* also Item 2).

2. *Therapeutic efficacy.* An early-intervention strategy must have a method for reasonably accurate case identification (*see* Item 1) and efficacious therapy. The cognitive and spectrum pathologies relevant to the prepsychotic phase have only recently been the focus of careful assessment in clinical trials. In persons with fully manifest schizophrenia psychosis, there is little or no therapeutic response to current psychosocial and pharmacologic treatments of primary negative symptoms and cognitive impairments *(21–23)*. This is the case even when robust effect is observed for psychosis, depression, and anxiety components of the clinical picture. Far too little work has been reported with biological relatives with spectrum traits to reach a conclusion on efficacy. There are many risks associated with antipsychotic drug treatments, and they have little or no efficacy for the prepsychotic components of the illness. Therefore, the hypothesis that administration of antipsychotic drugs to at-risk young people will prevent schizophrenia is weak. Any protocol at present must be carefully constructed and closely monitored by an institutional review board (IRB), as is the case with the first trial of new-generation antipsychotic drugs with nonpsychotic relatives of patients with schizophrenia *(24)*.

3. *Special ethical issues come into consideration.* Likely subjects for this aspect of early intervention would be consented by legal guardians (i.e., parents) and would participate with assent. As such, issues of a vulnerable population must be addressed. As to risk, stigma, expectation of a dread disease developing, alterations in the parent. child relationship, and other issues will have to be addressed with little empirical data. If the hypothesis relates to preventing or delaying the onset of psychosis, then long-term treatment with the attendant risk of the medications (e.g., weight gain, diabetic and lipid risk profiles, neurological) must be considered.

Put simply, detection and intervention early in the first psychotic episode and early in exacerbation/relapse phases of subsequent illness is presently straightforward, fairly effective, easily justified on clinical grounds, and poses few new ethical questions unless the proposed detection techniques lack sufficient specificity for schizophrenia. New knowledge on molecular mechanisms of the disease will, no doubt, produce safer and more effective drug treatment, but much can be done now. However, applying the same concepts to the prepsychotic phase of illness or to children at risk is presently highly speculative and appropriate only in carefully constructed research protocols. Challenges to implementation include a lack of validated case ascertainment procedures; no safe and efficacious drug has been established for the prepsychotic pathologic manifestations; and interventions must be tested in a vulnerable population. It is here that new knowledge on the molecular mechanisms of primary negative symptoms and cognitive impairments is needed to identify new molecular targets for drug development, and to discover gene-based case ascertainment.

CONCEPTS OF PREVENTION

The focus on psychosis as the core defining quality of schizophrenia (i.e., the reality distortion emphasis from Schneiderian first-rank symptoms through *DSM–IV*) has led some workers to confuse early intervention with prevention. For example, Falloon described treating early psychotic manifestations, and patients who did not progress to full diagnostic criteria were considered instances of prevention *(7,8)*. This is more appropriately viewed as muting the severity of expression rather than prevention. Others have hypothesized secondary and tertiary prevention associated with early intervention. Here the hope is that the more effective management of the first episode will have long-lasting beneficial effects on the disease process. However, because effective psychosocial and antipsychotic drug therapies are not known to alter the course of cognitive and negative symptom pathologies, it seems doubtful that disease progression *per se* is prevented. At a theoretical level, it is crucial to distinguish the prevention of adverse epiphenomena from the prevention of disease progression. For example, an effective early intervention might help a young patient avoid hospitalization, finish high school, and obtain a job. This may leave the person substantially better off in occupational and social outcomes than would have been the case if social relationships were interrupted by hospital care and stigmatizing symptoms, and high school failure restricted job opportunities. This example illustrates why the clinical prudence argument is strong, whereas the disease progression argument remains speculative.

The most important prevention challenge is to reduce the number of cases of schizophrenia in the population. In the absence of precise knowledge of etio-

pathophysiologic pathways to schizophrenia, primary prevention is based on risk factors. At times the data are sufficiently robust to be considered by individuals. Individuals who have schizophrenia, or who have a twin or even a first-degree relative with the disease, may wish to understand heritability data in order to make childbearing decisions. But less understandable and less robust risk factors are not likely to influence childbearing behavior. It is doubtful whether anyone avoids winter birth with schizophrenia prevention in mind, and men are not likely to consider the increased risk of mutations associated with advancing paternal age. Altogether missing are markers that are highly informative of an individual's risk. At present, with tongue in cheek, we can advise the woman anticipating pregnancy to secure a negative family history, avoid first-trimester starvation, second-trimester influenza, birth complications, and mate with a young man timing inception to avoid a winter birth (or summer birth if the deficit form of schizophrenia is of concern) *(25)*.

MOLECULAR BIOLOGY
AND EARLY INTERVENTION AND PREVENTION

A detailed outline of the human genome is now available and work on the human proteome is advancing. What can the schizophrenologist interested in treatment and prevention expect? Rather a great deal, but time to fruition may be lengthy given the clinical syndrome of schizophrenia will likely produce several polygenetic diseases with uncertainty as to whether any single gene or protein will contribute decisively to the overall pathologic picture. In this essay we will comment on advances in molecular pathology of schizophrenia, which may most quickly influence case ascertainment, early intervention with cognitive and negative pathologies, and primary prevention. Although schizophrenia is most validly conceptualized in a broad biopsychosocial medical model, the information that will most aggressively advance treatment and prevention in the near future will emerge from understanding gene/protein phenomena contributing to vulnerability or representing therapeutic targets.

As noted above, case ascertainment and efficacious therapeutics are two limiting factors in prepsychotic early intervention. At present, family history, electrophysiologic markers reflecting sensory gating, eye-tracking dysfunction, information processing reflected in late components of evoked potential waves, spectrum psychopathologies, and cognitive impairments can each distinguish at-risk cohorts from control cohorts. Much is yet to be learned about the most effective classification based on combined clinical and phenotype marker information, but it is clear that robust prediction of an individual's risk has not yet been achieved outside of twin pairs. There are now "hot spots" on many chromosomes where linkage and other genetic analyses suggest vulnerability genes for schizophrenia are

located *(26)*. Some locations can be considered confirmed, and the apparent overlap with bipolar affective disorder is substantial *(26)*. The difficult task of moving from genome approximate location to specific gene identification can be undertaken presently. We can anticipate that a number of allelic variations will be associated with risk for schizophrenia. It remains to be determined to what extent positive predictive power in case ascertainment can be achieved when genotyping information is added to the clinical and phenotype marker information. It is likely that new treatments addressing cognition, negative symptoms, and impaired neurointegrative function (i.e., phenotype markers) will be developed in advance of valid case ascertainment through genotyping.

At the same time that progress in genotyping for schizophrenia vulnerability is progressing, pharmacogenetics may also produce genotypes with drug response information. As drugs become available to ameliorate cognitive and negative pathologies, selection of cases likely to respond will, to some extent, offset shortcomings in positive predictive power for a schizophrenia outcome. The early-intervention paradigm will shift from schizophrenia therapeutics to a paradigm of pharmacologic modification of subtle deviations in normal functions with uncertain relationship to disease outcome. Young persons with observed deficits in cognition and/or affect and drive, who genotype as likely responders to a procognition drug or a negative symptom therapeutic agent, may be treated on an empirical basis even though risk for schizophrenia is uncertain. This shift must address profound ethical and clinical issues. However, the case for moving forward with this therapeutic research will be more compelling than the prepsychotic introduction of antipsychotic drugs in a primary-prevention paradigm.

Of several optimistic forecasts, the following is most probable. A drug with pro-cognitive effects will be developed and efficacy confirmed in persons with schizophrenia (*see* section on Drug Discovery). Assuming reasonable safety, investigators will hypothesize potential beneficial effects in young people with cognitive impairments, making the positive predictive power for schizophrenia in case ascertainment less important. Schizophrenia investigators will want to test efficacy in a cohort biased toward schizophrenia risk, and will define the cohort with genotyping, family history, physiologic phenotype markers, and spectrum-like pathologies. Most essential will be the cognitive impairments targeted for the therapeutic intervention. Initial studies will determine short-term efficacy. If efficacious, a secondary prevention hypothesis will be tested (i.e., can early intervention with cognitive enhancement prevent or delay the onset of psychosis in at-risk populations?). The ethical issues will be addressed by having a drug of demonstrated efficacy for cognitive pathology, extending its use to younger subjects by nature of their having increased risk for schizophrenia, and having the specific target for the pharmacotherapy. Molecular genetic information on risk will be modest, but will enhance sensitivity/specificity and positive predictive

power. Genotyping for therapeutic response will strengthen the scientific design and increase the likelihood of benefit for participating subjects. The experiments will be conducted with extensive ethics consultation, and will be nested in public debate. Advocates will see a parallel with the development of polio vaccine, and critics will find an analogy in the administration of growth hormone to boys at the 33rd percentile of height. The debate will properly center on the value/justification of enhancing normal range cognition vs therapy of disease impaired cognition. If sensitivity/specificity/positive predictive power become robust, the treatment of disease paradigm will prevail.

Primary prevention is more difficult to conceptualize, for any approach will be dependent on the exact information regarding etiopathophysiology. For example, the finding that advancing paternal age increases the risk of mutations (which in turn convey risk for schizophrenia) suggests that the incidence of schizophrenia could be reduced in the population by reducing impregnation by older men. This, of course, is not practical since the effect would be very small and men are not known to be sensible when engaged in mating behaviors. It does, however, illustrate that prevention methods will be cause-specific. As new knowledge of etiology and pathophysiology emerges from genomic and proteomic data, prevention science will develop an empirical basis for conceptualizing prevention strategies. Advances in gene therapies may permit modification of genes contributing to neurodevelopmental vulnerability to schizophrenia. When DNA data can define substantial risk, genetic counseling may contribute to prevention.

ADVANCING KNOWLEDGE
OF MOLECULAR ETIOPATHOPHYSIOLOGY

The reader is referred elsewhere for basic information on genomic and proteomic technologies and their application to the study of disease and the identification of molecular targets for drug discovery (27–37).

How might this area of science contribute to early intervention and prevention in schizophrenia? There are many possibilities. The following illustrates an approach being pursued by investigators at the Maryland Psychiatric Research Center.

The etiology of schizophrenia must ultimately be understood in terms of gene, and subsequently protein, expression. Even if DNA mutations specific to schizophrenia are found, the neurobiological consequences of the mutant proteins will have to be addressed in brain. Furthermore, it appears likely that many gene variants combine to convey vulnerability, and environmental factors may influence gene expression and posttranslational modifications of brain proteins. A single gene may encode for a plethora of protein products but the tissue-specific expression of processing enzymes are integral factors that dictate the protein products

present in each brain region. For these and other reasons, investigating schizophrenia at the level of qualitative and quantitative analysis of brain proteins in areas of specific neuroanatomic relevance to the disease is most decisive in principle. Proteomic technology using biochemical techniques involving electrophoresis and determining protein identity with mass spectroscopy is capable of identifying tens of thousands of proteins in postmortem brain tissue. Comparing a series of tissue samples from selected brain areas in schizophrenia with carefully matched control samples provides comparative data on a large number of proteins. Bioinformatic analysis using available databases can inform selection of proteins of interest for brain function. Differential expression in disease owing to alterations in physicochemical characteristics may result from posttranslational modification, or by substitution or deletion of one or more amino acids in the protein backbone. These later changes arise at the gene level from single-nucleotide polymorphisms. Given current understanding of genetic mechanisms, these polymorphisms potentially arise as a result of an allelic variation or mutation that may represent the molecular basis for diseases such as schizophrenia. The advantage in using proteomic technology is a direct identification of the protein(s) involved in a given disease and information about the allelic nature of the change. A further advantage is the possibility of moving more rapidly toward understanding the etiopathophysiology of the disease. However, at present a proteomic approach is technical difficult in human brain tissue. Alternatively, a genomic approach consisting of an analysis (e.g., linkage, association) in an affected population and identifying a region of a chromosome onto which a phenotype of interest maps can also be employed. Subsequently, the laborious task of sequencing a large stretch of genomic DNA would need to be undertaken to identify the gene with which the trait is linked. If one is lucky enough to identify and sequence the gene linked to the trait, then investigations into the nature of the changes in protein structure or function involved in the disease can begin. Thus, the advantage of this approach is less technically demanding assays in easy to obtain tissue (e.g., blood). The disadvantages of this approach are the extremely time-intensive nature of the sequencing process to identify the gene of interest, the dearth of information derived from this approach about the proteins involved in the disease process, and virtual lack of knowledge gained about single nucleotide polymorphisms or allelic variations that might be involved in the disease. Additional studies to validate finding(s) for schizophrenia as opposed to coincident phenomenon; e.g., neuroleptic treatment become critical regardless of which approach is taken. Although, well-planned animal experimentation may provide useful information to dissect primary, disease-specific findings from closely associated secondary events.

Identifying genes and their protein products involved in schizophrenia etiopathophysiology provide a platform for disease and drug discovery.

DISEASE NEUROBIOLOGY

Knowledge of the primary genetic/proteomic agent(s) responsible for the disease of schizophrenia can result in new molecular diagnostics that effectively detect the genetic predisposition for the disease. Additionally, basic neurobiological information about the role of the primary causative agent in early brain development and/or function could lead to an approach to reduce the primary liability of the disease. Understanding the biology of the molecular basis of schizophrenia may provide a target for the development of new gene-based therapeutic agents that could be used during fetal development or shortly thereafter during periods when the brain remains remarkably plastic. The combination of molecular-based diagnostics and novel gene-altering therapeutics may eventually result in an approach to primary prevention. It may become possible, for example, to perform an intervention that would allow delivery of genes directly into an at-risk fetus during the course of brain development that repairs the primary defect(s) involved in a disease like schizophrenia. However, the polygenic nature of the disease may make this approach less tenable. Alternative strategies for repairing genetic defects will sure be developed in the future. In the meantime, basic molecular knowledge on etiology will lead directly to the study of neurobiology of schizophrenia through bioinformatics (already established knowledge of gene and protein function) and experimentation (e.g., genetically altered rodent models). The field is poised to move from animal models based on theory to animal models based on molecular knowledge of schizophrenia.

DRUG DISCOVERY

Knowledge of the mutated gene/protein(s) involved in the disease process of schizophrenia will likely lead to information about protein partners associated with the causative agents. Whereas therapies directed at the primary molecular targets of schizophrenia may be impractical for a number of reasons, the proteins associated with these primary factors may represent more accessible and feasible targets for drug development. A point of clarification may be important at this juncture regarding the molecular targets involved in schizophrenia. If the disease is a disorder of brain development, delivering a therapy that is preventative may mean intervening during fetal or early postnatal brain development. Although this is clearly one of the molecular targets of the disease, a degree of impracticality is associated with developing a drug for this purpose. However, most probably the molecular basis of schizophrenia will also produce secondary changes in brain protein expression that result in the behavioral phenotype associated with schizophrenia. For example, antipsychotic agents provide relief from the positive symptoms of the disease, but dopamine may be a secondary target that partners with a primary molecular etiology. Similarly, identification of a secondary target that

partners with the primary causative agents of cognitive dysfunction and/or negative symptoms of schizophrenia could be therapeutic. Hence, molecular knowledge of etiology can lead to drug development even if the causative molecules are not the therapeutic targets themselves.

CONCLUSIONS

Presently available drug and psychosocial therapies can be introduced early in an initial or recurrent psychotic process with significant clinical advantage. Prepsychotic early intervention requires high positive predictive power in case ascertainment and experimental testing of the intervention at present, since efficacious treatment for schizophrenia-spectrum pathologies (i.e., cognitive, affect, and drive impairments) that define high-risk persons are not yet documented. Once safe and effective drugs are developed for cognitive and negative symptom impairments, the clinical paradigm and ethical issues will shift and experimental trials will be more compelling even if positive predictive power for a schizophrenia outcome is modest.

Primary prevention requires more precise knowledge of molecular etiopathophysiology if prevention techniques are to be developed with application in individual cases. It is here that proteomic and genomic technical and information advances offer greatest promise for new discovery. Knowledge of genetic causation and protein pathology can lead to primary prevention targets and downstream molecular partners for secondary treatment targets.

Although complex syndromes will produce several polygenic diseases, and the challenge for advancing molecular knowledge is profound, schizophrenia is one of the major disease problems for which the genomic/proteomic era offers great promise.

REFERENCES

1. Bustillo J, Buchanan RW, Carpenter WT Jr. Prodromal symptoms vs. early warning signs and clinical action in schizophrenia. Schizophr Bull 1995; 21(4):553..559.
2. Carpenter WT, Buchanan RW, Kirkpatrick B, Breier AF. Diazepam treatment of early signs of exacerbation in schizophrenia. Am J Psychiatry 1999; 156(2):299..303.
3. Phillips L, McGorry PD, Yung AR, et al. The development of prevention interventions for early psychosis: early findings and directions. Schizophr Res 1999; 36:331..332.
4. McGlashan TH. Treating schizophrenia earlier in life and the potential for prevention. Curr Psychiatry Rep 2000; 2:386..392.
5. Lehman AF, Steinwachs DM, Survey Co-Investigators of the PORT Project. Patterns of usual care for schizophrenia: initial results from the schizophrenia patient outcomes research team (PORT) client survey. Schizophr Bull 1998; 24(1):11..20.
6. Hafner H, van der Heiden W. Epidemiology of schizophrenia. Can J Psychiatry 1977; 42: 139..151.

7. Falloon IRH. Early intervention for first episodes of schizophrenia: a preliminary exploration. Psychiatry 1992; 55:4..15.
8. Wyatt R. Neuroleptics and the natural course of schizophrenia. Schizophr Bull 1991; 17: 325..351.
9. Lieberman J, Sheitman B, Kinon B. Neurochemical sensitization in the pathophysiology of schizophrenia: deficits and dysfunction in neuronal regulation and plasticity. Neuropsychopharmacology 1997; 17:205..229.
10. Wyatt RJ. Research in schizophrenia and the discontinuation of antipsychotic medications. Schizophr Bull 1997; 23(1):3..9.
11. Carpenter WT Jr. The risk of medication-free research. Schizophr Bull 1997; 23(1):11..18.
12. Carpenter WT, Schooler NR, Kane JM. The rationale and ethics of medication-free research in schizophrenia. Arch Gen Psychiatry 1997; 54:401..407.
13. Norman RMG, Malla AK. Duration of untreated psychosis: a critical examination of the concept and its importance. Psychol Med 2001; 31:381..400.
14. Lieberman JA, Fenton WS. Delayed detection of psychosis: causes, consequences, and effect on public health (Editorial). Am J Psychiatry 2000; 157(11):1727..1730.
15. DeHaan L, van der Gaag M, Wolthaus J. Duration of untreated psychosis and the long-term course of schizophrenia. Eur Psychiatry 2000; 15:264..267.
16. Barnes TRE, Hutton SB, Chapman MJ, Mutsatsa S, Puri BK, Joyce EM. West London first-episode study of schizophrenia. Clinical correlates of duration of untreated psychosis. Br J Psychiatry 2000; 177:207..211.
17. Craig TJ, Bromet EJ, Fennig S, Tanenberg-Karant M, Lavelle J, Galambos N. Is there an association between duration of untreated psychosis and 24-month clinical outcome in a first-admission series? Am J Psychiatry 2000; 157:60..66.
18. Hoff AL, Sakuma M, Razi K, Heydebrand G, Csernansky JG, DeLisi LE. Lack of association between duration of untreated illness and severity of cognitive and structural brain deficits at the first episode of schizophrenia. Am J Psychiatry 2000; 157:1824..1828.
19. Johnstone EC, Owens DG, Crow TJ, Davis JM. Does a four-week delay in the introduction of medication alter the course of functional psychosis? J Psychopharmacology 1999; 13(3): 238..244.
20. Adler LE, Freedman R, Ross RG, Olincy A, Waldo MC. Elementary phenotypes in the neurobiological and genetic study of schizophrenia. Biol Psychiatry 1999; 46:8..18.
21. Geddes JR, Freemantle N, Harrison P, Bebbington PE. Atypical antipsychotics in the treatment of schizophrenia-systematic overview and meta-regression analysis. Br Med J 2000; 321: 1371..1376.
22. Carpenter WT, Conley RR, Buchanan RW, Breier A, Tamminga CA. Clozapine conflict (Letter to the Editor in rebuttal to editorial by Herbert Meltzer, Am J Psychiatry 152:821..825). Am J Psychiatry 1996; 153:1505..1507.
23. Buchanan RW, Carpenter WT Jr. Evaluating negative symptom treatment efficacy. In: Richard S, Keefe E, McEvoy JP, eds. Negative Symptom and Cognitive Deficit Treatment Response in Schizophrenia. Washington, DC: American Psychiatric Press, 2001:1..18.
24. Tsuang MT, Stone WS, Seidman LJ, et al. Treatment of nonpsychotic relatives of patients with schizophrenia: four case studies. Biol Psychiatry 1999; 45:1412..1418.
25. Kirkpatrick B, Buchanan RW, Ross DE, Carpenter WT. A separate disease within the syndrome of schizophrenia. Arch Gen Psychiatry 2001; 58:165..171.
26. Berrettini WH. Are schizophrenic and bipolar disorders related? A review of family and molecular studies. Biol Psychiatry 2000; 48:531..538.

27. Wang JH, Hewick RM. Proteomics in drug discovery. Drug Discov Today 1999; 4:129..133.
28. Cunningham MJ. Genomics and proteomics: the new millenium of drug discovery and development. J Pharmacol Toxicol Methods 2000; 44:291..300.
29. Debouck C, Metcalf B. The impact of genomics on drug discovery. Ann Rev Pharmacol Toxicol 2000; 40:193..207.
30. Harris S, Foord SM. Transgenic gene knock-outs: functional genomics and therapeutic target selection. Pharmacognomics 2000; 1:433..443.
31. Naaby-Hansen S, Waterfield MD, Cramer R. Proteomics   post-genomic cartography to understand gene function. Trends Pharmacol Sci 2001; 22:376..384.
32. Edgar PF. Comparative analysis of the hippocampus implicates chromosome 6q in schizophrenia. Mol Psychiatry 2000; 5:85..90.
33. Voshol H, Bilbe G, Roberts RC, et al. A proteomics approach to study differential protein expression in brains of schizophrenic patients. Schizophr Res 2001; 49(Suppl):58.
34. Scangos G. Drug discovery in the postgenomic era. Nat Biotechnol 1997; 15(12):1220..1221.
35. Dollery CT. Drug discovery and development in the molecular era. Br J Clin Pharmacol 1999; 47(1):5..6.
36. Marcotte ER, Srivastava LK, Quirion R. DNA microarrays in neuropsychopharmacology. Trends Pharmacol Sci 2001; 22(8):426..436.
37. Mirnics K, Middleton FA, Lewis DA, Levitt P. Analysis of complex brain disorders with gene expression microarrays: schizophrenia as a disease of the synapse. Trends Neurosci 2001; 24(8): 479..486.

Index

A

AA, *see* Arachidonic acid
Academic performance, schizophrenia
    predictive value, 236, 237
Amygdala, volume in schizophrenia
    patients, 230, 232
Animal models, schizophrenia,
    obstetrical complication rat models,
        60, 61
    rat ventral hippocampus lesion mod-
        els, 59, 61
Arachidonic acid (AA), phospholipid
    membrane hypothesis of schizo-
    phrenia, 345
Attention deficits, schizophrenia predic-
    tive value, 238..240
Autonomic responsivity, early detection
    of schizophrenia, 218, 219

B

Brainstem, vulnerable brainstem hypothesis
    in diathesis..stress model, 126..128

C

CAARMS, *see* Comprehensive Assess-
    ment of At-Risk Mental States
Case-control study, overview, 260, 261
Chromosome linkage analysis, *see* Link-
    age analysis, schizophrenia
Clozapine, schizotaxia management in
    adults, 288, 289
Communication deviance,
    diathesis..stress model stress source,
        119
    schizotaxia findings, 98, 99
Community rejection/disapproval, stress
    source in diathesis..stress model,
    121, 122

Comprehensive Assessment of At-Risk
    Mental States (CAARMS), prodro-
    mal symptom assessment, 86
Computed tomography (CT),
    brain morphometry findings in rela-
        tives of schizophrenia patients,
        189, 190
    etiology and timing of brain abnor-
        malities in relatives, 197..199
CT, *see* Computed tomography

D

Declarative memory, schizophrenia
    findings in patients and relatives,
    139, 140
Dermatoglyphic abnormalities, schizo-
    phrenia prediction value, 229, 230
DHA, *see* Docosahexaenoic acid
Diathesis..stress model,
    high-risk children characteristics,
        124..126
    interventions, 127
    schizopherogenic brain abnormality
        relationship with stress, 117, 118
    stress sources,
        community rejection/disapproval,
            121, 122
        familial influences,
            communication deviance, 119
            expressed emotion and affective
                style, 119
            harsh and punitive treatment,
                119..121
        urban poverty, 122, 123
    vulnerable brainstem hypothesis,
        126..128
Docosahexaenoic acid (DHA), phospho-
    lipid membrane hypothesis of
    schizophrenia, 345

Dopamine, schizophrenia neurotransmission defects, 339.342

Drug abuse, schizophrenia risk prediction, 242

E

Eicosapentaenoic acid (EPA),
    phospholipid membrane hypothesis of schizophrenia, 345
    schizophrenia management, 297

Emotion processing, see Socioemotional deficits, schizophrenia

EPA, see Eicosapentaenoic acid

ERPs, see Event-related potentials

ETD, see Eye-tracking dysfunction

Event-related potentials (ERPs), early detection of schizophrenia,
    overview of components, 214
    P50 sensory gating, 215, 216
    P300 abnormalities, 216, 217

Executive function,
    schizophrenia findings in patients and relatives, 137, 138
    schizotaxia findings, 99

Eye-tracking dysfunction (ETD), early detection of schizophrenia, 212, 213

F

Family environment, schizophrenia studies,
    comparison of rearing factors within high-risk design, 33, 34
    dysfunctional families,
        high-risk studies, 31, 32
        low-risk studies, 29, 30
    genetically vulnerable children and impact of rearing environment, 30.35
    neurocognitive risk indicator studies and family treatment strategies, 150..152
    parental loss effects,
        high-risk studies, 32
        low-risk studies, 30

pregnancy, see Pregnancy

schizopherogenic family concept, 116

shift to genetic factors in etiology theory, 116, 117

stress sources in diathesis. stress model,
    communication deviance, 119
    expressed emotion and affective style, 119
    harsh and punitive treatment, 119... 121

Fetal brain damage, see Second trimester disruption

fMRI, see Functional magnetic resonance imaging

Functional magnetic resonance imaging (fMRI),
    emotion processing studies, 170, 171
    etiology and timing of brain abnormalities in relatives, 197..199
    relatives of schizophrenia patient findings, 192, 194..196
    schizophrenia patient findings, 184, 185, 187

G

Genetic counseling,
    genetic testing,
        direct DNA testing, 329.331
        diseases and availability, 325
        ethical issues, 332.334
        presymptomatic testing guidelines, 331, 332
        prospects, 335
    Internet resources, 334
    purposes, 325, 326
    stages,
        burden and benefit evaluation, 328
        consult and evaluation, 328
        diagnosis confirmation, 326, 327
        family history, 327
        follow-up, 329
        plan of action formulation, 328, 329
        recurrence risk assessment, 327, 328

Genetic epidemiology studies, schizo-
    phrenia,
    adoption studies, 5, 6, 263
    family studies, 4, 115, 227, 263, 264
    twin studies, 4, 5, 115, 227, 263
Genetic linkage, *see* Linkage analysis,
    schizophrenia
Glucose dysregulation, schizophrenia,
    346. 348
Glutamate, schizophrenia neurotransmis-
    sion defects, 342, 343

H

HD, *see* Huntington•s disease
Hillside RAP program, *see* Prodrome in
    schizophrenia
Hippocampus,
    dysfunction in schizophrenia, 59
    volume,
        relatives of schizophrenia patients,
        191
        schizophrenia patients, 230, 232
Huntington•s disease (HD),
    presymptomatic testing guidelines,
    331, 332

I

IE, *see* Intervention effectiveness
Immigration,
    schizophrenia risk prediction, 242
    stress and migration as schizophrenia
    risk factors, 57
Incidence,
    definition, 259
    schizophrenia, 255
Influenza, fetal exposure and schizophre-
    nia risks, 23, 24, 52, 53, 265
Inhibitory control, schizophrenia findings
    in patients and relatives, 141, 142
Intelligence quotient (IQ),
    schizophrenia findings in patients and
    relatives, 135, 136
    schizophrenia predictive value, 233...
    236, 238

Intervention effectiveness (IE), calcula-
    tion, 266
IQ, *see* Intelligence quotient

L

Learning and memory tasks, schizotaxia
    findings, 99
Life events, schizophrenia risk predic-
    tion, 242, 244
Linkage analysis, schizophrenia,
    chromosome 1, 11
    chromosome 2, 11
    chromosome 5, 11, 12
    chromosome 6, 12
    chromosome 8, 12
    chromosome 10, 13
    chromosome 11, 13
    chromosome 13, 13
    chromosome 15, 13, 14
    chromosome 22, 14
    glucose metabolism genes, 347
    LOD scores, 10
    neurocognitive risk indicator studies,
    149, 150
    overview, 10, 11, 14, 180, 181
    X chromosome, 14

M

Magnetic resonance imaging (MRI),
    brain morphometry findings,
        etiology and timing of brain abnor-
        malities in relatives, 197..199
        relatives of schizophrenia patients,
        190..193, 197
        schizophrenia patients, 182..184
    functional imaging, *see* Functional
        magnetic resonance imaging
Magnetic resonance spectroscopy (MRS),
    etiology and timing of brain abnor-
        malities in relatives, 197..199
    relatives of schizophrenia patient
        findings, 196
    schizophrenia patient findings, 185...
    187

Maternal malnutrition, effects on schizo-
    phrenia development, 53
Medial temporal lobe, dysfunction in
    schizophrenia, 59, 60
Mental control-encoding, schizophrenia
    findings in patients and relatives,
    138, 139
MFP model, see Multifactorial polygenic
    model
Minor physical anomalies (MPA),
    schizophrenia prediction value,
    229, 230
Mismatch negativity (MMN), impair-
    ment in early detection of schizo-
    phrenia, 217, 218
MMN, see Mismatch negativity
MPA, see Minor physical anomalies
MRI, see Magnetic resonance imaging
MRS, see Magnetic resonance spectros-
    copy
Multifactorial polygenic (MFP) model,
    schizophrenia heredity, 9

N

Negative predictive value, definition,
    226
Negative symptoms, schizophrenia, 3
Neurobiologic endophenotype, defini-
    tion, 188, 189
Neuromotor development, schizophrenia
    predictive value, 232, 233
Neurophysiological endophenotypes,
    early detection of schizophrenia,
    autonomic responsivity, 218, 219
    event-related potentials,
        mismatch negativity impairment,
            217, 218
        overview of components, 214
        P50 sensory gating, 215, 216
        P300 abnormalities, 216, 217
    ocular motor dysfunction,
        eye-tracking dysfunction, 212, 213
        saccadic eye movements, 213, 214
    overview, 211
    prepulse inhibition of startle reflex, 218
    prospects for study, 218, 219
Neuropsychological assessment,
    confounding factors in schizophrenia,
        134
    risk indicators in schizophrenia,
        composite indicator importance,
            144, 145
        criteria, 134, 135, 225, 226
        implications for intervention and
            prevention,
            family treatment strategies,
                150..152
            genetic linkage studies, 149, 150
        overview in specific cognitive
            domains, 142, 143
        relationship among indicators, 145,
            146
        specificity, 143, 144
    schizophrenia findings in patients and
        relatives,
        declarative memory, 139, 140
        executive function, 137, 138
        heterogeneity in findings, 146, 147
        inhibitory control, 141, 142
        intelligence quotient, 135, 136
        mental control-encoding, 138, 139
        perceptual motor speed, 138
        relative type differences, 148
        sex differences, 147, 148
        stability of neurocognitive deficits,
            146
        sustained attention-vigilance, 137
        verbal fluency, 140, 141
    schizotaxia,
        communication deviance, 98, 99
        executive function, 99
        learning and memory tasks, 99
        motor ability, 97, 98
        perceptual motor speed, 98
        short-term memory, 98
        sustained attention, 98
Niacin skin flush, attenuation in schizo-
    phrenia, 343, 344

O

Obstetrical complications,
   brain abnormalities in schizophenia, 28
   discrepant findings in schizophenia
      research, 28
   genetic susceptibility linkage, 48..51,
      62, 264, 265
   rat models, 60, 61
   types related to schizophenia develop-
      ment, 27, 28, 44..48, 227..229
   vulnerable children, 29
Ocular motor function, see Eye-tracking
      dysfunction; Saccadic eye movements
Odds ratio (OR), calculation, 260, 261
OR, see Odds ratio

P

P50, see Event-related potentials
P300, see Event-related potentials
PAR, see Population attributable risk
Perceptual motor speed,
   schizophrenia findings in patients and
      relatives, 138
   schizotaxia findings, 98
PET, see Positron emission tomography
Phospholipid membrane hypothesis,
      schizophrenia, 344..346
Poliovirus, fetal exposure and schizo-
      phrenia risks, 53
Population attributable risk (PAR),
   calculation, 262
   small high-risk groups, 270
Population prevention effect (PPE),
      calculation, 267
Positive predictive value, definition, 226
Positive symptoms, schizophrenia, 3
Positron emission tomography (PET),
   etiology and timing of brain abnor-
      malities in relatives, 197..199
   relatives of schizophrenia patient
      findings, 192, 194
   schizophrenia patient findings, 184,
      185

PPE, see Population prevention effect
PPI, see Prepulse inhibition
Pregnancy, see also Obstetrical compli-
      cations; Second trimester disrup-
      tion,
   malnutrition effects on schizophrenia
      development, 53
   season of birth as schizophrenia risk
      factor, 54, 55, 265, 266
   stress and migration as schizophrenia
      risk factors, 57
   urban birth as schizophrenia risk
      factor, 55..57, 239, 242
Prepulse inhibition (PPI), early detection
      of schizophrenia, 218
Prevalence, schizophrenia, 3
Prevention intervention,
   adherence, implementation, and par-
      ticipation, 274, 275
   case identification,
      behavioral manifestations, 356, 357
      phenotypic markers, 356
   early intervention concepts, 255..258
   ethics, 357
   General Growth Mixture Model test-
      ing of impact, 273
   indicated interventions, 267..269
   molecular biology prospects,
      disease neurobiology, 363
      etiopathophysiology studies, 361, 362
      therapeutics development, 359...
         361, 363, 364
   prevention concepts, 358, 359
   prospects for study, 276, 277
   research cycle, 258, 259
   sample size considerations in testing,
      275, 276
   selective interventions, 267..269
   timing,
      early risk factor targeting, 272, 273
      period of high incidence, 271, 272
      transition periods, 274
   universal interventions, 267..270

Prodrome in schizophrenia,
    comorbid disorders, 317, 318
    definitions, 76
    diagnostic criteria, 86
    duration, 75
    heterogeneity, 310, 311
    intervention,
        developmental concerns, 311
        Hillside RAP program,
            clinical subgroups, 314, 315,
                318, 319
            description, 312, 313
            early treatment findings, 317
            initial selection strategy, 313
            preliminary clinical outcome,
                315, 316, 319
        rationale, 89, 90, 308
        second-generation antipsychotic
            medications, 309, 310
        trials, 86..88
    neurocognitive deficits, 305, 306
    pathophysiology theories, 76, 77, 304,
        305
    premorbid phases,
        early and mid-premorbid phases,
            77..79
        late premorbid phase, 79, 80
    prospective descriptions with predic-
        tive validity, 85, 86
    retrospective descriptions, 80..85
    socioemotional deficits, 168..173
    symptoms,
        assessment, 86, 89
        CASID cluster, 306..308
        schizophrenia risk prediction, 244...
            246
Prospective cohort study, overview, 261

Q

QTL, see Quantitative trait loci
Quantitative trait loci (QTL), schizophre-
    nia heredity, 9

R

Relative risk (RR), calculation, 260, 261
Risperidone,
    indications, 289
    prodrome in schizophrenia interven-
        tion, 88
    schizotaxia management in adults,
        289, 290
RR, see Relative risk
Rubella, fetal exposure and schizophre-
    nia risks, 53

S

Saccadic eye movements, early detection
    of schizophrenia, 213, 214
Scale of Prodromal Symptoms (SOPS),
    prodromal symptom assessment, 86
Schizophrenia-spectrum disorders,
    psychotic spectrum disorders, 7
    schizotaxia, see Schizotaxia
    schizotypal personality disorder, see
        Schizotypal personality disorder
Schizotaxia,
    clinical features,
        neuropsychological performance,
            97..100
        overview, 93..95
        psychiatric signs and symptoms,
            96, 97
        psychosocial functioning, 99..101
    clinical implications, 106, 107
    definition, 76, 93, 94
    diagnostic criteria establishment, 104,
        105, 107, 291..293
    genetic epidemiology, 8, 293
    indicators, overview, 268, 269
    outcomes in children, 291, 294, 295
    schizotypal personality disorder rela-
        tionship,
        comorbidity, 103, 104
        rationale for differentiation, 101...
            103, 106

treatment,
  adults,
    clozapine, 288, 289
    prospects, 290
    psychological interventions,
        287, 288
    rationale, 286, 287
    risperidone, 289, 290
  children,
    antipsychotic medications, 296,
        297
    ethics, 293. 295
    progressive outcome treatment
        goals, 294
    stable outcome treatment goals,
        295
  validation as syndrome, 104,
        105, 348
Schizotypal personality disorder (SPD),
  epidemiology, 8
  Finnish recruit study of second tri-
      mester disruption effects, 25, 26
  neuroimaging studies, 188
  schizotaxia relationship,
    comorbidity, 103, 104
    rationale for differentiation, 101...
        103, 106
Season of birth, schizophrenia risk fac-
    tor, 54, 55, 265, 266
Second trimester disruption,
  behavioral indicants of fetal brain
      damage,
    childhood neuromotor deficits and
        adult schizophenia, 26
    infant neuro-behavioral defi-
        cits and adult schizophenia,
        26, 27
  Finnish recruit study of schizotypal
      personality disorder, 25, 26
  infection effects on schizophenia
      development,
    influenza, 23, 24, 52, 53

poliovirus, 53
rubella, 53
Selective serotonin reuptake inhibitors
    (SSRIs), high-risk adolescent
    population treatment, 274
Sensitivity, risk predictors, 226, 357
SES, see Socioeconomic status
Short-term memory, schizotaxia find-
    ings, 98
Single major locus (SML) model, schizo-
    phrenia heredity, 9
Single photon emission computed to-
    mography (SPECT),
  etiology and timing of brain abnor-
      malities in relatives, 197..199
  schizophrenia patient findings, 184,
      185
SIPS, see Structured Interview for Pro-
    dromal Symptoms
SML model, see Single major locus
    model
Socioeconomic status (SES),
  schizophrenia risk studies, 34, 35
  urban poverty as stress source in di-
      athesis. stress model, 122, 123
Socioemotional deficits, schizophrenia,
  functional magnetic resonance imag-
      ing studies, 170, 171
  nonverbal social deficits,
    expression of emotion, 161, 162
    recognition of emotion, 162..164
  overview, 159, 160
  precursors to schizophrenia in child-
      hood and adolescence, 165..168
  prodromal period, 168..173
  social cognition, 164
SOPS, see Scale of Prodromal Symp-
    toms
SPD, see Schizotypal personality disorder
Specificity, risk predictors, 226, 357
SPECT, see Single photon emission
    computed tomography

Speech development, schizophrenia
        predictive value, 236, 237
SSRIs, *see* Selective serotonin reuptake
        inhibitors
Stress management, prodrome in schizo-
        phrenia intervention, 87
Structured Interview for Prodromal
        Symptoms (SIPS), prodromal
        symptom assessment, 86
Sustained attention,
    schizophrenia findings in patients and
        relatives, 137
    schizotaxia findings, 98

T

TDI, *see* Thought Disorder Index
Thought Disorder Index (TDI), elevation
        in schizophrenia and disorders, 264
Two-hit model, schizophrenia etiology,

first hit, *see* Second trimester disruption
        overview, 23, 35, 36
second hit, *see* Family environment,
        schizophenia studies; Obstetri-
        cal complications

U

Urban birth, schizophrenia risk factor,
        55.57

V

Verbal fluency, schizophrenia findings in
        patients and relatives, 140, 141

W

WCST, *see* Wisconsin Card Sorting Test
Wisconsin Card Sorting Test (WCST),
        schizophrenia findings in patients
        and relatives, 137, 139, 142, 143,
        146